STUDY GUIDE TO ACCOMPANY

Introductory Medical–Surgical Nursing

SIXTH EDITION

STUDY GUIDE TO ACCOMPANY

Introductory Medical–Surgical Nursing

SIXTH EDITION

JEANNE C. SCHERER, RN, BSN, MS

Former Assistant Director and Medical–Surgical Coordinator
Sisters School of Nursing
Buffalo, New York

BARBARA K. TIMBY, RNC, BSN, MA

Nursing Professor
Medical–Surgical Nursing
Glen Oaks Community College
Centreville, Michigan

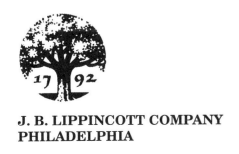

J. B. LIPPINCOTT COMPANY
PHILADELPHIA

Coordinating Editorial Assistant: Sarah L. Andrus
Cover Designer: Ilene Griff
Production Manager: Janet Greenwood
Production Editor: Mary Kinsella
Production Service: Berliner, Inc.
Printer/Binder: Courier/Kendalville
Cover Printer: Lehigh Press

ISBN: 0-397-55098-7

⊗ This Paper Meets the Requirements of ANSI/NISO 239.48-1992 (Permanence of Paper).

6 5 4 3 2 1

Any procedure or practice described in this book should be applied by the healthcare practitioner under appropriate supervision in accordance with professional standards of care used with regard to the unique circumstances that apply in each practice situation. Care has been taken to confirm the accuracy of information presented and to describe generally accepted practices. However, the authors, editors, and publisher cannot accept any responsibility for errors or omissions or for any consequences from application of the information in this book and make no warranty express or implied, with respect to the contents of the book.

PREFACE

The *Study Guide to Accompany Introductory Medical-Surgical Nursing,* previously referred to as the *Student Work Manual for Introductory Medical-Surgical Nursing,* has been redesigned to accompany the completely revised and updated sixth edition of *Introductory Medical–Surgical Nursing.*

The major objectives of the Study Guide are (1) to assist the user in increasing proficiency in nursing practice, (2) to provide one method of preparing for the NCLEX-PN examination, and (3) to help the user internalize medical-surgical nursing knowledge.

The *Study Guide to Accompany Introductory Medical–Surgical Nursing* is designed around the following elements:

- The *Study Guide* correlates to the textbook chapter by chapter.
- Every question is based solely on information found within the text. This eliminates the need for the student to seek information from other reference sources.
- Answers to the multiple-choice questions are found in the appendix and are grouped by chapter number.

New elements contained in the *Study Guide* are:

- NCLEX-STYLE MULTIPLE-CHOICE QUESTIONS. These have been written to encompass every aspect of medical–surgical nursing—assessment, planning, implementation, and evaluation. Each multiple-choice question is constructed in the manner proposed for the CAT NCLEX-PN examination. Working through these questions will assist the user in preparation for the NCLEX-PN examination.
- NURSING PROCESS AND CLIENT NEED. The steps of the Nursing Process and the Client Need are given after each question to familiarize the user with the categorization of specific nursing actions and client needs and to assist in preparation for the NCLEX-PN examination.
- CRITICAL THINKING EXERCISES. At the end of each chapter are critical thinking exercises based on the material contained in the chapter. Critical thinking exercises aid in broadening knowledge of a subject and help increase proficiency in nursing practice by presenting realistic clinical situations and asking the reader to consider the problem carefully and propose one or more solutions. These exercises provide the user with practice in analyzing and utilizing information critical to the practicing medical–surgical nurse. Answers to these questions may be entered in the space provided below each question. Writing a detailed and thorough answer to each question is encouraged. When a long answer is necessary, the reader is encouraged to use extra paper. The solutions to each critical thinking exercise may be found by closely reading the appropriate chapter.

Jeanne C. Scherer
Barbara K. Timby

CONTENTS

Unit I   Nursing Roles and Responsibilities

Unit II   Psychosocial Aspects of Client Care

Unit III   Concepts of Health and Illness

Unit IV   Common Medical–Surgical Problems

Unit V   Caring for Clients with Respiratory Disorders

Unit VI   Caring for Clients with Cardiovascular Disorders

Unit VII   Caring for Clients with Hematopoietic and Lymphatic Disorders

Unit VIII   Caring for Clients with Immune Disorders

Unit IX   Caring for Clients with Neurologic Disorders

Unit X   Caring for Clients with Sensory Problems

Unit XI   Caring for Clients with Gastrointestinal Problems

Unit XII   Caring for Clients with Endocrine Problems

Unit XIII Disturbances of Sexual Structures or Reproductive Function

Unit XIV Caring for Clients with Urinary and Renal Problems

Unit XV Caring for Clients with Musculoskeletal Problems

Unit XVI Caring for Clients with Integumentary Problems

STUDY GUIDE TO ACCOMPANY

Introductory Medical–Surgical Nursing

SIXTH EDITION

I Nursing Roles and Responsibilities

1/ Current Trends in Nursing and Health Care

The health care system is becoming quite specialized, complex, and expensive. Consequently, many individuals are bewildered and confused as to how, where, and to whom to turn for their health needs. For those who are uninsured or underinsured, the options tend to be limited, fragmented, or unaffordable. Several approaches have been implemented to keep the health care system efficient and cost effective, yet meet the needs of persons within the community. As health team members, nurses are filling a much-needed void by expanding their scope of practice to provide services for improving the well-being of healthy individuals, helping clients avoid preventable illnesses, and caring for those who become sick or injured.

The following questions deal with the content of Chapter 1.

I. MULTIPLE CHOICE QUESTIONS

Circle the number of the most appropriate answer.

1. A client with a family history of hypertension is interested in reducing the risks of developing cardiovascular disease. The best initial resource the nurse could recommend is
   1. a primary care provider, like the client's family physician, who may assess the client's current health
   2. a secondary care provider, like a general hospital, where the client may undergo diagnostic tests
   3. a tertiary care provider, like a cardiologist, who specializes in treating heart diseases
   4. a long-term care facility, like a rehabilitation clinic, for individuals recovering from heart ailments

   Nursing Process: Implementation
   Client Need: Safe, Effective Care Environment

2. A client who lives alone is scheduled for discharge from a hospital following the surgical repair of a fractured hip. The client still needs assistance with ambulation and performing activities of daily living. The type of care that would be most appropriate for the nurse to recommend in this case is a person or individual who provides

   1. primary care
   2. secondary care

   3. tertiary care
   ⅃ 4. long-term care

   Nursing Process: Implementation
   Client Need: Safe, Effective Care Environment

3. A private physician refers a client with a history of heart disease to a cardiologist, a specialist in diagnosing and treating heart disorders. It would be most correct for the nurse to describe the type of care provided by a cardiologist as

   1. primary care
   ⅃ 2. secondary care

   3. tertiary care
   4. long-term care

   Nursing Process: Implementation
   Client Need: Safe, Effective Care Environment

4. While listening to a speaker at a conference on health care trends, which one of the following is an inaccurate statement of a goal to which the United States Public Health Service has committed this country by the year 2000?

   1. to increase the span of healthy life for Americans
   2. to reduce health disparities among Americans

   ⅃ 3. to provide free health care for all Americans
   4. to provide preventive services for all Americans

   Nursing Process: Evaluation
   Client Need: Health Promotion/Maintenance

5. The best evidence that a client has understood a nurse's explanation of a health maintenance organization (HMO) is the statement that a member of an HMO prepays a fixed fee that

   ⅃ 1. covers the cost of all health care
   2. acts as a deductible towards health care costs

   3. is applied to health care costs
   4. is refunded if there are no health care claims

   Nursing Process: Evaluation
   Client Need: Health Promotion/Health Maintenance

6. A nurse would be most correct in informing a client who is interested in joining an HMO that its major emphasis is on the

   1. study of factors affecting health and disease
   2. provision of government-subsidized health care

   ⅃ 3. delivery of comprehensive health care
   4. establishment of satellite clinics

   Nursing Process: Implementation
   Client Need: Safe, Effective Care Environment

7. The best evidence that a client understands the cost-effective strategy utilized by a preferred provider organization (PPO) is the statement that PPOs

   ⅃ 1. discount charges in exchange for customer referrals
   2. control costs by promoting health and wellness programs

   3. reduce expenses by performing early preventive treatment
   4. lower fees by employing fewer health care professionals

   Nursing Process: Evaluation
   Client Need: Health Promotion/Health Maintenance

8. A nurse would be most correct in explaining to the family of an older client that there is an incentive to discharge Medicare clients as soon as possible to comply with a financial strategy developed by the federal government referred to as

    1. Health and Human Services (HHS)
    2. Hospital Control Authority (HCA)
    3. Diagnostic Related Groups (DRGs)
    4. Progressive Care Considerations (PCC)

    Nursing Process: Implementation
    Client Need: Safe, Effective Care Environment

9. When a client asks a nurse to clarify the significance of diagnostic related groups (DRGs), the best explanation is that DRGs were developed as a method to

    1. study the patterns of common disorders
    2. reduce health care services to healthy individuals
    3. lower infectious disease mortality rates
    4. reduce the costs for caring for Medicare clients

    Nursing Process: Implementation
    Client Need: Safe, Effective Care Environment

10. Which one of the following is a common public perception of the DRG system? DRGs have

    1. increased commercial health insurance costs for most clients
    2. prolonged the length of hospitalization for some clients
    3. contributed to the premature discharge of some clients
    4. neglected proper supervision of health care of many clients

    Nursing Process: Implementation
    Client Need: Safe, Effective Care Environment

II. CRITICAL THINKING EXERCISES

1. What examples could you provide of how nursing has demonstrated remarkable flexibility for implementing the strategies of health care reforms?

2. In what specific ways could clients be encouraged to prevent diseases and promote their health to higher levels?

3. What are some advantages and disadvantages in belonging to an HMO?

4. Assume that you have been asked to serve on a hospital's planning committee. What trends or directions could you suggest to improve the delivery of health care?

5. In what ways are nurses being utilized through expanded roles to meet the health needs of individuals in America?

2/ The Nursing Process

The *nursing process* is a systematic method for solving a client's health problems. It acts as the framework for nursing action. The five essential steps in the nursing process, which consist of *assessment, analysis,* sometimes called *diagnosis, planning, implementation,* and *evaluation,* are used to develop and implement a plan of care that meets the needs of a specific client.

The following questions deal with the content of Chapter 2

I. MULTIPLE CHOICE QUESTIONS

Circle the number of the most appropriate answer.

A nurse is assigned to admit Mr. Adams to a health care agency. It is this client's first experience.

1. When the client asks why the nurse is making inquiries about his symptoms and past history, it would be most correct for the nurse to respond by saying,

    1. "Perhaps, you forgot to tell the physician something."
    2. "The information is used to plan your nursing care."
    3. "The insurance company requires detailed information."
    4. "You may be needing special tests or diagnostic procedures."

    Nursing Process: Implementation
    Client Need: Safe, Effective Care Environment

2. The nurse in charge asks the admitting nurse for the client's subjective data. Of the following groups of information, which one is the best response to the charge nurse's request?

    1. Mr. Adams is 5' 11" tall and weighs 200 lbs.
    2. Mr. Adams' skin is warm and intact.
    3. Mr. Adams has chest pain that is relieved with rest.
    4. Mr. Adams' pulse is strong and regular.

    Nursing Process: Implementation
    Client Need: Safe, Effective Care Environment

3. While assessing Mr. Adams, which one of the following would be the best approach for obtaining objective data?

    1. watching the client's facial expressions
    2. observing if the client looks relaxed
    3. inspecting the client's body
    4. asking the client questions

    Nursing Process: Planning
    Client Need: Physiological Integrity

4. At the end-of-shift report, a newly employed nursing assistant asks why so much information, referred to as a data-base, is obtained when a client like Mr. Adams is first admitted. The best explanation is that the data-base

    1. is the source from which the client's initial and ongoing problem list is compiled
    2. eliminates the need to continue collecting further data of a similar nature
    3. saves the physician time when performing a history and physical examination
    4. conveys that the nursing personnel are concerned about the client's problems

    Nursing Process: Implementation
    Client Need: Safe, Effective Care Environment

5. The nurse on the next shift takes Mr. Adams' vital signs. Which one of the following nursing actions shows that the nurse is making appropriate use of the earlier data-base assessment findings? The nurse
   1. records the current vital signs on a flow sheet
   2. compares the current vital signs with those on admission
   3. analyzes the current vital signs to determine if they are normal
   4. reports the current vital signs to the nurse in charge

   Nursing Process: Implementation
   Client Need: Physiological Integrity

6. Mr. Adams asks the practical nurse who is caring for him to clarify the difference between the role of the practical nurse and the registered nurse. One difference in relation to the nursing process that might be identified is that the registered nurse
   1. does not provide bedside care to clients
   2. communicates directly to the physician
   3. administers all the medications for clients
   4. develops the initial plan for nursing care

   Nursing Process: Implementation
   Client Need: Safe, Effective Care Environment

Individual Questions

7. The practical nurse reports all the data that indicate actual or potential health problems after assessing a client. When discussing the planning step in the nursing process with the nurse in charge, which activities are included?
   1. analyzing the data and implementing the care
   2. sorting the data and developing a plan for care
   3. establishing priorities and short-term goals
   4. carrying out the plan and evaluating outcomes

   Nursing Process: Implementation
   Client Need: Safe, Effective Care Environment

8. The practical nurse and the registered nurse look at the list of the client's initial problems. They include: Anxiety, Ineffective Individual Coping, Social Isolation, and Ineffective Breathing Pattern. Which problem requires immediate attention?
   1. Anxiety
   2. Ineffective Individual Coping
   3. Social Isolation
   4. Ineffective Breathing Pattern

   Nursing Process: Implementation
   Client Need: Safe, Effective Care Environment

9. All nursing team members are asked to review the care plans for their assigned clients and make recommendations for improvements. If all of the following short-term goals appeared, which one is the most incomplete?
   1. The client will lose 2 lbs. by 3/25.
   2. The client will drink more fluid by 3/14.
   3. The client will have a bowel movement by 3/18.
   4. The client will walk in the hall by 3/20.

   Nursing Process: Evaluation
   Client Need: Safe, Effective Care Environment

10. When the practical nurse assists the registered nurse in developing the plan for care, they are careful that the nursing orders contain all the following criteria except
    1. the nursing orders are clear and specific to personnel
    2. the nursing orders are compatible with medical orders
    3. the nursing orders are limited to a few selective nursing measures
    4. the nursing orders contain every intervention that may solve the problem

    Nursing Process: Implementation
    Client Need: Safe, Effective Care Environment

11. During the process of evaluation, which one of the following steps takes place first?

    1. determining if new problems have developed
    2. comparing the client's current status with the goal
    3. changing the predicted time for achievement
    4. selecting alternative plans for action

    Nursing Process: Evaluation
    Client Need: Safe, Effective Care Environment

II. CRITICAL THINKING

1. A friend tells you that he has been losing weight. Using the steps in the nursing process, explain how you would investigate the problem and help resolve it.

2. Your goal is to achieve at least a 90% on the next nursing examination. Write a list of measures in the style of nursing orders to help meet that goal.

3/ Interviewing and Physical Assessment

Assessment consists of gathering information about the client's health. The initial assessment includes two parts: 1) the interview, during which the client's health history and other subjective data are obtained, and 2) a physical examination for the purpose of obtaining objective data.

The following questions deal with the content of Chapter 3.

I. MULTIPLE CHOICE QUESTIONS

Circle the number of the most appropriate answer.

Ms. Wilson is scheduled to be admitted to the hospital. Before Ms. Wilson arrives, the practical nurse reviews the procedure for admitting a client.

1. From among the actions listed, which one is most essential before the nurse admits a new client?

    1. locate an oral thermometer
    2. develop a list of questions

    3. notify the client's physician
    4. consult with the charge nurse

    Nursing Process: Implementation
    Client Need: Safe, Effective Care Environment

2. Ms. Wilson tells the nurse that the reason she is seeking health care is because she has been having difficulty breathing, especially at night. The nurse would be most correct in documenting this information under the category of the client's

    1. chief complaint
    2. psychosocial history

    3. review of systems
    4. past health history

    Nursing Process: Implementation
    Client Need: Safe, Effective Care Environment

3. The nurse obtains all of the following information. Which of the following would the nurse document under the category of the client's psychosocial history?

    1. Ms. Wilson is 5'2" and weighs 122 lbs.
    2. Ms. Wilson is allergic to wheat and corn products.

    3. Ms. Wilson is the divorced mother of 2 children.
    4. Ms. Wilson had her appendix removed at the age of 13.

    Nursing Process: Implementation
    Client Need: Safe, Effective Care Environment

4. Taking a cue from the fact that Ms. Wilson says she has trouble breathing, the nurse asks whether she has had a cough, a recent fever, or if she experiences any wheezing. The nurse would be most correct in explaining to Ms. Wilson that this focus assessment helps to

    1. prepare her for diagnostic tests
    2. add depth to her earlier information

    3. utilize assistive personnel more efficiently
    4. identify her teaching needs before discharge

    Nursing Process: Implementation
    Client Need: Safe, Effective Care Environment

5. When obtaining Ms. Wilson's past health history, it would be appropriate for the nurse to ask
   1. what, if anything, triggers her symptoms
   2. what kind of childhood disease she had
   3. her to describe her breathing episodes
   4. the kinds of diseases that run in her family

   Nursing Process: Assessment
   Client Need: Safe, Effective Care Environment

6. Ms. Wilson looks startled when the nurse asks her to identify the cause and age when her parents died. The client's cooperation may be facilitated if the nurse explains that
   1. many disorders follow hereditary patterns.
   2. it helps to review the records of deceased relatives.
   3. many health records are often incomplete.
   4. this information is now reported to the Bureau of Vital Statistics.

   Nursing Process: Implementation
   Client Need: Safe, Effective Care Environment

7. The best explanation that the nurse can give Ms. Wilson concerning what will take place during a review of body systems is that during this aspect of the admission process she will be
   1. physically examined over all aspects of her body
   2. evaluated as to whether there is an undiagnosed disease
   3. asked health-related questions
   4. prepared for further testing

   Nursing Process: Implementation
   Client Need: Safe, Effective Care Environment

Individual Questions

8. The nurse plans to perform a physical assessment. The following supplies are gathered: examination gown and drape, stethoscope, and penlight. Which additional item should the nurse plan to obtain?
   1. electrocardiogram machine
   2. syringe for drawing blood
   3. vinyl or latex rubber gloves
   4. an exercise treadmill

   Nursing Process: Planning
   Client Need: Safe, Effective Care Environment

9. A client asks the nurse to explain what is meant by "auscultation." The best answer would be that auscultation means
   1. looking
   2. feeling
   3. listening
   4. tapping

   Nursing Process: Implementation
   Client Need: Safe, Effective Care Environment

10. The nurse taps the client's abdomen and listens as the sound changes from a dull sound to a hollow sound. When documenting these findings, the nurse consults a text on physical assessment to identify the correct term to describe the information. The term the nurse is looking for is
    1. decibel
    2. audiometric
    3. resonance
    4. gurgles

    Nursing Process: Implementation
    Client Need: Safe, Effective Care Environment

11. When the nurse wants to feel for vibrations—for example, over the heart where it underlies the chest—the best assessment technique to use is

    1. auscultation
    2. palpation
    3. inspection
    4. percussion

    Nursing Process: Assessment
    Client Need: Safe, Effective Care Environment

12. A nursing assistant asks the practical nurse to explain the term tympany which was used in documenting physical assessment findings. The best explanation is that it refers to a

    1. hollow sound
    2. dull sound
    3. tinkling sound
    4. loud sound

    Nursing Process: Implementation
    Client Need: Safe, Effective Care Environment

13. Before palpating the client's abdomen, the nurse should plan to

    1. use a stethoscope to listen to sounds within the abdomen.
    2. use a tape measure and measure the girth of the abdomen.
    3. tap the abdomen to outline the size of underlying structures.
    4. ask the client to use the restroom to empty the bladder.

    Nursing Process: Planning
    Client Need: Safe, Effective Care Environment

14. When examining a female client, which one of the following is considered an abnormal finding in the breasts?

    1. spooning
    2. ataxia
    3. aphasia
    4. dimpling

    Nursing Process: Evaluation
    Client Need: Physiological Integrity

II. CRITICAL THINKING EXERCISES

1. How would the physical assessment of a female client differ from that of a male?

2. What assessment data would be appropriate when examining a client's skin?

3. What would it mean if a nurse documented that a client had a positive Babinski?

4. What information would be important to document when assessing a client's mental status?

4/   Legal and Ethical Issues

Nurses must be knowledgeable about the laws affecting their practice and the rights of clients. Laws are followed in the course of public duty; ethics are upheld as a result of personal integrity. Nursing practice must be both lawful to maintain the public's trust and ethical to sustain its high regard.

The following questions deal with the content of Chapter 4.

I. MULTIPLE CHOICE QUESTIONS

Circle the number of the most appropriate answer.

A team conference has been scheduled to discuss laws and ethical issues that affect nursing and client care. The nurses who will be attending the team conference are asked to prepare for it by reviewing their state's definition of nursing, the scope of nursing practice within that state, and the titles that may be used by qualified nurses.

1. The best resource for the information described above would be found in the state's
   1. original constitution
   2. nursing practice act
   3. code of civil laws
   4. health regulations

   Nursing Process: Implementation
   Client Need: Safe, Effective Care Environment

2. A nurse would be most correct in identifying which one of the following as the source that empowers the federal and state governments to ensure the health and safety of its citizens?
   1. civil laws
   2. criminal laws
   3. administrative laws
   4. property laws

   Nursing Process: Implementation
   Client Need: Safe, Effective Care Environment

3. A nurse at the conference asks the conference leader to clarify the difference between an intentional tort and an unintentional tort. The best answer is that an intentional tort is one in which a person commits a deliberately aggressive act and an unintentional tort is one in which
   1. a person is harmed accidentally
   2. an injured person was negligent
   3. a person is injured but not killed
   4. an injured person files a lawsuit

   Nursing Process: Implementation
   Client Need: Safe, Effective Care Environment

4. The best example of assault that the leader of the conference could give is a situation in which a nurse
   1. raises a hand to gesture that the client may be struck
   2. pinches an unconscious client's skin to assess the level of consciousness
   3. administers a sedative to a client who persists in turning on the signal light
   4. reports that a client has been stubborn and demanding

   Nursing Process: Implementation
   Client Need: Safe, Effective Care Environment

5. After explaining the difference between assault and battery, the conference leader asks nurses in attendance to provide a situation that could be considered a basis for battery. If all of the following situations are offered, the best example is one in which a nurse

   1. accuses a client of giving false information
   2. gives prescribed medications to the wrong client
   3. reveals information about a client to a neighbor
   4. fails to obtain a client's consent for treatment

   Nursing Process: Evaluation
   Client Need: Safe, Effective Care Environment

6. A nurse at the conference explains that she has been assigned to write a paper involving a case study on one of the clients for whom she cared. She asks the conference leader how best to protect the client's confidentiality and avoid being charged with invasion of privacy. The best suggestion is to

   1. ask the instructor to shred the paper after it is graded
   2. place the written report in a sealed envelope
   3. use the client's initials or a fictitious name
   4. use pronouns, like he or she, when referring to the client

   Nursing Process: Planning
   Client Need: Safe, Effective Care Environment

7. One of the nurses asks if offering negative opinions about the level of a physician's expertise would be unlawful. The best answer is that this type of action is considered a form of

   1. scandal
   2. libel
   3. slander
   4. assault

   Nursing Process: Implementation
   Client Need: Safe, Effective Care Environment

8. A nurse shares a story about a colleague who was sued for malpractice. He asks the leader and others at the conference how the jury decides if the defendant's actions did not comply with the standard for care. In response to the question, one of the resources that the jury might use is

   1. information reported on television
   2. the testimony of expert witnesses
   3. their own prior life experiences
   4. what they may have read in a book

   Nursing Process: Implementation
   Client Need: Safe, Effective Care Environment

9. The conference leader explains the historical background on medical lawsuits. When describing the precedent for holding hospitals accountable for the quality of care provided by its employed nurses, the conference leader is most correct in calling it the principle of

   1. *caveat emptor*
   2. *respondeat superior*
   3. breach of promise
   4. implied consent

   Nursing Process: Implementation
   Client Need: Safe, Effective Care Environment

10. The leader of the conference asks those attending to evaluate if a nurse would be held responsible if a client fell after disregarding the nurse's instructions to call when needing assistance. The best analysis is that

    1. the nurse would be held totally and exclusively accountable
    2. the court may hold that the client contributed to the injury
    3. the court may hold that the hospital is liable for damages
    4. the nurse would have to prove that the client was competent

    Nursing Process: Evaluation
    Client Need: Safe, Effective Care Environment

11. The conference leader asks the nurses for suggestions on ways to protect oneself if or when becoming involved in a malpractice lawsuit. Of the following suggestions offered, which one is the best?
    1. Make sure the hospital's insurance carrier covers employees.
    2. Deposit money in a personal account to cover liability cases.
    3. Acquire personal, professional liability insurance.
    4. Divest oneself of all financial assets to avoid paying damages.

    Nursing Process: Planning
    Client Need: Safe, Effective Care Environment

Individual Questions

12. In most cases, prior to applying physical restraints, it is essential that the nurse determine if
    1. there is a written medical order for their use
    2. the client will become violent and unmanageable
    3. the family has an objection to their use
    4. the client will recognize who applied them

    Nursing Process: Assessment
    Client Need: Safe, Effective Care Environment

13. During a nursing audit, all of the following are noted in the medical records of hospitalized clients. Based upon the principles of charting, which one is the best example for documenting a client's mental status?
    1. confused and disoriented
    2. when asked to identify location, responded "Holiday Inn"
    3. belligerent and uncooperative
    4. seems to be incoherent and unclear as to present situation

    Nursing Process: Evaluation
    Client Need: Safe, Effective Care Environment

14. When discussing incident reports at the team conference, which one of the following comments made by one of the nurses reflects misinformation? Incident reports are
    1. used to prevent future accidents
    2. filed within the medical record
    3. compiled whenever an injurious situation occurs
    4. used as a reference in case of future litigation

    Nursing Process: Evaluation
    Client Need: Safe, Effective Care Environment

15. Which one of the following nursing actions demonstrates that the nurse is protecting the client's right to confidentiality? The nurse
    1. pulls the privacy curtain about the client before providing nursing care
    2. seeks the client's permission before releasing information to a relative
    3. consults with the client on alternative plans for health treatment
    4. asks the client about his feelings concerning resuscitation

    Nursing Process: Implementation
    Client Need: Safe, Effective Care Environment

16. After consulting with a client, the physician writes a "Do not resuscitate" (DNR) order on a chart. If this client should experience a cardiac arrest, which one of the following actions supports the client's right to self-determination? The nurse
    1. summons the emergency code team
    2. administers life-saving medications immediately
    3. opens the airway and gives the client some breaths
    4. assesses the client for signs of death

    Nursing Process: Implementation
    Client Need: Safe, Effective Care Environment

17. A nurse is concerned about the safety of clients cared for by a nurse who frequently comes to work under the influence of alcohol. The most ethical action to take would be to

    1. assign the nurse to answer the phone and do paper work
    2. co-assign another nurse to the same clients when this occurs
    3. document and report the nurse's behavior to the supervisor
    4. ask to be transferred to another nursing unit in the hospital

    Nursing Process: Implementation
    Client Need: Safe, Effective Care Environment

18. When ethical dilemmas arise and it is difficult to determine which of two decisions is in the best interest of the client, the best resource to consult for legal and ethical issues would be

    1. a clergyman
    2. a lawyer
    3. a nursing colleague
    4. an ethics committee

    Nursing Process: Implementation
    Client Need: Safe, Effective Care Environment

II. CRITICAL THINKING EXERCISES

1. How would you explain the differences between laws and ethics?

2. What federal agencies have been authorized to ensure the health and safety of American citizens?

3. What is the role and responsibilities of a state's board of nursing?

4. If a friend asked what nurses do to protect themselves from being sued, what would be your response?

5. What charting practices help to ensure a good legal defense in a malpractice lawsuit?

II Psychosocial Aspects of Client Care

5/ Caring for Young Adults

The practice of nursing involves providing care to individuals across the life cycle from birth to old age. Therefore, it is important for nurses to know how to prepare clients for the physical changes and common life experiences that occur at various stages throughout life. To do this, nurses must be knowledgeable about the unique changes in health and social relationships that are characteristic of each period in life. The first stage of adult life, called the period of young adulthood, is like no other. It roughly spans the years between 18 and 35.

The following questions deal with the content of Chapter 5.

I. MULTIPLE CHOICE QUESTIONS

Circle the number of the most appropriate answer.

Jack, who is age 20 and unmarried, has had an emergency appendectomy which was accompanied by complications.

1. When conducting the admission interview, which one of the following categories could the nurse expect that Jack will have difficulty in providing information?

   1. chief complaint
   2. psychosocial history
   3. present history
   4. past history

   Nursing Process: Assessment
   Client Need: Health Promotion/Maintenance

2. Because of Jack's stage of development, the nurse could expect to find that he

   1. is lax about scheduling regular physical examinations
   2. performs regular testicular self-examinations
   3. is familiar with community health care resources
   4. has adequate health insurance for his current needs

   Nursing Process: Evaluation
   Client Need: Health Promotion/Maintenance

3. Which one of the following behaviors that Jack admits to is most likely to place him at highest risk for life-threatening health consequences? Jack says he

   1. does not regularly floss his teeth
   2. eats jelly donuts for breakfast
   3. has unprotected sex with many partners
   4. sleeps approximately 6 hours each night

   Nursing Process: Evaluation
   Client Need: Health Promotion/Maintenance

4. If Jack is typical of most young adults, which of the following physical characteristics is the nurse most likely to observe when performing a physical assessment?

   1. His hand grip is weakening.
   2. His wisdom teeth are erupting.
   3. He needs to shave every 2 days.
   4. He has multiple skin blemishes.

   Nursing Process: Implementation
   Client Need: Health Promotion/Maintenance

5. When planning Jack's care, as well as the care of other young adults, the nurse may overlook the fact that young adults may

   1. not manifest typical signs of an infection
   2. feel insecure and need emotional support
   3. not heal as quickly as older adults
   4. require more sleep than adolescents

   Nursing Process: Planning
   Client Need: Health Promotion/Maintenance

Individual Questions

6. Which developmental task is considered unique to babies under the age of 18 months? Infants must

   1. learn to be toilet trained.
   2. begin feeding themselves
   3. get attention for their needs.
   4. double their weight in 6 months.

   Nursing Process: Evaluation
   Client Need: Health Promotion/Maintenance

7. A nurse is asked how to respond to a mother of a child who is 1 year old and has begun toilet training efforts. The best suggestion would be that the mother

   1. place the child on the training seat at frequent intervals
   2. give the child some type of incentive like raisins or candy
   3. wait until the child matures, which may be another 12 months
   4. watch the child closely for signs that he needs to eliminate

   Nursing Process: Implementation
   Client Need: Health Promotion/Maintenance

8. At a conference, nurses are asked to develop a list of experiences that are common during the period of young adulthood. If all of the following are mentioned, which one is incorrect? Young adults generally

   1. challenge the views of their parents
   2. live separately from their parents
   3. establish their own lifestyle
   4. marry or form new peer relationships

   Nursing Process: Implementation
   Client Need: Safe, Effective Care Environment

9. An office nurse prepares a 20-year-old female for an examination. Which of the following physical characteristics could the nurse expect to find if the client is typical of others in this age group? The

   1. client is missing several molar teeth
   2. client has dark skin plaques on her face
   3. client's height has not changed in 4 years
   4. client's menstrual periods are irregular

   Nursing Process: Evaluation
   Client Need: Health Promotion/Maintenance

10. A 25-year-old client confides that she has no close female friends and has had only three dates in her life. The nurse would be most correct in believing that unless this client expands her social relationships, the outcome of her developmental state will be one of

   1. mistrust
   2. inferiority

   3. role confusion
   4. isolation

   Nursing Process: Evaluation
   Client Need: Psychosocial Adaptation

11. If a young adult's social development is typical, which one of the following is apt to be true?

   1. Relationships with former classmates become closer.
   2. There are very few changes in previous relationships.

   3. Peer conformity loses the importance it once had.
   4. Relationships with brothers and sisters become stronger.

   Nursing Process: Evaluation
   Client Need: Health Promotion/Maintenance

II. CRITICAL THINKING EXERCISES

1. Why is it critical to accomplish the developmental tasks of a particular stage rather than earlier or later in life?

2. Maria, age 28, is being admitted to the hospital for the treatment of pneumonia. What nursing measures would be appropriate for meeting her physical, emotional, and social needs?

3. Ronald, a 32-year-old father of two school-age children, has injured his back. He is self-employed and has no health insurance. He has been advised to remain inactive for the next 6 weeks. How might this injury affect him during the period of young adulthood?

4. Robert, age 21, is being seen by the physician for the diagnosis and treatment of a sexually transmitted disease. What characteristics of young adults makes Robert particularly vulnerable to this type of health problem?

6/   Caring for Middle-Aged Adults

Middle age, from about age 35 to 65, is characterized as the established years. This developmental stage generally terminates with retirement. Just as young adulthood has its satisfactions as well as its stresses, so also does middle life have a mixture of the two.

The following questions deal with the content of Chapter 6.

I. MULTIPLE CHOICE QUESTIONS

Circle the number of the most appropriate answer.

1. A nurse interviews a middle-aged client. If the client reports all of the following, which one is most typical for this period of life? The client says he is

   1. an advisor for the Boy Scouts of America
   2. finishing the requirements for a bachelor's degree

   3. preparing to purchase his first home
   4. seeing a counselor for some personal problems

   Nursing Process: Evaluation
   Client Need: Health Promotion/Maintenance

2. A middle-aged client describes all of the following situations for which he is responsible. Which one is a stressor that occurs uniquely during the middle-aged years?

    1. working full time
    2. completing college
    3. caring for one's parents
    4. doing home maintenance

    Nursing Process: Evaluation
    Client Need: Health Promotion/Maintenance

3. Which one of the following behaviors would indicate to the nurse that a middle-aged client is acquiring the characteristic of generativity? The client

    1. pursues opportunities for self-fulfillment
    2. begins to deal emotionally with losses
    3. invests energy in sustaining relationships
    4. doubts his ability to handle crises

    Nursing Process: Evaluation
    Client Need: Health Promotion/Maintenance

4. Which one of the following would be appropriate for the nurse to assess to determine if a middle-aged client has acquired the negative characteristic of stagnation? The client's

    1. financial arrangements
    2. present health history
    3. plans for future projects
    4. religious philosophy

    Nursing Process: Assessment
    Client Need: Health Promotion/Maintenance

5. A middle-aged client asks the nurse to explain the term presbycusis which he heard used by the physician. The nurse would be most correct in telling the client that this word refers to

    1. impaired taste
    2. blurred vision
    3. stooped posture
    4. diminished hearing

    Nursing Process: Implementation
    Client Need: Safe, Effective Care Environment

6. A middle-aged client tells the nurse that he has a fairly sedentary lifestyle. If all of the following findings are made during a physical assessment, which one is most likely related to the client's statement? The client's

    1. height has declined since young adulthood
    2. joint motion is somewhat restricted
    3. stool volume is reduced to a degree
    4. facial skin is showing signs of wrinkling

    Nursing Process: Evaluation
    Client Need: Health Promotion/Maintenance

7. A middle-aged client asks the nurse to identify conditions which she is at highest risk for developing at this stage in her life. The nurse would be most correct by telling the client that after menopause women are especially at risk for developing

    1. a peptic ulcer
    2. migraine headaches
    3. leukemia
    4. osteoporosis

    Nursing Process: Implementation
    Client Need: Health Promotion/Maintenance

8. A middle-aged client is worried that because she is slow to recall some information, she may be developing Alzheimer's disease, a chronic brain disorder. Which of the following statements would be most reassuring to the client? "Memory changes do occur during middle age, but

    1. they are not necessarily evidence of significant pathology"
    2. Alzheimer's disease can only be confirmed by an autopsy"
    3. you may wish to consult a neurologist to be sure"
    4. I'm sure you have absolutely nothing to worry about"

    Nursing Process: Implementation
    Client Need: Psychosocial Integrity

9. While assisting with the examination of a middle-aged client, the physician says, "You have several keratotic lesions on your back." Afterwards the client asks the nurse to explain what the physician meant. The best explanation is that a keratotic lesion is a(n)

   1. elevated, darkly pigmented, skin plaque
   2. flat, reddish skin lesion, with many crevices
   3. raised, white discoloration of the skin
   4. soft, round lump of tissue beneath the skin

   Nursing Process: Implementation
   Client Need: Health Promotion/Maintenance

10. A middle-aged male client is concerned about how age will affect his sexuality. Which one of the following statements is most correct?

    1. "Males do not experience any sexual changes as they age."
    2. "Your frequency and vigor of intercourse may decrease."
    3. "Your performance will be the same, but your desire will not."
    4. "You may achieve an erection, but have difficulty ejaculating."

    Nursing Process: Implementation
    Client Need: Health Promotion/Maintenance

11. The nurse is interviewing a 50-year-old female client. Which one of the following questions would be most appropriate for determining if the client has begun going through menopause?

    1. "When was your last child born?"
    2. "How regular are your periods?"
    3. "Do you experience hot flashes?"
    4. "Are you irritable or depressed?"

    Nursing Process: Assessment
    Client Need: Safe, Effective Care Environment

12. A middle-aged female client asks the nurse, "Besides not being able to have any more children, are there any other effects I may experience as a result of menopause?" The nurse would be most correct in stating,

    1. "The cessation of menstruation is the only sign of menopause"
    2. "Your breasts may become smaller and less supple"
    3. "You may notice a clear, mucus discharge instead of monthly bleeding"
    4. "There may be occasional uterine cramping, but you won't have a period"

    Nursing Process: Implementation
    Client Need: Health Promotion/Maintenance

13. A nurse overhears a colleague explain to a middle-aged client that when menopause begins, the menstrual periods may be short and scant some months, and heavy and prolonged during others. Which one of the following is a correct analysis of the nurse's statement? It is

    1. inaccurate because menstruation suddenly ceases at menopause
    2. inaccurate because there are no changes in the volume of menstrual flow
    3. accurate because the periods become irregular and erratic
    4. accurate because the periods are correlated with the emotions

    Nursing Process: Evaluation
    Client Need: Safe, Effective Care Environment

14. A middle-aged female client confides to the nurse that although she has a husband, she anticipates that she will be quite lonely when her children marry and leave home. Which one of the following responses is most accurate? During middle age, social relationships

    1. often expand as sons- and daughters-in-law are added
    2. with children are replaced by adding new friends
    3. do diminish, but many find other activities to fill the void
    4. remain unchanged from those established in earlier years

    Nursing Process: Implementation
    Client Need: Health Promotion/Maintenance

15. A 54-year-old man makes an appointment with the physician because he has been having episodes at work during which he becomes short of breath and lightheaded. Before being seen by the physician, he tells the nurse that he has just recently been promoted at his place of employment. Based on the information provided by this client, which one of the following is the most logical explanation for his symptoms?

    1. His place of employment probably contains toxic substances.
    2. His performance anxiety can be producing physical symptoms.
    3. He may need more oxygen now that he has reached middle age.
    4. He is being affected by passive smoking in the environment.

    Nursing Process: Evaluation
    Client Need: Psychosocial Integrity

16. A middle-aged client reports that all of the following events have occurred in the past 2 months. Which one is most likely the motivating factor in his making an office appointment for a physical examination?

    1. He read about a new contagious tropical disease
    2. he won a trip to Florida in an office raffle.
    3. he attended the funeral of his best friend.
    4. he started taking high-potency vitamins.

    Nursing Process: Evaluation
    Client Need: Psychosocial Integrity

17. Which one of the following health practices would be most appropriate for the nurse to advise middle-aged clients?

    1. avoid carbonated drinks
    2. stop smoking cigarettes
    3. eat a high-protein diet
    4. take vitamin supplements

    Nursing Process: Implementation
    Client Need: Health Promotion/Maintenance

II. CRITICAL THINKING EXERCISES

1. How might acquiring a chronic illness, such as diabetes, affect a person during the middle stage of adulthood?

2. Anne Holcombe, who is 35 years old, needs to have her gallbladder removed. She was divorced 2 months ago and is unemployed at this time. How would Ms. Holcombe's circumstances affect her physical, emotional, and social well-being?

3. A teenage client tells the nurse that he thinks his parents are going through a mid-life crisis. Explain the meaning that is implied by this expression and give some examples of behavior that is characterized by this term.

7/   Caring for Older Adults

Senescence is the last stage in the life cycle. The years 65 and over are used as a reference point for describing the older adult. Older people are valuable contributors to life at home, in the workplace, and in the community. They offer others with less maturity the benefit of their wisdom from an accumulation of life experiences. Health care workers play a vital role in helping older adults maintain their health to remain productive members of society.

The following questions deal with the content of Chapter 7.

I. MULTIPLE CHOICE QUESTIONS

Circle the number of the most appropriate answer.

Several nurses who are interested in the nursing care of older adults attend a workshop at a local hospital.

1. At one of the workshop sessions, several theories on aging are discussed. If all of the following are mentioned, which one is used to explain the fact that the weight and height of older adults decreases with age?

    1. free radical damage
    2. faulty DNA replication
    3. the stress response
    4. autophagocytosis

    Nursing Process: Implementation
    Client Need: Safe, Effective Care Environment

2. In an effort to study the cause and effects of aging, the nurses are informed about research in which cells are examined for a particular substance that seems to increase as individuals age. To what is the leader of the workshop referring?

    1. cytoplasm
    2. lipofuscin
    3. the nucleolus
    4. the Golgi apparatus

    Nursing Process: Implementation
    Client Need: Safe, Effective Care Environment

3. Before the conference begins, the workshop leader gives a pretest. The nurses are asked to identify a theory used by some to explain the process of aging and eventual death which was proposed by the physician, Hans Selye, in 1930. Of the following choices, which one is correct?

    1. the stress response
    2. Kreb's cycle
    3. oxidation and reduction
    4. glycogenesis

    Nursing Process: Implementation
    Client Need: Safe, Effective Care Environment

4. When discussing the stress response, the workshop leader asks if any of the nurses can give an example of the stage of resistance. The most correct example would be the onset of

   1. symptoms
   2. inflammation

   3. exhaustion
   4. degeneration

   Nursing Process: Implementation
   Client Need: Safe, Effective Care Environment

5. If Selye's theory concerning the stress response is used as a model for explaining aging and death during the workshop, which one of the following stages would correspond to the stage during which death occurs? The

   1. stage of exhaustion
   2. stage of resistance

   3. alarm stage
   4. prodromal stage

   Nursing Process: Implementation
   Client Need: Safe, Effective Care Environment

6. The workshop leader lists several body systems and asks which one is probably the most critical to preserving health. The best response is the

   1. sensory system
   2. neurological system

   3. immune system
   4. reproductive system

   Nursing Process: Implementation
   Client Need: Safe, Effective Care Environment

7. Someone at the conference asks what causes cells to become damaged by free radicals. One of the best explanations for this is chronic exposure to

   1. environmental toxins
   2. biological parasites

   3. synthetic fibers
   4. infectious organisms

   Nursing Process: Implementation
   Client Need: Safe, Effective Care Environment

8. If the nurses are asked to select from the list that follows the characteristic that most Americans attribute to older adults, the most likely choice is

   1. healthy
   2. productive

   3. rigid
   4. fearful

   Nursing Process: Implementation
   Client Need: Safe, Effective Care Environment

Individual Questions

9. When a friend who works in a nursing home comes to the nurse asking advice on the types of programs appropriate for older adults, the best response the nurse could give is to make sure the activity provides a sense of

   1. adventure and excitement
   2. enjoyment and amusement

   3. humor and entertainment
   4. usefulness and self-worth

   Nursing Process: Planning
   Client Need: Psychosocial Integrity

10. A client asks a nurse if there is any substance that can promote cellular integrity. The best answer the nurse can give is that health and longevity can be theoretically prolonged by consuming foods or other sources containing

    1. aspartame
    2. beta-carotene

    3. gamma globulin
    4. polysaccharides

    Nursing Process: Implementation
    Client Need: Safe, Effective Care Environment

11. An older adult asks the nurse why his physician has recommended that he take a capsule of vitamin E daily. One explanation is that vitamin E theoretically

    1. keeps bones from demineralizing
    2. builds healthy red blood cells

    3. protects cells from injury
    4. provides a source of energy

    Nursing Process: Implementation
    Client Need: Health Promotion/Maintenance

12. The nurse would be most correct in identifying which one of the following as a developmental task that usually takes place during older adulthood?

    1. maintaining health
    2. investing savings

    3. adjusting to losses
    4. doing community service

    Nursing Process: Evaluation
    Client Need: Health Promotion/Maintenance

13. While caring for an older adult in a nursing home, which statement conveys to the nurse that the client has developed ego integrity?

    1. "I just finished making my will."
    2. "I've had a long and happy life."

    3. "I'd like to learn how to knit."
    4. "I plan to visit South America."

    Nursing Process: Evaluation
    Client Need: Health Promotion/Maintenance

14. An older client tells the nurse, "If I only had my life to live over again, I'd do things a whole lot differently." Which negative attribute associated with older adulthood is most likely being manifested by this statement?

    1. shame
    2. guilt

    3. inferiority
    4. despair

    Nursing Process: Evaluation
    Client Need: Health Promotion/Maintenance

15. While caring for an older adult, the client tells the nurse he just doesn't feel well. The client's temperature is slightly elevated and the nurse calls the client's physician. The nurse's action is

    1. appropriate because older adults require aggressive treatment
    2. appropriate because mild symptoms are often very significant in older adults

    3. inappropriate because an elevated temperature is not unusual for an older adult
    4. inappropriate because older adults tend to be overtreated for mild symptoms

    Nursing Process: Evaluation
    Client Need: Physiological Integrity

16. During a physical assessment of a 70-year-old client, which structure should the nurse assess to determine if the client has kyphosis?

    1. abdomen
    2. genitalia

    3. spine
    4. scalp

    Nursing Process: Assessment
    Client Need: Safe, Effective Care Environment

17. When assessing an older client's nutrition and dietary patterns, if the client is typical of older adults, the nurse is most likely to find that the client's diet is high in

    1. beef, pork, and poultry
    2. rice, noodles, and pasta
    3. eggs, cheese, and milk
    4. lettuce, cabbage, and corn

    Nursing Process: Assessment
    Client Need: Safe, Effective Care Environment

18. Before discharging an older adult client, which one of the following would be most appropriate to cover in the teaching plan?

    1. a list of foods that are high in carbohydrates
    2. how to limit calories to match reduced needs
    3. the names of chemical food additives to avoid
    4. the locations of stores that give seniors discounts

    Nursing Process: Planning
    Client Need: Health Promotion/Maintenance

19. Which one of the following observations best indicates that the Alzheimer's disease which an older client has is progressively becoming worse? The client

    1. falls frequently
    2. wants to go home
    3. cries for no reason
    4. no longer speaks

    Nursing Process: Assessment
    Client Need: Physiological Integrity

20. When interviewing older adult clients, which of the following actions should the nurse take to accommodate for age-related changes?

    1. complete the interview in as short a time as possible
    2. devote more time for asking and answering questions
    3. obtain information from the family rather than the client
    4. use very simple terms when asking medical questions

    Nursing Process: Planning
    Client Need: Psychosocial Integrity

21. During an interview, an older client is very slow to respond to the questions and sometimes gives an illogical answer. Which one of the following would be most appropriate for the nurse to investigate before assuming that the client has a problem with understanding or interpreting information?

    1. hearing
    2. vision
    3. speech
    4. comfort

    Nursing Process: Assessment
    Client Need: Physiological Integrity

22. A 68-year-old client for whom a nurse is caring has diabetes mellitus. The nurse understands that this condition places the client at risk for

    1. poor healing
    2. poor nutrition
    3. forming blood clots
    4. forming kidney stones

    Nursing Process: Evaluation
    Client Need: Safe, Effective Care Environment

23. To accommodate for an older adult's age-related skin changes, it would be most appropriate for the nurse to schedule bathing

    1. on a daily basis
    2. once a week
    3. every 2 days
    4. twice a month

    Nursing Process: Planning
    Client Need: Physiological Integrity

24. One of the older adult clients in a nursing home asks for a sweater even though the room temperature is 75°F. Which of the following analyses is most correct? Many older adults feel chilled because

    1. they burn calories faster
    2. their perception is impaired

    3. they perspire more heavily
    4. their metabolism is lower

    Nursing Process: Evaluation
    Client Need: Physiological Integrity

25. Which nursing action should the nurse plan to take for an older client who experiences postural hypotension?

    1. have the client rise slowly from a lying position
    2. take the client's blood pressure on both arms

    3. keep oxygen equipment at the bedside for periodic use
    4. offer the client oral fluids throughout the day

    Nursing Process: Planning
    Client Need: Safe, Effective Care Environment

26. The nurse reads in an older male client's medical record that he has an enlarged prostate gland. Which one of the following should the nurse expect to occur? The client may

    1. be unable to achieve an erection
    2. need to get up at night to urinate

    3. have drainage from his urethra
    4. may experience pain during urination

    Nursing Process: Assessment
    Client Need: Physiological Integrity

27. When a nurse assess an older female client prior to being seen by the physician, several bruises are noted about her body. She confides that when her son asked her for money and she refused, he lost his temper and struck her several times. The most appropriate action the nurse should take is to

    1. call the Commission on Aging
    2. notify Adult Protective Services

    3. suggest the son get counseling
    4. tell the client to call the police

    Nursing Process: Implementation
    Client Need: Safe, Effective Care Environment

28. When teaching an older adult, the best plan is to

    1. give instructions just prior to discharge
    2. give the client a booklet to read

    3. find out what the client already knows
    4. wait until the client asks a question

    Nursing Process: Planning
    Client Need: Health Promotion/Maintenance

29. Which one of the following would provide the best arrangement for meeting the hygiene needs of an active older adult client?

    1. helping the client into a bath tub
    2. arranging for the client to shower

    3. having the client bathe at the sink
    4. giving the client a complete bed bath

    Nursing Process: Planning
    Client Need: Safe, Effective Care Environment

30. A nurse does all of the following. Which one is most likely to help older adult clients remain oriented? The nurse

    1. provides calendar in each client's room
    2. asks clients to tell stories about their youth

    3. supplies clients with novels and mystery books
    4. encourages clients to participate in their care

    Nursing Process: Implementation
    Client Need: Psychosocial Integrity

II. CRITICAL THINKING EXERCISES

1. Emma Franklin, age 76, is nearly blind. Her two children are married and live in other states. Her closest friend is her 68-year-old neighbor, Mary. What reasons might Emma have for opposing the suggestion that she move into a nursing home?

2. Evelyn Morgan, age 70, can no longer maintain her home independently. She plans to sell it and move into an apartment in a retirement community. What are some advantages and disadvantages that Evelyn may experience as a result of this change in living arrangements?

3. William O'Reilly, age 75, tells the office nurse where he receives medical care that he is really lonely since his wife died 6 months ago. What suggestions could the nurse give Mr. O'Reilly to improve the quality of his life?

8/   Caring for Dying Clients

The role of health care workers in supporting dying clients and their loved ones often is neglected because emphasis is placed on the details of therapy that, although necessary and important, do not in themselves convey human caring. Nurses have the opportunity to be involved with clients and families at the time of death—an opportunity that can enable them to help others during one of life's crucial experiences, as well as to grow personally in their understanding and acceptance of death as part of life.

The following questions deal with the content of Chapter 8.

I. MULTIPLE CHOICE QUESTIONS

Circle the number of the most appropriate answer.

Gordon Phillips, age 45, has just been told that his lung cancer is not responding to drug therapy and he is not expected to live more than another 6 months.

1. When Mr. Phillips hears the information, he says, "There's got to be a mistake. I want the tests repeated." According to the stages described by Dr. Elisabeth Kübler-Ross, the nurse would be most correct in assuming that Mr. Phillips is manifesting

    1. mistrust
    2. shock
    3. denial
    4. fear

    Nursing Process: Evaluation
    Client Need: Psychosocial Integrity

2. Mr. Phillips says, "I hope I die quickly and don't suffer." Which one of the following replies is most likely to interfere with therapeutic communication between the client and the nurse? The nurse says,

    1. "You shouldn't talk like that."
    2. "You're sounding very depressed."
    3. "Tell me about your concerns."
    4. "There are ways to ease your discomfort."

    Nursing Process: Implementation
    Client Need: Psychosocial Integrity

3. The most definitive sign that Mr. Phillips has become resigned to the fact that his condition is terminal is when he

    1. asks for a second opinion
    2. arranges his funeral service
    3. requests to be discharged
    4. calls his estranged wife

    Nursing Process: Evaluation
    Client Need: Psychosocial Integrity

Sarah Overstreet, age 73, has diabetes and heart disease. She has been a client in a nursing home for 3 years. The nurse has noticed a sudden change in her condition and alerts her family that she may be dying.

4. When assessing Ms. Overstreet's skin as she nears death, which finding is the nurse likely to detect? The skin may appear

    1. pale or mottled
    2. flushed and hot
    3. yellow and cool
    4. swollen and taut

    Nursing Process: Assessment
    Client Need: Physiological Integrity

5. Which one of the following would be most appropriate for the nurse to assess to determine if Ms. Overstreet's cardiac output is low?

   1. tendon reflexes
   2. lung sounds

   3. bowel sounds
   4. urine output

   Nursing Process: Assessment
   Client Need: Physiological Integrity

6. The nursing assistant reports to the nurse that Ms. Overstreet is drooling and seems to be unable to swallow her own saliva. The best action the nurse can recommend is that the nursing assistant

   1. place the client on her back
   2. place the client on her side.

   3. place an emesis basin beneath her mouth
   4. place an absorbent pad beneath her chin

   Nursing Process: Planning
   Client Need: Physiological Integrity

7. Ms. Overstreet's daughter cries and says to the nurse, "I don't want to see my mother suffer, but I don't know what I'll do without her." The nurse tells the client's daughter that sometimes dying clients forestall death until they know

   1. that there is nothing that can cure them
   2. their funeral arrangements have been made

   3. their loved ones can deal with their death
   4. that they are loved and will be missed

   Nursing Process: Implementation
   Client Need: Health Promotion/Maintenance

Individual Questions

8. After discussing hospice care with a client who has a terminal illness, which one of the following statements indicates that the client has accurate information about the care provided by this organization? The client says, "To be accepted for hospice care, I must

   1. have special health insurance"
   2. be able to afford private nurses"

   3. have only 6 months to live"
   4. agree to refuse hospitalization"

   Nursing Process: Evaluation
   Client Need: Health Promotion/Maintenance

9. A dying client tells the nurse that he feels cold. Which one of the following would be most appropriate to do first?

   1. place a heating pad under the client
   2. apply more clothing or a light blanket

   3. offer the client some hot soup to drink
   4. raise the temperature in the room

   Nursing Process: Implementation
   Client Need: Physiological Integrity

10. A dying client's lips are dry from mouth breathing. If all of the following were available, which one would not be appropriate to use?

   1. vaseline
   2. petroleum jelly

   3. zinc oxide ointment
   4. glycerin

   Nursing Process: Implementation
   Client Need: Physiological Integrity

11. When planning the care of a dying client, the practical nurse suggests that staff interact with the client at least every 2 hours. This best rationale for this nursing action is that

   1. the client could die without someone knowing it
   2. dying clients tend to become socially isolated

   3. anything less would be grounds for negligence
   4. attention keeps the client alert and oriented

   Nursing Process: Planning
   Client Need: Psychosocial Integrity

12. A dying client asks a nurse, who is Presbyterian, to read from the Book of Mormon. The best action the nurse can take would be to

    1. contact someone from the Church of Latter Day Saints
    2. ask the client if the Bible could be substituted

    3. delegate the request to the hospital chaplain
    4. read the passage as the client has requested

    Nursing Process: Implementation
    Client Need: Safe, Effective Care Environment

13. What would be the most appropriate action the nurse could take after the family comes to view the body of a deceased client?

    1. ask the family to which funeral home the body should be sent
    2. take the family to a private area and answer their questions

    3. encourage each of them to kiss the deceased and then go home
    4. determine which family member will take the client's property

    Nursing Process: Implementation
    Client Need: Psychosocial Integrity

14. Which one of the following statements made by a dying client is the best indication that he or she is in the bargaining stage? The client says,

    1. "I'll never complain about dying if I can just complete this year of teaching"
    2. "I'd be very grateful if you could get me some pineapple juice"

    3. "I think I could get back to the classroom if I could just get over this nausea"
    4. "I'd like to negotiate for a higher salary, but I won't live long enough to earn it"

    Nursing Process: Evaluation
    Client Need: Psychosocial Integrity

15. A nursing assistant reports to the practical nurse that her client with a terminal illness pounded her fist and screamed, "Why me?" after talking with the physician. The best explanation for the client's behavior is that it indicates a stage in the dying process called

    1. denial
    2. depression

    3. anger
    4. bargaining

    Nursing Process: Evaluation
    Client Need: Psychosocial Integrity

16. A client brings a copy of a living will to the hospital. The nurse would be most correct in informing the client that a living will

    1. must be notarized to be legal
    2. is not considered a legal document

    3. is binding under current laws
    4. requires the signatures of two witnesses

    Nursing Process: Implementation
    Client Need: Safe, Effective Care Environment

17. A client is resuscitated following sudden cardiac arrest. The nurse can assume the client has had a near-death experience if he said he

    1. cannot recall being resuscitated
    2. felt himself floating above his body

    3. heard choirs of angels singing hymns
    4. accepts that death is a part of life

    Nursing Process: Assessment
    Client Need: Psychosocial Integrity

18. A terminally ill client is experiencing increasing levels of pain. Which one of the following plans would be best for promoting the client's comfort? Pain medication should be given

    1. when the client requests it
    2. when the pain is most severe
    3. on a routine schedule
    4. just before bedtime

    Nursing Process: Planning
    Client Need: Physiological Integrity

19. A dying client tells the nurse that he is concerned that he may become addicted to the narcotics used for relieving his pain. Which one of the following is the best response?

    1. "Promoting your comfort has a higher priority."
    2. "Addiction only occurs when using street drugs."
    3. "Don't worry, you can get these drugs legally."
    4. "There are other drugs for treating addiction."

    Nursing Process: Implementation
    Client Need: Safe, Effective Care Environment

20. During a team conference on the care of a client who is dying of autoimmune deficiency syndrome (AIDS), all of the following goals are formulated. Which one has the highest priority?

    1. The client will reach the stage of acceptance.
    2. The client's fears will be relieved.
    3. The client's discomfort will be reduced.
    4. The client will complete unfinished business.

    Nursing Process: Planning
    Client Need: Physiological Integrity

II. CRITICAL THINKING EXERCISES

1. Raoul Martinez has developed liver failure following hepatitis. He has refused a liver transplant which is his only hope for becoming cured. What options are available to Mr. Martinez for terminal nursing care?

2. Violet Thomas' father is comatose due to an inoperable brain tumor. He is being kept alive with intravenous fluids and mechanical ventilation. What suggestions could the nurse make when Ms. Thomas asks what measures she can take to prevent similar treatment if she is ever unable to communicate her wishes?

9/   Nurse–Client Relationships

The establishment of a good nurse-client relationship helps the nurse deal with the client's problems—both physical and emotional. The nurse who concentrates on clients and their feelings, recognizes and understands clients' physical and emotional needs, establishes physical contact, performs technical skills with competence, and is supportive will more likely create a therapeutic atmosphere.

The following questions deal with the content of Chapter 9.

I. MULTIPLE CHOICE QUESTIONS

Circle the number of the most appropriate answer.

During National Nurse's Week, the hospital conducts several continuing learning conferences. Several nurses are attending today's presentation on promoting therapeutic nurse-client relationships.

1. The phases of the nurse-client relationship are reviewed at the conference. The nurses would be most correct in stating that the period during which the client identifies the problems for which help is being sought takes place in the

    1. introductory phase
    2. planning phase

    3. working phase
    4. terminating phase

    Nursing Process: Implementation
    Client Need: Safe, Effective Care Environment

2. When the nurse-client relationship is discussed at the conference, which criterion best determines the circumstances for ending a nurse-client relationship? The relationship terminates when

    1. the client reaches a maximum state of well-being
    2. there is mutual agreement that the client has improved

    3. the client's health insurance will no longer pay the costs
    4. there are no other health problems that can be resolved

    Nursing Process: Implementation
    Client Need: Safe, Effective Care Environment

A nursing manager has been invited to speak at a workshop for nurses on aspects of the nurse-client relationship.

3. The guest speaker tells the group of nurses that one of the best ways to show empathy is to use a technique called sharing perceptions. The best example of this communication technique is when the nurse says,

    1. "How are you feeling?"
    2. "You seem anxious."

    3. "Is your pain relieved?"
    4. "I don't understand."

    Nursing Process: Implementation
    Client Need: Psychosocial Integrity

4. Nurses at the workshop are advised to avoid asking clients questions that begin with "why," a nontherapeutic technique referred to as demanding an explanation. When asked how a question like "Why didn't you take your medication?" could be rephrased, the most therapeutic example would be

    1. "Perhaps there is a misunderstanding about when and how often to take your medication."
    2. "There must be a good explanation for why you have not taken your medicine."

    3. "Do you understand when and how many of your pills you must take every day?"
    4. "You know you should be taking one of your pills every 4 hours until they are gone."

    Nursing Process: Implementation
    Client Need: Psychosocial Integrity

5. Which one of the following nonverbal communication techniques discussed at the conference is the one most likely to be misinterpreted by clients?

   1. silence
   2. touch
   3. space
   4. grimace

   Nursing Process: Implementation
   Client Need: Psychosocial Integrity

Kyle Benson, age 56, has had chronic angina for several years. He has been prescribed medication, but admits that sometimes he forgets to take it. He is admitted to the hospital for an evaluation of the status of his heart disease.

6. Mr. Benson becomes angry over the fact that his lunch tray was late and the food was cold. Which analysis of Mr. Benson's behavior is most correct? The client's anger may be

   1. misdirected due to his anxiety
   2. a result of compromising standards
   3. due to a perfectionistic attitude
   4. a consequence of a rigid personality

   Nursing Process: Evaluation
   Client Need: Psychosocial Integrity

7. During Mr. Benson's emotional outburst, the best action the nurse can take is to

   1. leave him alone to work through his anger
   2. explain that anger may harm his heart
   3. listen to his complaints nonjudgmentally
   4. request that the dietitian visit him

   Nursing Process: Implementation
   Client Need: Psychosocial Integrity

8. Mr. Benson is scheduled for a heart catheterization. Because the nurse believes he is moderately anxious, which one of the following actions is most appropriate for the nurse to take? The nurse

   1. repeats the test explanation several times
   2. restricts his visitors to just the family
   3. suggests that he stay up late so he sleeps better
   4. transfers him to a room across from the nursing desk

   Nursing Process: Implementation
   Client Need: Safe, Effective Care Environment

Individual Questions

9. A nurse observes a colleague's interaction with a client. If all of the following occur, the one aspect that needs improvement is that the nurse

   1. makes frequent eye contact with the client
   2. nods and says, "Go on"
   3. sits in a chair at the client's bedside
   4. glances at the clock several times

   Nursing Process: Evaluation
   Client Need: Safe, Effective Care Environment

10. A nurse overhears a colleague tell a worried preoperative client, "Relax. Everything will work out just fine." The best analysis of this interaction is that it is

    1. therapeutic because it relieves the client's anxiety
    2. therapeutic because it demonstrates the nurse's confidence
    3. nontherapeutic because it intimidates the client
    4. nontherapeutic because it trivializes the client's fears

    Nursing Process: Evaluation
    Client Need: Safe, Effective Care Environment

11. A client who is Native American asks that his drinking water be kept in a special pottery jar. To promote a therapeutic nurse–client relationship, it would be best to

    1. suggest that it would be safer to send the jar home
    2. ask the client if the jar is made from safe materials
    3. place the water in the pottery jar as requested
    4. seek an explanation for the client's request

    Nursing Process: Implementation
    Client Need: Safe, Effective Care Environment

12. A client, who is scheduled to have intestinal surgery and will have an abdominal opening through which stool will pass, expresses his concern to the nurse that he will be rejected by his family and friends. If all of the following are possible, which plan would be most helpful in resolving the client's fears?

    1. arrange a meeting with a person who had similar surgery
    2. reassure the client that everyone will treat him the same
    3. show the client the equipment that he will use postoperatively
    4. give the client a booklet about the prospective surgery

    Nursing Process: Planning
    Client Need: Psychosocial Integrity

13. A client will be undergoing a mastectomy (removal of a breast) and is concerned about her rehabilitation and adjustment afterwards. Which volunteer program would be most helpful to this client?

    1. Renewed Hearts
    2. Lost Cord Society
    3. The Body Shop
    4. Reach to Recovery

    Nursing Process: Planning
    Client Need: Safe, Effective Care Environment

14. A nursing assistant asks for suggestions on how to help develop trust. The best response the nurse can give is that trust develops

    1. only after knowing a client a long time
    2. when a client's fears have been relieved
    3. by being available and attentive to clients
    4. by organizing and carrying out nursing care

    Nursing Process: Implementation
    Client Need: Safe, Effective Care Environment

15. Which one of the following techniques would be most appropriate for determining whether an anxious client understands the procedure to which he has consented?

    1. ask the client if he would like to change his mind
    2. give the client a printed test of questions to answer
    3. watch the client's body language during the explanation
    4. ask the client to paraphrase the information

    Nursing Process: Evaluation
    Client Need: Safe, Effective Care Environment

II. CRITICAL THINKING EXERCISES

1. Anne Hinkley is a student nurse who has been assigned to care for Alex Foster, age 24, who is recovering from a sports injury. After giving Mr. Foster a backrub, Mr. Foster tries to kiss Ms. Hinkley and asks her for a date. What factors may have led the client to misinterpret the intentions of the student nurse?

2. Kent Walters is a new nursing graduate. He has been asked to admit a female client, a procedure that will involve a physical examination. Since the two are opposite genders, what techniques will promote emotional comfort and propriety while carrying out this task?

3. Mr. Liu Tanaka, age 22, is being hospitalized for the first time after discovering a lump in his testicle. He will undergo several diagnostic tests in the next few days. What common fears might Mr. Tanaka be experiencing and how can the nurse relieve them?

4. John Andrews, a student nurse, confides that he gets very anxious when the clinical instructors start asking questions about his plans for his assigned client's care. What suggestions might be helpful in relieving John's anxiety?

10/   Caring for Culturally Diverse Clients

Transcultural nursing, a term coined by Madeline Leininger in the 1970s, refers to providing nursing care within the context of another's culture. Culture-specific care requires that nurses learn how the differences in anatomy and physiology, health needs, and beliefs affect a culturally diverse client's health decisions, nursing care, and responses to treatment interventions. Ignorance of a cultural group's unique biopsychosocial characteristics results in health care that is less than optimum.

The following questions deal with the content of Chapter 10.

I. MULTIPLE CHOICE QUESTIONS

Circle the number of the most appropriate answer.

A team conference is arranged to discuss cultural diversity.

1. At the conference the nurses debate whether the "melting pot" theory is valid. Which one of the following facts is the best evidence for disputing it?
    1. Thousands of individuals from all over the world immigrate each year to the United States.
    2. There are culturally distinct pockets of ethnic communities throughout the United States.
    3. The United States controls immigration through a strict quota system.
    4. Many individuals marry others who are not from their country of origin.

    Nursing Process: Implementation
    Client Need: Safe, Effective Care Environment

2. The nurses attending the conference discuss the effects of ethnocentrism. One of the best examples raised during the discussion is that Americans tend to
    1. be stunned when others behave dissimilarly
    2. be fascinated by unique and unusual practices
    3. oppose paying tax dollars for foreign aid
    4. encourage open immigration for oppressed groups

    Nursing Process: Implementation
    Client Need: Safe, Effective Care Environment

Individual Questions

3. When performing a physical assessment on a dark-skinned client, which structure of the integument would provide the most valid site for assessing cyanosis?

   1. lips
   2. skin
   3. mouth
   4. nails

   Nursing Process: Assessment
   Client Need: Physiological Integrity

4. A nurse reports that his client, who is African-American, is jaundiced because his sclerae appear yellow. Which one of the following is another valid analysis of the data? The sclerae of some non-Caucasians may appear yellow due to

   1. an effect of chronic kidney disease
   2. excess consumption of orange juice
   3. toxic absorption of clothing dyes
   4. an accumulation of fatty deposits

   Nursing Process: Evaluation
   Client Need: Physiological Integrity

5. A nurse performs a physical assessment. Which one of the following findings indicates that the client has keloids? The client

   1. has yellow sclerae
   2. has a barrel chest
   3. long, flabby earlobes
   4. thick, elevated scars

   Nursing Process: Assessment
   Client Need: Safe, Effective Care Environment

6. When working in a newborn nursery, in what location would the nurse expect to see Mongolian spots?

   1. lower back and buttocks
   2. upper back and shoulders
   3. bridge of the nose
   4. between the eyes

   Nursing Process: Assessment
   Client Need: Safe, Effective Care Environment

7. A nurse observes that a client's hair is extremely thick and curly. Which one of the following would be best for the nurse to use for hair care?

   1. pocket comb with narrow teeth
   2. hair brush with wire bristles
   3. pick with widely spaced teeth
   4. curling iron on a cool setting

   Nursing Process: Planning
   Client Need: Physiological Integrity

8. In response to a question from a nursing assistant, which one of the following statements is correct information regarding the epicanthal eye folds, a common physical characteristic among Asians? The epicanthal eye fold

   1. improves visual acuity
   2. filters ultraviolet rays from sunlight
   3. makes it difficult to wear contact lenses
   4. has no effect on vision

   Nursing Process: Implementation
   Client Need: Safe, Effective Care Environment

9. When inspecting the oral cavity of a client who is a Native American, which one of the following is a common inherited characteristic? The

   1. tongue is furrowed
   2. mucosa is spotted
   3. uvula is split in two
   4. hard palate is V-shaped

   Nursing Process: Assessment
   Client Need: Safe, Effective Care Environment

10. Which one of the following comments should alert the nurse that the client may have an inherited enzyme deficiency?

    1. "When I drink milk, I get terrible abdominal cramps."
    2. "When I eat strawberries, I break out in hives."
    3. "When I cook grilled fish, I sneeze and cough."
    4. "When I chop raw onions, my hands itch."

    Nursing Process: Assessment
    Client Need: Physiological Integrity

11. A nurse is caring for a foreign student from China. If all of the following drugs were prescribed, which one should the nurse withhold until consulting with the physician since some ethnic groups commonly lack an enzyme needed to metabolize it?

    1. penicillin (Pentids)
    2. acetaminophen (Tylenol)
    3. quinine (Quine)
    4. cimetidine (Tagamet)

    Nursing Process: Implementation
    Client Need: Physiological Integrity

12. When reviewing a client's health history, which one of the following is a commonly inherited disease among individuals who trace their origins to Africa?

    1. rheumatoid arthritis
    2. multiple sclerosis
    3. sickle cell disease
    4. cystic fibrosis

    Nursing Process: Assessment
    Client Need: Physiological Integrity

13. A nurse is caring for Ms. Whitefeather, a member of the Pima Indian tribe. The nurse recommends that she receive regular health examinations because this group of American Indians has a high incidence of developing

    1. gallbladder disease
    2. diabetes mellitus
    3. thyroid cancer
    4. peptic ulcer disease

    Nursing Process: Implementation
    Client Need: Health Promotion/Maintenance

14. Which one of the following ethnic substances should the nurse advise an Asian-American client to avoid in order to reduce the client's hypertension?

    1. raw fish
    2. soy sauce
    3. rice noodles
    4. mung beans

    Nursing Process: Implementation
    Client Need: Health Promotion/Maintenance

15. A nurse is part of a United State Public Health team that will be studying health problems among Native Americans. Which one of the following conditions is most likely to be included in the study?

    1. birth defects
    2. alcoholism
    3. malnutrition
    4. heart disease

    Nursing Process: Assessment
    Client Need: Physiological Integrity

16. A Latino client with ovarian cancer attributes her disease to castigo de Dios. The nurse would be most correct in interpreting this to mean

    1. the evil eye
    2. living in poverty
    3. eating spicy food
    4. punishment from God

    Nursing Process: Assessment
    Client Need: Safe, Effective Care Environment

17. While caring for a client, which action by the nurse best demonstrates respect for the client's culture? The nurse

    1. consults the client on the plan for care
    2. replaces a religious medal after a test
    3. asks if any form of contraception is used
    4. pulls the privacy curtain before an exam

    Nursing Process: Implementation
    Client Need: Safe, Effective Care Environment

18. When planning measures for health promotion with an Asian-American client, which one of the following would be most culturally acceptable to the client?

    1. daily exercise
    2. taking vitamins
    3. restricting food
    4. increasing fluids

    Nursing Process: Planning
    Client Need: Health Promotion/Maintenance

19. When a nurse observes a Latino client drinking an herbal tea brought by a curandero, it would be most appropriate to

    1. prohibit the client from any further use
    2. consult with the physician about its safety
    3. ask the client about its curative properties
    4. send a sample to the laboratory for analysis

    Nursing Process: Implementation
    Client Need: Health Promotion/Maintenance

20. A pregnant client reports to the nurse at a prenatal clinic that her first child was delivered by a partera. Which one of the following would be the most appropriate action for the nurse to take at this time?

    1. commend her current decision to seek obstetrical care
    2. inform her that lay midwives are not safe practitioners
    3. explain that nonprofessional care is associated with a high infant mortality rate
    4. emphasize that a physician can provide better care of her and her unborn baby

    Nursing Process: Implementation
    Client Need: Health Promotion/Maintenance

II. CRITICAL THINKING EXERCISES

1. Ms. Firoozeh Patel, a visitor in the United States from India, falls and breaks a hip. Ms. Patel does not speak English; but her daughter does. How might the nursing staff communicate with this client?

2. The medical record indicates that Ms. Hernandez, age 38, needs to have her uterus removed to treat fibroid tumors. Ms. Hernandez and her husband are recent Mexican immigrants. How might the nurse best facilitate compliance with the physician's recommendation?

3. Ricardo Alvarez moved to the United States from Cuba 10 years ago. Mr. Alvarez, now age 40, has been having rectal bleeding. What may cause him to delay seeking medical attention?

III Concepts of Health and Illness

11/ Interaction of Body and Mind

Despite the skepticism over alternative health beliefs and practices, there are many examples of how the mind influences the functions of the body. Scientists have only recently begun to understand just how powerful the mind can be as both a weapon and a tool. Gradually, the role of the mind, though not completely understood, is being accepted as a factor that influences physiology for better and worse.

The following questions deal with the content of Chapter 11.

I. MULTIPLE CHOICE QUESTIONS

Circle the number of the most appropriate answer.

Two student nurses who are interested in utilizing emotional as well as physical treatment approaches are attending a conference on holistic health care.

1. At the conference, the nursing students learn about how the mind influences the body. From the following list, they are asked to identify which one is the best example of this phenomenon. The best answer is

    1. skin heals following a surgical procedure
    2. red cells are produced following blood loss
    3. salivation occurs when seeing food prepared
    4. coughing occurs after inhaling smoke

    Nursing Process: Implementation
    Client Need: Safe, Effective Care Environment

2. The placebo effect is discussed at the conference. When sharing the information with other nurses who could not attend the conference, the student nurses' best explanation of this term is that it refers to a

    1. therapeutic response to an inactive substance
    2. therapeutic response to an active substance
    3. positive response to a negative stimulus
    4. negative response to a positive stimulus

    Nursing Process: Implementation
    Client Need: Safe, Effective Care Environment

3. Various alternative treatment approaches are discussed at the conference. Which one of the following nontraditional techniques could be used to provide the client with electronic information on his or her success at controlling a symptom?

    1. psychocybernetics
    2. acupuncture
    3. acupressure
    4. biofeedback

    Nursing Process: Planning
    Client Need: Physiological Integrity

4. At the conference, the nurses are given a list of nursing measures that may be used therapeutically to relieve discomfort and improve a client's feeling of well-being. All of the following might appear on the list except

    1. engaging in conversation
    2. listening to music
    3. fasting from food
    4. promoting laughter

    Nursing Process: Implementation
    Client Need: Safe, Effective Care Environment

5. The conference leader explains the role of the psyche. Which one of the following is the best description of the superego? It is the component of personality that Freud described as the

    1. pleasure seeker
    2. disciplinarian
    3. integrator
    4. terminator

    Nursing Process: Implementation
    Client Need: Safe, Effective Care Environment

Individual Questions

6. If asked to identify the body system that most likely orchestrates the physiological changes accompanying the stress response, the best answer is the

    1. hematopoeitic system
    2. integumentary system
    3. autonomic nervous system
    4. central nervous system

    Nursing Process: Implementation
    Client Need: Safe, Effective Care Environment

7. A client is learning to use biofeedback to control his hypertension. When he is first attached to the equipment, it would be most appropriate for the nurse to instruct him to

    1. use whatever means he can to quiet a beeping alarm that correlates with his blood pressure
    2. press a signal button sounding an alarm when he feels his blood pressure rising
    3. give himself an electrical shock if his blood pressure becomes dangerously elevated
    4. monitor his blood pressure and report measurements that are outside the acceptable range

    Nursing Process: Implementation
    Client Need: Health Promotion/Maintenance

8. A client has had a seige of diarrhea, but no reason has been found to explain its cause. If the client discloses all of the following, which one is the most likely factor affecting the client's health at this time?

    1. The client's spouse died 3 months ago.
    2. The client sleeps 6 hours each night.
    3. The client is allergic to antibiotics.
    4. The client's vacation plans were cancelled.

    Nursing Process: Assessment
    Client Need: Psychosocial Integrity

9. Which one of the following would the nurse expect to find when a client has been under prolonged stress?

   1. increased white blood cells
   2. accelerated wound healing
   3. decreased blood glucose
   4. sleep pattern disturbance

   Nursing Process: Assessment
   Client Need: Physiological Integrity

10. If a client reacts to stress through the parasympathetic pathway, which one of the following observations will the nurse most likely make? The client will demonstrate

    1. generalized inactivity
    2. exceptional hyperactivity
    3. increased muscle tone
    4. decreased bowel sounds

    Nursing Process: Assessment
    Client Need: Physiological Integrity

11. A client confides to the nurse that her unemployed husband always has some unreasonable excuse for why he is not hired following a job interview. Which one of the following best explains the husband's behavior according to Freudian psychology?

    1. her husband must have been rigidly toilet trained as an infant
    2. her husband is over-reacting to a particularly stressful event
    3. Everyone responds to stress in a unique manner or pattern.
    4. Everyone uses coping mechanisms to protect self-image.

    Nursing Process: Implementation
    Client Need: Psychosocial Integrity

12. A client asks the nurse to identify under what circumstances it is unhealthy to use psychological coping mechanisms. The response that is most correct is when these mechanisms interfere with

    1. psychological growth
    2. finding happiness
    3. the rights of others
    4. medical treatment

    Nursing Process: Implementation
    Client Need: Safe, Effective Care Environment

13. When an alcoholic client is asked to describe his pattern of alcohol consumption, he tells the nurse that he is a "social drinker." The nurse would be most accurate in describing the client's response to other co-workers as one of

    1. repression
    2. regression
    3. denial
    4. undoing

    Nursing Process: Implementation
    Client Need: Psychosocial Integrity

14. A nurse observes that a client who has been raped cannot recall any of the circumstances surrounding the attack. The nurse might infer that this client is using which one of the following coping mechanisms to protect herself from the reality of the sexual trauma?

    1. denial
    2. rationalization
    3. displacement
    4. repression

    Nursing Process: Evaluation
    Client Need: Psychosocial Integrity

15. After a physician confronts a client about his noncompliance in taking prescribed medication, the client criticizes the nurse for applying a blood pressure cuff too tightly. This client is most likely demonstrating which one of the following coping mechanisms?

    1. suppression
    2. displacement

    3. somatization
    4. compensation

    Nursing Process: Evaluation
    Client Need: Psychosocial Integrity

II. CRITICAL THINKING EXERCISES

1. Samuel Gordon is being treated for lung cancer. What reasons might explain why Mr. Gordon becomes nauseated and vomits when driving to the hospital for his chemotherapy treatment.?

2. To control her motion sickness as a child, Sally Turner's parents told her that if she held a penny in each hand she would not vomit; the suggestion frequently was successful. Explain this phenomenon from the perspective of the *placebo effect.*

3. A client experiences bursts of rapid heart rate, causing very uncomfortable sensations of palpitations, light headedness, and shortness of breath. Since the symptoms are not life-threatening and the physician feels that there are likely to be more risks than benefits in using drugs, biofeedback is recommended. Explain how this technique is used.

4. A client tells the nurse that after she jogs each morning, she has a high level of energy and elated feeling. What explanations can be offered for this client's reaction?

12/ Caring for Clients with Stress-Related Disorders

Questions remain as to whether stress-related disorders are genetically inherited, learned, or a combination of both. Research indicates that many stress-related disorders run in families. However, individuals learn stress responses and coping mechanisms from their interactions with significant others.

The following questions deal with the content of Chapter 12.

I. MULTIPLE CHOICE QUESTIONS

Circle the number of the most appropriate answer.

Mr. Alonzo Ferantino is being cared for on a medical nursing unit. The nurses have observed that this client has hypertension and has not been sleeping well. As a result of his care, there is a decision to call a team conference to learn more about the topic of stress-related disorders.

1. Besides hypertension, which is caused by a dominant sympathetic nervous system response to stress, a nursing assistant asks a nurse to identify other examples of disorders in this same category. The list might include all of the following except

   1. low back pain
   2. bruxism
   3. insomnia
   4. gallstones

   Nursing Process: Implementation
   Client Need: Safe, Effective Care Environment

2. If Mr. Ferantino is typical of others with stress-related disorders, which one of the following is a common symptom he experiences?

   1. tightness in the chest
   2. numbness in the legs
   3. decreased urination
   4. persistent weight loss

   Nursing Process: Assessment
   Client Need: Physiological Integrity

3. During the conference, the profile of individuals who develop stress-related disorders is discussed. Of all the following comments, which one is most correct? Stress-related disorders
    1. follow a major infection
    2. tend to run in families
    3. occur in unstable individuals
    4. tend to increase with age

    Nursing Process: Assessment
    Client Need: Safe, Effective Care Environment

4. Each of four case histories involving disorders of the gastrointestinal tract and accessory digestive organs are reviewed at a team conference. For which client is stress likely a primary factor in the disorder?
    1. Frances Reams, who has irritable bowel syndrome
    2. Oliver Jones, who has an inflamed gallbladder
    3. Stanley Rogers, who has rectal hemorrhoids
    4. Jean Evans, who has acute pancreatitis

    Nursing Process: Implementation
    Client Need: Safe, Effective Care Environment

5. If the nurse used the Social Readjustment Rating Scale as a tool for predicting which clients are at greatest risk for acquiring a stress-related disorder, which one of the following events has been correlated with the maximum amount of stress?
    1. returning to school
    2. getting a promotion
    3. sexual difficulties
    4. death of a spouse

    Nursing Process: Assessment
    Client Need: Psychosocial Integrity

6. If a client tells the nurse that he abuses all of the following substances, which one is most likely to cause symptoms similar to those experienced by individuals with stress-related disorders produced by the sympathetic nervous system?
    1. marijuana
    2. morphine
    3. heroin
    4. cocaine

    Nursing Process: Assessment
    Client Need: Psychosocial Integrity

7. All of the following are essential to quality care. Which one is a priority when planning the nursing care of a client with a stress-related disorder?
    1. teaching the client ways to make healthy lifestyle changes
    2. explaining the prescribed diagnostic tests and procedures
    3. ensuring that the client's meals are served hot and on time
    4. clarifying information that may be unfamiliar to the client

    Nursing Process: Planning
    Client Need: Physiological Integrity

8. A nurse observes all of the following behaviors of a client who is scheduled for a diagnostic test in the outpatient department. Which one is most characteristic of someone who is experiencing stress? The client is seen to
    1. read an assortment of educational pamphlets
    2. make several phone calls at a pay telephone
    3. get several drinks of water from the fountain
    4. pace about the waiting room in a continuous fashion

    Nursing Process: Assessment
    Client Need: Psychosocial Integrity

9. Which approach would be the best plan to implement for a client who must eliminate caffeine in order to control stress-related symptoms?

    1. restrict all sources of caffeine immediately
    2. substitute hot chocolate in place of coffee
    3. gradually reduce caffeine over several days
    4. replace caffeine with tea or cola soft drinks

    Nursing Process: Planning
    Client Need: Physiological Integrity

10. A client asks the nurse for a cup of warm milk before retiring. Which information from the nurse is most correct? Drinking milk at this time of the day is

    1. inappropriate because it contains lactose, a type of sugar for sustaining energy
    2. inappropriate because it contains calcium, a mineral for promoting the transmission of nerve impulses
    3. appropriate because it contains protein, a nutrient for cellular growth and repair
    4. appropriate because it contains L-tryptophan, a chemical that promotes sleep

    Nursing Process: Implementation
    Client Need: Health Promotion/Maintenance

11. A client tells the nurse that the reason he has not had a bowel movement since his admission to the hospital is because he finds it stressful to use a public toilet. Which action would be best for restoring a normal pattern for bowel elimination for this client?

    1. place a portable commode at the client's bedside
    2. ensure that the client has privacy while using the toilet
    3. pull the privacy curtains when the client uses a bedpan
    4. obtain a medical order to administer a laxative

    Nursing Process: Planning
    Client Need: Health Promotion/Maintenance

12. Which one of the following nursing measures is best for reducing the anxiety a client is manifesting? The nurse

    1. keeps the area well-lit to promote orientation and safety
    2. administers care without bothering the client with decisions
    3. speaks in a modulated voice and makes explanations brief
    4. advises visitors to come only during scheduled hours

    Nursing Process: Implementation
    Client Need: Psychosocial Integrity

13. After several unsuccessful approaches at relieving a client's anxiety, a nursing assistant asks the practical nurse for further advice. If the nurse suggests that a visualization technique be used, the best instruction would be to have the client

    1. think about a pleasurable place or experience
    2. look at a magazine with colorful photographs
    3. gaze out the hospital window toward the park
    4. watch a program on television that he enjoys

    Nursing Process: Implementation
    Client Need: Health Promotion/Maintenance

14. A client has been taking all of the drugs listed below for several months. To prevent symptoms from appearing that are similar to anxiety, it would be most appropriate for the nurse to inform the client to never discontinue which one of the following drugs abruptly?

    1. alprazolam (Xanax), a minor tranquilizer
    2. ranitidine (Zantac), a histamine blocker
    3. estradiol (Estrace), a synthetic estrogen
    4. chlorothiazide (Diuril), a diuretic

    Nursing Process: Implementation
    Client Need: Health Promotion/Maintenance

15. A client tells the nurse that he experiences gastrointestinal symptoms like gas and bloating when he is under stress. Which one of the following measures would be most appropriate for the nurse to recommend?

    1. take a full half-hour to eat each meal
    2. avoid using pepper when seasoning food
    3. refrain from drinking through a straw
    4. drink carbonated beverages between meals

    Nursing Process: Planning
    Client Need: Health Promotion/Maintenance

II. CRITICAL THINKING EXERCISES

1. Ursula Froelich experiences heart palpitations that are due to stress. What kind of advice could a nurse give Ms. Froelich and others like her regarding over-the-counter drugs?

2. Kenneth Yablonski describes himself as having a *Type A* personality. Explain what Mr. Yablonski means and contrast it with what has been identified as a *Type B* personality.

3. Gary Teeters suffers from stress-related symptoms. If Mr. Teeters reveals a history of drinking alcohol to excess, explain what effect this may have on his condition.

13/ Caring for Clients with Psychosomatic Disorders

The mind and the body are not separate; what affects one very often affects the other. The effect of the mind on the body and the illnesses that may be produced because of the mind's influence on the body are not yet fully understood.

The following questions deal with the content of Chapter 13.

I. MULTIPLE CHOICE QUESTIONS

Circle the number of the most appropriate answer.

The nursing staff is frustrated by the challenge of caring for a client with ulcerative colitis, a disease that is sometimes classified as a psychosomatic disorder. Consequently, a team conference is being organized to review more about the nature of psychosomatic disorders.

1. A nurse is asked to describe one of the most distinguishing characteristics of psychosomatic disorders. Of the following, which response is most correct?

    1. They go from an acute stage to one that is chronic.
    2. They affect older adults more so than younger adults.
    3. They occur among individuals who exaggerate the significance of their symptoms.
    4. They have cycles during which symptoms are absent and then reoccur.

    Nursing Process: Implementation
    Client Need: Safe, Effective Care Environment

2. The team leader asks if anyone can provide the term used to describe the period during which symptoms that had been inactive are remanifested? The term to which the conference leader is referring is

    1. exenteration
    2. exacerbation
    3. remission
    4. proliferation

    Nursing Process: Implementation
    Client Need: Safe, Effective Care Environment

3. At the conference, the nurses are informed that during an assessment, the onset of the symptoms associated with a psychosomatic disorder is most likely to coincide with a period during which clients are

    1. not consuming healthy nutrients
    2. recovering from an infection
    3. experiencing emotional problems
    4. unusually fatigued from activity

    Nursing Process: Assessment
    Client Need: Safe, Effective Care Environment

4. From a list of statements that follow, the conference leader asks the nurses to identify which one fits the description of a malingerer. The one which is most correct is that a malingerer is one who

    1. has a real illness but does not recognize the symptoms
    2. refuses medical treatment despite symptoms of a disorder
    3. deliberately fakes illness to achieve a secondary gain
    4. has an illness but exaggerates the symptoms for attention

    Nursing Process: Implementation
    Client Need: Safe, Effective Care Environment

Individual Questions

5. From a psychiatric nursing textbook, a nurse reviews the characteristics of malingering. The nurse is most likely to find that the motivational factor underlying malingering is that the client's symptoms are manifested for all of the following reasons except

   1. to obtain drugs
   2. to avoid work

   3. to acquire money
   4. to find relief

   Nursing Process: Implementation
   Client Need: Safe, Effective Care Environment

6. A client asks what pathophysiological mechanism is responsible for the symptoms associated with a psychosomatic disorder. The best response is that psychosomatic disorders occur due to an impairment in the

   1. immune system's feedback loop
   2. endocrine system's hormone levels

   3. protein synthesis by DNA molecules
   4. regulation of growth and repair

   Nursing Process: Implementation
   Client Need: Safe, Effective Care Environment

7. A nurse who has done extensive reading on psychosomatic disorders reports to others at a team conference that a psychosocial need that is often unfulfilled among individuals with these disorders is the need for

   1. autonomy
   2. industry

   3. dependence
   4. identity

   Nursing Process: Implementation
   Client Need: Safe, Effective Care Environment

8. When observing a client with a psychosomatic disorder which finding is most characteristic? The client

   1. avoids expressing anger
   2. tends to be noncommunicative

   3. demonstrates an air of optimism
   4. doubts the sincerity of others

   Nursing Process: Assessment
   Client Need: Psychosocial Integrity

9. Which one of the following would be most therapeutic when developing the plan of care for a client with a psychosomatic disorder?

   1. spending time with the client when no physical tasks are required
   2. encouraging the client to be as self-reliant and independent as possible

   3. withholding attention beyond that which is required for giving physical care
   4. monitoring the client closely for rapidly fluctuating signs and symptom

   Nursing Process: Planning
   Client Need: Psychosocial Integrity

10. If all of the following problems are listed on the initial care plan of a client with a psychosomatic disorder, which one requires the practical nurse's priority for attention?

   1. High Risk for Impaired Social Interaction
   2. Ineffective Individual Coping

   3. Impaired Skin Integrity
   4. High Risk for Ineffective Management of Therapeutic Regimen

   Nursing Process: Planning
   Client Need: Physiological Integrity

II. CRITICAL THINKING EXERCISES

1. A nurse comments that clients with psychosomatic disorders are often ambivalent. How does this term apply to individuals with these types of disorders?

2. The nurse determines that a client with a psychosomatic disorder needs nutritional health teaching. Using the food pyramid developed by the USDA, explain what a normal adult should consume each day.

14/ Homeostasis and Homeostatic Mechanisms

Nursing, as a health profession, helps people to reach and maintain optimal health or wellness. It also is concerned with preventing disease and caring for those who are ill. Wellness and illness are relative states that are constantly changing. A state of wellness or illness depends on the body's ability to meet biologic, physiologic, and sociologic needs and make suitable adaptations to internal and external stresses as they arise.

The following questions deal with the content of Chapter 14.

I. MULTIPLE CHOICE QUESTIONS

Circle the number of the most appropriate answer.

As part of their class in physiology, the professor has arranged for a class of nursing students to attend a conference for health professionals on the topic of homeostasis. After attending the conference, each student will present separate topics on some aspect of their learning to a group of high school students from a health occupations class on career day.

1. When a beginning student nurse asks one of the more advanced students in the nursing program to define the term homeostasis, the best explanation is that it refers to a

    1. condition that leads to a medical disorder
    2. state of physiologic chaos or disharmony
    3. method of keeping the body in a neutral state
    4. relatively stable state of equilibrium or balance

    Nursing Process: Implementation
    Client Need: Safe, Effective Care Environment

2. A student nurse is asked to identify the location of the sodium-potassium pump that plays a vital role in maintaining homeostasis. The correct answer is that this structure is within

    1. each cell's membrane
    2. each ventricle of the heart
    3. the salivary glands
    4. the membranes of the lung

    Nursing Process: Implementation
    Client Need: Safe, Effective Care Environment

3. The students are given a questionnaire to assess their own level of knowledge. One of the questions asks, "What structure of the body provides the body's major defense against invading microorganisms?". The most correct answer is the

    1. liver
    2. skin
    3. lungs
    4. stomach

    Nursing Process: Implementation
    Client Need: Safe, Effective Care Environment

4. For the clinical presentation, one student nurse has decided to discuss the healthful benefits that result from the many microorganisms that live on and in the body. Which one of the following is an example this student could provide? Microorganisms

    1. keep the skin elastic
    2. synthesize vitamin K
    3. neutralize body acids
    4. absorb carbon dioxide

    Nursing Process: Implementation
    Client Need: Safe, Effective Care Environment

5. A student nurse explains at one of the career day presentations that the brain and spinal cord are protected by several membranes, the toughest of which is the

   1. nucleus pulposus
   2. pia mater

   3. arachnoid layer
   4. dura mater

   Nursing Process: Implementation
   Client Need: Safe, Effective Care Environment

Individual Questions

6. A nurse would be most correct in identifying the substances that incapacitate microorganisms and foreign tissue as

   1. antibodies
   2. antigens

   3. antibiotics
   4. antipyrines

   Nursing Process: Implementation
   Client Need: Safe, Effective Care Environment

7. If a client asked a nurse to explain the purpose of vomiting, the best answer is that vomiting

   1. controls binge eating
   2. serves no protective purpose

   3. eliminates irritating substances
   4. prevents gastric distention

   Nursing Process: Implementation
   Client Need: Safe, Effective Care Environment

8. After assessing that an assigned client has a fever, the nurse counts the client's pulse. The nurse's action is

   1. unnecessary since the two assessments are not physiologically related
   2. unnecessary since the heart has nothing to do with temperature regulation

   3. necessary to detect the effect of the fever on cardiac activity
   4. necessary to determine the effect of cardiac activity on temperature regulation

   Nursing Process: Assessment
   Client Need: Physiological Integrity

9. A nurse observes that a client is experiencing muscle wasting and weight loss. Which one of the following is a valid analysis of these data? The client is experiencing the effects of

   1. anabolism
   2. catabolism

   3. metabolism
   4. cannibalism

   Nursing Process: Evaluation
   Client Need: Physiological Integrity

10. When explaining the process of hemostasis to a client, the nurse would be correct in identifying which one of the following steps as occurring first?

    1. clot lysis
    2. clot formation

    3. platelet aggregation
    4. vasoconstriction

    Nursing Process: Implementation
    Client Need: Safe, Effective Care Environment

11. The nurse would be most correct in explaining to a client that clots are dissolved by a substance called

    1. plasmin
    2. plasminogen

    3. immunoglobulin
    4. urobilin

    Nursing Process: Implementation
    Client Need: Safe, Effective Care Environment

12. A client asks a nurse to inspect a cut on his hand which occurred while he was carving meat 2 days ago. If the nurse observes all of the following, which one is not a normal characteristic of an inflammatory response?

    1. The edges of the wound appear red.
    2. There is white drainage within the wound.
    3. There is swelling in the area of the cut.
    4. The wound is tender when touched.

    Nursing Process: Assessment
    Client Need: Physiologic Integrity

13. When reviewing the laboratory test results of a client who had blood drawn for a complete blood count, which one of the following findings supports the conclusion that the client is experiencing an inflammatory response? The

    1. leukocyte count is elevated
    2. erythrocyte count is elevated
    3. thrombocyte count is reduced
    4. myelocyte count is reduced

    Nursing Process: Assessment
    Client Need: Safe, Effective Care Environment

14. A nurse inspects the incision of a client postoperatively. Which type of exudate would be important to report immediately?

    1. sanguineous
    2. serous
    3. mucoid
    4. purulent

    Nursing Process: Assessment
    Client Need: Physiological Integrity

15. Which one of the following best indicates to the nurse that a wound is healing by second intention?

    1. The wound edges are approximated.
    2. There is gauze packing in the wound.
    3. The wound is closed with staples.
    4. There are 5 sutures present.

    Nursing Process: Assessment
    Client Need: Safe, Effective Care Environment

II. CRITICAL THINKING EXERCISES

1. Virginia Hopkins and her husband are interested in various types of contraceptives that are available. Using your knowledge of feedback loops, explain how oral contraceptives prevent pregnancy.

2. Virgil Bache and Stephen Klein both had the same surgical procedure on the same day. Mr. Bache is scheduled to be discharged sooner than Mr. Klein. Discuss some factors that may affect the rate of tissue repair.

IV Common Medical-Surgical Problems

15/ Caring for the Client with an Infectious Disease

A wide variety of microorganisms are present in our environment, some of which are harmful. At certain times, microorganisms may reside in or on the body without causing disease. At other times, microorganisms do invade the body and cause disease.

The following questions deal with the content of Chapter 15.

I. MULTIPLE CHOICE QUESTIONS

Circle the number of the most appropriate answer.

Ms. Ames is admitted to the hospital with a draining abscess of her left ankle and heel.

1. At a team conference the head nurse tells the staff that it is most important that all health team members plan to handle the fomites in Ms. Ames' room according to hospital policy. A nurse assistant asks what the word fomite means. The correct response is that fomites are

   1. living objects acting as reservoirs of infection
   2. single-celled bacteria
   3. a member of the rickettsiae family
   4. inanimate objects acting as reservoirs of infection

   Nursing Process: Planning
   Client Need: Safe, Effective Care Environment

2. When caring for Ms. Ames, the nurse must remember that
   1. most microorganisms are not pathogenic unless the client is acutely ill
   2. an infection is not serious until it enters the bloodstream
   3. the skin must be kept alkaline in order to prevent superficial infections
   4. defense against invading microorganisms is provided by unbroken and healthy skin and mucous membranes

   Nursing Process: Implementation
   Client Need: Safe, Effective Care Environment

3. The nurse participates in a team conference concerned with nursing management of Ms. Ames. When asked to explain the two major defense mechanisms provided by the mononuclear phagocyte system, her correct response is phagocytosis and the
   1. manufacture of antigens
   2. immune response
   3. production of cold agglutinins
   4. pathogenic response

   Nursing Process: Implementation
   Client Need: Safe, Effective Care Environment

4. The nurse is asked to assist in developing a plan of care for Ms. Ames who has developed septicemia, a term used when microorganisms
   1. are found in the blood
   2. invade surrounding tissues
   3. become localized in a specific area
   4. promote the production of antibodies

   Nursing Process: Implementation
   Client Need: Safe, Effective Care Environment

Mr. Lyons is admitted to the hospital with an infection. He is acutely ill. The cause or type of infection is unknown at the present time.

5. When planning nursing management for Mr. Lyons the nurse must be aware that prolonged illness and a decreased food intake can result in a state of catabolism, which uses ____ as a source for energy.
   1. carbohydrates
   2. fats
   3. glucose
   4. body protein

   Nursing Process: Planning
   Client Need: Physiological Integrity

6. Mr. Lyons has anorexia. To encourage him to eat, it may be necessary to contact the dietitian who may recommend
   1. having visitors bring in food
   2. telling the client that he won't get well unless he eats
   3. a diet suited to the client's condition and food preferences
   4. a clear liquid diet

   Nursing Process: Implementation
   Client Need: Physiological Integrity

7. Mr. Lyons is placed in isolation. To reduce the effects of social isolation the nurse can
   1. explain to Mr. Lyons why isolation is necessary
   2. communicate and interact with Mr. Lyons as often as possible
   3. ask other clients to visit Mr. Lyons
   4. have Mr. Lyons visit with other clients with infections

   Nursing Process: Implementation
   Client Need: Psychosocial Integrity

8. Mr. Lyons' chart states that he has a mycoplasma infection. When participating in a team conference the nurse can describe this type of microorganism to others by describing mycoplasmas as being

   1. ciliated single-celled microorganisms
   2. microorganisms transmitted by arthropods
   3. organisms of the plant kingdom
   4. single-celled and pleomorphic

   Nursing Process: Implementation
   Client Need: Safe, Effective Care Environment

Individual Questions

9. When reviewing the assessment of a client with an infectious disease, the nurse notes the term nosocomial infection, which is an infection

   1. that has spread throughout the body
   2. acquired from another individual
   3. acquired in the hospital
   4. present prior to admission to the hospital

   Nursing Process: Collecting Data
   Client Need: Safe, Effective Care Environment

10. A client has a rickettsial disease. In planning care for this client the nurse must be aware that rickettsial diseases are transmitted

    1. from human to human
    2. by contaminated water
    3. by arthropods
    4. by animals

    Nursing Process: Planning
    Client Need: Safe, Effective Care Environment

11. When planning nursing care for a client with an infection, the nurse must be aware of the fact that the term reservoir applies to the

    1. route by which the infectious agent escapes from the infected host
    2. type of agent that transmits the infection
    3. environment in which the infectious agent is able to survive and reproduce
    4. type of contact by which the infectious agent is transmitted

    Nursing Process: Planning
    Client Need: Safe, Effective Care Environment

12. On a client's chart, the word interferon is noted. Interferon is a protein substance produced by white blood cells and probably other body cells in response to

    1. viral infections
    2. malignant tumors
    3. bacterial infections
    4. a change in the body pH

    Nursing Process: Implementation
    Client Need: Safe, Effective Care Environment

13. When assessing a client with a generalized infection, the nurse must be aware of the fact that the signs and symptoms of this type of infection are

    1. specific
    2. variable
    3. rarely serious
    4. almost always vague

    Nursing Process: Collecting Data
    Client Need: Safe, Effective Care Environment

14. When a client is placed on strict isolation, the nurse must identify the correct procedure regarding the infection control measures necessary to
    1. prevent the spread of highly contagious and virulent infections
    2. prevent an infection from spreading to other parts of the client's body
    3. slow the multiplication of pathogenic microorganisms
    4. prevent the spread of infection spread by way of the respiratory trac

    Nursing Process: Collecting Data
    Client Need: Safe, Effective Care Environment

15. When planning to explain a communicable disease to a client, the nurse correctly states that the signs and symptoms of some communicable diseases, as, for example, measles,
    1. are always vague and unpredictable
    2. are rarely serious
    3. may be fairly uniform and predictable
    4. are unknown

    Nursing Process: Planning
    Client Need: Safe, Effective Care Environment

16. The physician orders protective isolation for a client with an infectious disease. A nurse working on the unit states that this term is unfamiliar. Another term the nurse can give for protective isolation is
    1. enteric precautions
    2. blood and secretion precautions
    3. reverse isolation
    4. strict isolation

    Nursing Process: Implementation
    Client Need: Safe, Effective Care Environment

17. A nurse assistant asks the purpose of protective isolation. The correct response is that this form of isolation is used to
    1. prevent the spread of infection to nursing personnel
    2. protect clients with impaired resistance to infection
    3. prevent the spread of microorganisms causing a respiratory infection
    4. promote good isolation technique

    Nursing Process: Implementation
    Client Need: Safe, Effective Care Environment

18. A thorough history obtained from a client with a community-acquired infection may identify the source of infection, which in turn may
    1. correctly identify the causative microorganism
    2. indicate the type of antibiotic therapy necessary for treatment
    3. prevent the infection from becoming more serious
    4. indicate public health measures that may be necessary to prevent the spread of the disease

    Nursing Process: Collecting Data
    Client Need: Safe, Effective Care Environment

19. When universal precautions are implemented there is special handling of
    1. bed linens and eating utensils
    2. blood and body fluids
    3. instruments and dressings
    4. contaminated dressings and syringes

    Nursing Process: Implementation
    Client Need: Safe, Effective Care Environment

20. When explaining a skin test for tuberculosis to a client, the nurse includes the fact that the test site will be examined for a reaction in
    1. 10 to 15 minutes
    2. 1 to 2 hours
    3. 24 hours
    4. 48 to 72 hours

    Nursing Process: Implementation
    Client Need: Safe, Effective Care Environment

21. When reviewing a chart, the nurse notes that the client has been receiving large doses of a corticosteroid preparation for a prolonged period of time, which may result in a(n)
    1. increased production of thrombocytes
    2. decreased production of white blood cells
    3. increased production of antibodies
    4. decreased production of antigens

    Nursing Process: Collecting Data
    Client Need: Physiological Integrity

22. Ms. Williams is placed on strict isolation which will require that everyone entering the room must wear a
    1. gown and gloves
    2. mask and gloves
    3. mask, gown, cap, and gloves
    4. sterile gown and gloves

    Nursing Process: Implementation
    Client Need: Safe, Effective Care Environment

23. When blood and body fluid precautions are necessary, particular care is taken to
    1. avoid needlestick injury
    2. dispose of body fluids in glass containers
    3. use only sterile linens
    4. keep visitors from entering the room

    Nursing Process: Implementation
    Client Need: Safe, Effective Care Environment

24. When planning nursing care for the client with an infection, it is important to remember that fever and sweating
    1. increase the body's need for fluids
    2. increases the urinary output
    3. results in a rise in serum electrolytes
    4. decreases the respiratory rate

    Nursing Process: Planning
    Client Need: Physiological Integrity

II. CRITICAL THINKING EXERCISES

1. You are working in a nursing home and have been asked to give a team conference on universal precautions to the nursing assistants. What arguments would you give to stress the importance of following universal precautions when caring for clients in this facility?

2. Mr. Reynolds who has AIDS is terminally ill. He is hemorrhaging from esophageal varices and is vomiting bright red blood. The nurse caring for him asks you to help change his bedding. Besides gloves, what other protective devices or apparel would you wear?

3. Mr. Dalton comes to the emergency department complaining of a high fever and "feeling very sick." During questioning he tells you that he has no other symptoms. You note that he has a large cut healing on his left index finger. What questions would you ask him about the cut on his finger?

4. A nurse assistant asks you why hospitalized clients seem to be more prone to infection. What reasons would you give for this problem?

5. A client with a small child tells you that she does not want her child immunized. What reasons could you give for the the importance of adequate immunization of all children?

16/   Caring for Clients with Cancer

Meeting the needs of those with cancer are varied and complex and depend on their reactions to the diagnosis, the location of the cancer, impairment of body functions that may result from the disease or its treatment, the stage of the disease, and the prognosis.

The following questions deal with the content of Chapter 16.

I. MULTIPLE CHOICE QUESTIONS

Circle the number of the most appropriate answer.

Ms. Allen, age 59, has cervical cancer.

1. Mr. Allen states that he does not really know what the term cancer means. The most correct answer is that cancer is a name for a large group of diseases that are characterized by
   1. cells that multiply rapidly, invading and destroying normal tissues
   2. death in a high percentage of cases
   3. a course of treatment lasting 4-5 years
   4. production of a toxin that causes a spread of abnormal cells

   Nursing Process: Implementation
   Client Need: Physiological Integrity

2. Ms. Allen is scheduled for internal radiation therapy. When planning nursing care it is most important to be aware of the fact that this type of radiation therapy has the advantage of
   1. being less expensive
   2. having few side effects
   3. delivering the highest dose of radiation within the tumor
   4. not exposing the client to the hazards of radiation

   Nursing Process: Planning
   Client Need: Safe, Effective Care Environment

3. Ms. Allen is observed for signs and symptoms of radiation sickness, which include
   1. diarrhea, nervousness, increased appetite
   2. vomiting, chills, diaphoresis
   3. fluid volume excess, bradycardia, constipation
   4. weight gain, irregular pulse, decreased respiratory rate

   Nursing Process: Collecting Data
   Client Need: Physiological Integrity

4. To avoid nausea and vomiting after radiation therapy, the nurse and dietitian can plan
   1. a diet high in fats and proteins
   2. a low-carbohydrate diet
   3. omission of food at least 1 hour before and after therapy
   4. a liquid diet to be served immediately after therapy

   Nursing Process: Planning
   Client Need: Physiological Integrity

5. Ms. Allen develops severe diarrhea and is observed for signs and symptoms of
   1. a fluid volume deficit
   2. hyperkalemia
   3. a fluid volume excess
   4. hypernatremia

   Nursing Process: Collecting Data
   Client Need: Physiological Integrity

6. To prevent uric acid crystalluria and possible kidney failure Ms. Allen is encouraged to
   1. drink up to 3000 mL of fluid daily
   2. eat a well-balanced diet
   3. eat foods high in protein
   4. ambulate as often as possible

   Nursing Process: Implementation
   Client Need: Physiological Integrity

A team conference on cancer is held for all members of a medical unit.

7. A staff member asks how malignant tumors spread. The correct answer is that malignant tumors may spread by
   1. autoinnoculation
   2. white blood cells
   3. nerve cells
   4. transportation by the lymph or vascular system

   Nursing Process: Implementation
   Client Need: Safe, Effective Care Environment

8. A nurse assistant asks for an explanation of the difference between malignant and benign tumors. The correct explanation is that malignant tumors
   1. infiltrate surrounding tissues
   2. are encapsulated
   3. remain localized
   4. always require radiation therapy

   Nursing Process: Implementation
   Client Need: Safe, Effective Care Environment

9. A client receiving PCA for pain is discussed at the conference. A nurse assistant asks why this method is used instead of injections every 3 to 4 hours. The most correct response is that it has been shown that with the use of PCA
   1. addiction is less likely to occur
   2. drug tolerance is less likely to occur
   3. frequent, small doses of a narcotic best controls pain
   4. large doses provide longer analgesic effects

   Nursing Process: Implementation
   Client Need: Safe, Effective Care Environment

Mr. Olson, age 61, is admitted to the hospital for surgical removal of a possible malignant tumor of the colon.

10. Which one of the following is included in an initial physical assessment of Mr. Olson? A
    1. head-to-toe appraisal of his physical status
    2. review of his chart for planned laboratory tests
    3. determination of the stage of his disease
    4. review of his family's financial status

    Nursing Process: Collecting Data
    Client Need: Physiological Integrity

11. Mr. Olson is receiving chemotherapy with a drug that may cause stomatitis. To reduce the discomfort associated with stomatitis the nurse can
    1. help Mr. Olson select a diet high in roughage
    2. offer fruit juices and water at frequent intervals
    3. encourage the use of a commercial mouthwash after meals
    4. offer frequent warm-water mouth rinses

    Nursing Process: Implementation
    Client Need: Physiological Integrity

12. When developing a nursing care plan, it is important to remember that many antineoplastic drugs
    1. cause few side effects
    2. affect cells that divide at a rapid rate
    3. affect only tumor cells and not normal cells
    4. can only be given orally

    Nursing Process: Planning
    Client Need: Physiological Integrity

13. The drug given to Mr. Olson has the ability to depress the bone marrow, requiring close observation of Mr. Olson for
    1. signs of cerebral metastasis
    2. a rise in the white blood cell count
    3. bleeding tendencies
    4. a rise in the platelet count

    Nursing Process: Collecting Data
    Client Need: Physiological Integrity

14. Mr. Olson develops anorexia and has brief periods of nausea and vomiting following each chemotherapy treatment. Which one of the following assessments is included in his daily care plan?
    1. weigh Mr. Olson every 2 weeks
    2. check each meal tray and record the amount of food eaten
    3. monitor Mr. Olson's blood pressure every 8 hours
    4. check Mr. Olson's respiratory status

    Nursing Process: Collecting Data
    Client Need: Physiological Integrity

15. During outpatient chemotherapy treatments Mr. Olson becomes acutely ill and must be readmitted to the hospital. If he remains physically able to care for himself the nurse can
    1. encourage him to let the nurses assume most of the responsibility for his ADL
    2. talk to his family and suggest they supervise his activities
    3. allow him to be active within the limits of his ability
    4. allow him to assume all responsibility for his ADL

    Nursing Process: Implementation
    Client Need: Health Promotion/Maintenance

Individual Questions

16. When developing a plan of care for a terminally ill client, adequate amounts of food and fluid are considered to keep the client
    1. from developing side effects of therapy
    2. more aware of his or her surroundings
    3. pain-free
    4. comfortable and improve the quality of life

    Nursing Process: Planning
    Client Need: Physiological Integrity

17. A client who expresses fear and concern that pain associated with cancer may later become unbearable can be told that
    1. the time to worry about pain is when it occurs
    2. medications are available to relieve pain
    3. the physician will be told if pain occurs
    4. not all clients with cancer have pain

    Nursing Process: Implementation
    Client Need: Psychosocial Integrity

18. The client receiving repeated injections of a narcotic analgesic for pain is assessed for
    1. an increased respiratory rate
    2. tachycardia
    3. weight gain
    4. constipation

    Nursing Process: Collecting Data
    Client Need: Physiological Integrity

19. A terminally ill client is prescribed Brompton's mixture. Following administration, the client is evaluated for the relief of

    1. severe restlessness
    2. the side effects of chemotherapy
    3. severe pain
    4. diarrhea

    Nursing Process: Evaluation
    Client Need: Physiological Integrity

20. When a client is receiving radiation therapy the skin over the radiated area is inspected daily for signs of

    1. redness, ulceration, infection
    2. tumor regression
    3. dryness, hair loss, scaling
    4. radioactivity

    Nursing Process: Collecting Data
    Client Need: Physiological Integrity

21. A client develops stomatitis during chemotherapy and has difficulty eating. Which one of the following may be used to increase food intake?

    1. giving foods preferred by the client
    2. frequent, small feedings of high-caloric foods
    3. a high-fiber, high-vitamin diet
    4. a low-residue diet

    Nursing Process: Implementation
    Client Need: Physiological Integrity

22. Which one of the following may be used to remove accumulated debris from the teeth when the client has stomatitis?

    1. cold-water mouth rinses after meals
    2. glycerin mouth rinses between meals
    3. rinsing the mouth with undiluted hydrogen peroxide
    4. toothpaste on a cotton swab

    Nursing Process: Implementation
    Client Need: Physiological Integrity

23. If a client receiving an intramuscular antibiotic develops thrombocytopenia during chemotherapy,

    1. intravenous drugs are avoided
    2. prolonged pressure is applied at the site of intramuscular injections
    3. rectal temperatures are taken
    4. complete bedrest is instituted until the platelet count is normal

    Nursing Process: Implementation
    Client Need: Physiological Integrity

II. CRITICAL THINKING EXERCISES

1. Mr. Aldrich is terminally ill with metastatic cancer. His family asks for information about Hospice. What explanation can be given to the family?

2. Mr. Monroe, age 47, has lung cancer. His physician recommends radiation therapy as a palliative measure. His wife asks why the physician has recommended radiation. How can the purpose of this method of treatment be explained without addressing the fact that her husband has inoperable cancer and is terminal?

3. Ms. Levy is having radiation therapy following a mastectomy. She asks many questions because she wants to know why she has to do or not do certain things while she is having therapy. What reasons would you give her for not washing off the skin markings and not applying ointments or creams to the area being radiated?

4. Mr. Proctor is terminally ill with cancer. He appears depressed and withdrawn, and answers questions briefly or not at all. He rarely initiates a conversation. How could this problem be resolved?

5. Ms. Jenner is scheduled for outpatient chemotherapy. Her physician told her that she will probably lose all or most of her hair. What suggestions can be given to Ms. Jenner before she begins chemotherapy?

6. Mr. Kraft has a malignant tumor of his large intestine that has metastasized to his liver. The family does not want him to know that he has cancer. A few days later the family tells you that they wonder if they made the right decision. How would you approach this problem?

17/   Caring for Clients in Pain

There is no way a nurse can determine the amount of pain experienced by a client. The only information the nurse has is what comes from the client—an expression, a statement, an emotional reaction.

The following questions deal with the content of Chapter 17.

I. MULTIPLE CHOICE QUESTIONS

Circle the number of the most appropriate answer.

The topic of a team conference is pain.

1. When preparing for the team conference, the nurse is asked to explain endorphins and enkephalins. The correct description of these two chemical substances is that they

   1. mimic the actions of morphine
   2. are produced by the peripheral nervous system
   3. are found chiefly at motor nerve endings
   4. are hormones produced by the adrenal gland

   Nursing Process: Implementation
   Client Need: Safe, Effective Care Environment

2. The team conference leader asks, "What is the most serious consequence of sudden, severe pain?" The most correct response is

   1. shock
   2. respiratory depression
   3. metabolic alkalosis
   4. hypertension

   Nursing Process: Implementation
   Client Need: Safe, Effective Care Environment

3. A nurse attending the conference asks if anyone can give a definition of drug tolerance. The correct response is that drug tolerance is a(n)

   1. decrease in the dose is necessary to prevent addiction
   2. allergy to the drug has developed
   3. increase in the dose is required to produce the desired result
   4. cross-resistance to the drug has developed

   Nursing Process: Implementation
   Client Need: Safe, Effective Care Environment

4. A nurse assistant asks why nurses ask clients where their pain is located. The most correct response to this question is that

    1. the location of the pain must be charted
    2. the injection site depends on the location of pain

    3. this is a method of evaluating a response to an analgesic
    4. a potentially serious condition may go unnoticed

    Nursing Process: Implementation
    Client Need: Physiological Integrity

Ms. Marshall is seen in the emergency department for severe pain following an injury to her left arm. She is extremely nervous and fearful. The physician orders an analgesic stat and states that an open reduction of her fracture will be performed in about 4 hours.

5. Which one of the following can the nurse use to decrease anticipation of pain when preparing an injection for Ms. Marshall?

    1. Inform her that the injection will not hurt
    2. Ask if injections cause her pain

    3. Tell her to relax
    4. Prepare the injection out of her line of vision

    Nursing Process: Implementation
    Client Need: Physiological Integrity

6. After the narcotic analgesic is given to Ms. Marshall, the nurse can plan to

    1. keep the head of her bed elevated
    2. check her respiratory rate 30-45 minutes later

    3. leave her alone so she can rest
    4. check her blood pressure in 5 minutes

    Nursing Process: Planning
    Client Need: Physiological Integrity

7. Ms. Marshall states that she is afraid of the pain she may experience after surgery. When planning how to relieve Ms. Marshall's anxiety the nurse must remember that

    1. postoperative pain is almost always less than anticipated
    2. clients rarely have pain after surgery because of new ways to give analgesics

    3. a previous experience of pain may influence her response to pain after surgery
    4. an open reduction of a fracture rarely causes postoperative pain

    Nursing Process: Planning
    Client Need: Psychosocial Integrity

Individual Questions

8. When planning nursing care for the client with a cordotomy, it must be remembered that this surgical procedure is performed to

    1. reduce the blood supply to painful areas
    2. decrease the number of painful stimuli

    3. interrupt sensory nerve pathways in the spinal cord
    4. interrupt motor nerve pathways in the spinal cord

    Nursing Process: Planning
    Client Need: Physiological Integrity

9. When planning care for the client with pain, the nurse must remember that analgesics are best given

    1. early in the morning and at hs
    2. before pain reaches a maximum intensity

    3. at the time pain reaches maximum intensity
    4. after the client is made comfortable

    Nursing Process: Planning
    Client Need: Physiological Integrity

II CRITICAL THINKING EXERCISES

1. Mr. Akers is using PCA for postoperative pain. He presses the administration button frequently, and his family is concerned that he may be giving himself an overdose of the medication. What explanation would you give the family?

2. A nurse co-worker tells you that he believes Mr. Nash is becoming addicted to the morphine he is receiving for pain associated with terminal colon cancer. The nurse states that everyone should try and lengthen the time between the administration of each dose of the narcotic. What is your response to this nurse?

3. Ms. Matthews tells you that she has pain in her left leg and asks for something for pain. You have had 3 days off and do not know this client. What would you do?

4. The physician prescribed a TENS unit for Mr. Payne. What basic explanations regarding the TENS unit would you give to this client?

5. Ms. Evans' pain is being controlled by PCA. The family asks why she is allowed to administer her own medicine for pain. How would you explain the advantages of this method of providing pain relief?

18/ Substance Abuse

Substance (or drug) abuse has become one of the leading problems worldwide. The terms *drug* and *substance* often are used interchangeably. Substance (or drug) abuse is the use of a natural or synthetic substance to alter mood or behavior in a manner that differs from its generally accepted use. Every client seen in the home, clinic, or hospital setting must be considered a *potential* candidate for substance abuse and withdrawal symptoms.

The following questions deal with the content of Chapter 18.

I. MULTIPLE CHOICE QUESTIONS

Circle the number of the most appropriate answer.

Ms. Perkins is admitted for a left knee replacement. Her husband states that his wife has been drinking heavily prior to admission and is an alcoholic.

1. Following surgery the nurse observes Ms. Perkins for signs of alcohol withdrawal which usually develop in

   1. a few hours to 3 days or more
   2. a week to 10 days
   3. 1 to 3 weeks
   4. more than 3 weeks

   Nursing Process: Collecting Data
   Client Need: Psychosocial Integrity

2. When assessing Ms. Perkins pre- and postoperatively, the nurse observes for early signs and symptoms of alcohol withdrawal which include

   1. hypertension, bradycardia, tremors
   2. abdominal distention, jaundice, restlessness
   3. diarrhea, sleepiness, dehydration
   4. disorientation, diaphoresis, hallucinations

   Nursing Process: Collecting Data
   Client Need: Psychosocial Integrity

3. If signs of acute alcohol withdrawal occur, Ms. Perkins

   1. should have wrist and ankle restraints applied
   2. will require extra oral fluids
   3. must be protected from injury
   4. must be transferred to ICU

   Nursing Process: Implementation
   Client Need: Safe, Effective Care Environment

4. Ms. Perkins has agreed to take disulfiram (Antabuse) following discharge from the hospital. The nurse can explain that when she takes this drug, even small amounts of alcohol will cause

   1. severe nausea, vomiting, diarrhea
   2. abdominal cramping, sweating, skin rash
   3. double vision, nausea, fainting
   4. erratic behavior, hallucinations, anxiety

   Nursing Process: Implementation
   Client Need: Health Promotion/Maintenance

5. When counseling Ms. Perkins, the nurse can explain that the use of CNS depressants (such as barbiturates or tranquilizers) with alcohol can potentiate the effects of the depressant, possibly resulting in

   1. alcohol withdrawal syndrome
   2. an increase in the pulse and respiratory rates
   3. respiratory depression and coma
   4. kidney failure

   Nursing Process: Implementation
   Client Need: Psychosocial Integrity

A hospital emergency department sees many different types of emergencies, including clients with effects related to substance abuse.

6. When assessing a client for the signs and symptoms of possible acute heroin or other narcotic toxicity, the nurse looks for

   1. respiratory depression, stupor, hypotension
   2. hypertension, tachycardia, warm skin
   3. aggressiveness, dyspnea, dilated pupils
   4. apnea, hypocapnia, cardiac arrhythmias

   Nursing Process: Collecting Data
   Client Need: Psychosocial Integrity

7. When assessing a client for the signs and symptoms of possible acute cocaine toxicity, the nurse looks for

   1. stupor to coma, hallucinations, bradycardia
   2. respiratory depression, pinpoint pupils, emesis
   3. agitation, respiratory distress, cardiac arrhythmias
   4. hypothermia, diaphoresis, dry mucous membranes

   Nursing Process: Collecting Data
   Client Need: Psychosocial Integrity

8. When assessing a client for the signs and symptoms of possible acute amphetamine toxicity, the nurse looks for

   1. stupor, clammy skin, pinpoint pupils
   2. hypotension, bradycardia, irritability
   3. tachycardia, diffuse skin rash, coma
   4. hypertension, hostility, extreme agitation

   Nursing Process: Collecting Data
   Client Need: Psychosocial Integrity

9. Following assessment, which of the following symptoms of substance abuse would be treated first?

   1. severe coughing, decreased urine output, abdominal pain
   2. blurred vision, behavior changes, hyperthermia
   3. respiratory depression, hypotension, cardiac arrhythmias
   4. vomiting, ataxia, hallucinations

   Nursing Process: Implementation
   Client Need: Physiological Integrity

10. If a client has taken a substance capable of CNS depression, the nurse should

   1. evaluate the respiratory status at frequent intervals
   2. administer a mixture of oxygen and carbon dioxide by mask
   3. monitor the client's mental status every 4 to 6 hours
   4. insert a nasogastric tube

   Nursing Process: Implementation
   Client Need: Physiological Integrity

II. CRITICAL THINKING EXERCISES

1. In a busy emergency department, a man is brought in by the police. He had been at a rock concert where LSD was being sold. What emergency measures would you take until he is seen by the physician?

2. You are obtaining an admission history from Ms. Reed who is admitted for thrombophlebitis. She tells you that she has been taking a tranquilizer for years for treatment of anxiety and panic attacks. What additional information would you try to obtain? Explain the significance of long-term use of tranquilizers when formulating a plan of care.

3. Your brother tells you that he thinks his best friend, Ben, is an alcoholic. He asks you what can be done to help Ben overcome this problem. What advice can you give your brother?

4. Mr. Stevens, who is admitted to the hospital for multiple medical problems, gives a history of substance abuse, primarily heroin. He admits to taking heroin immediately before he came to the hospital. When would the nurse expect symptoms of withdrawal to begin? What are the early symptoms of heroin withdrawal?

19/ Water, Acid–Base, and Electrolyte Imbalances

About 60% of the adult human body is water. Electrolytes are in the water of both cellular and extracellular spaces. The normal composition of body fluids is dependent on the concentration of electrolytes as well as acids and alkalis.

The following questions deal with the content of Chapter 19.

I. MULTIPLE CHOICE QUESTIONS

Circle the number of the most appropriate answer.

1. When comparing the intake and output ratio, the nurse must take into account insensible fluid loss which is fluid lost through the

    1. kidneys   3. bowel
    2. skin and lungs   4. bladder

    Nursing Process: Collecting Data
    Client Need: Physiological Integrity

2. To determine whether a client has a fluid volume deficit the nurse can
   1. check skin turgor and elasticity
   2. palpate the abdomen for tenderness
   3. weigh the client weekly
   4. determine the total daily caloric intake

   Nursing Process: Collecting Data
   Client Need: Physiological Integrity

3. The client with a known fluid volume deficit is assessed for
   1. fever
   2. dry mucous membranes
   3. hypertension
   4. increased urine output

   Nursing Process: Collecting Data
   Client Need: Physiological Integrity

4. If a client has a mild fluid volume deficit the nurse can
   1. select a diet high in proteins
   2. force fluids high in concentrated glucose
   3. decrease the dietary potassium intake
   4. offer oral fluids that provide water and electrolytes

   Nursing Process: Implementation
   Client Need: Physiological Integrity

5. The urine specific gravity of a client with a fluid volume deficit is 1.030 which indicates
   1. dilute urine
   2. the urine contains crystals
   3. concentrated urine
   4. bacteria is present in the urine

   Nursing Process: Evaluation
   Client Need: Physiological Integrity

6. When assessing a client with a known fluid volume excess, the nurse looks for
   1. dry mucous membranes
   2. peripheral edema
   3. rapid weight loss
   4. rapid, weak pulse

   Nursing Process: Collecting Data
   Client Need: Physiological Integrity

7. A client with a fluid volume excess is placed on fluid restrictions. The nurse can plan to
   1. keep the client on complete bedrest with the head of the bed kept flat
   2. notify the physician if the output exceeds 500 mL per day
   3. offer small amounts of fluids at evenly spaced intervals
   4. offer a diet high in sodium, low in potassium, and high in protein

   Nursing Process: Planning
   Client Need: Physiological Integrity

8. When examining the client with a fluid volume excess who is in a sitting position, the nurse checks the neck veins for
   1. distention
   2. a palpable pulse
   3. collapse
   4. fluid waves

   Nursing Process: Collecting Data
   Client Need: Physiological Integrity

9. A client receiving diuretic therapy and excreting large volumes of urine is assessed for signs and symptoms of
   1. respiratory acidosis
   2. respiratory alkalosis
   3. metabolic acidosis
   4. metabolic alkalosis

   Nursing Process: Collecting Data
   Client Need: Physiological Integrity

10. When assessing a client suspected of having metabolic acidosis, the nurse looks for
    1. hypotension, poor skin turgor, bradycardia
    2. tachycardia, dry mucous membranes, constipation
    3. confusion, lethargy, drowsiness
    4. hypertension, cardiac arrhythmias, increased urine output

    Nursing Process: Collecting Data
    Client Need: Physiological Integrity

11. When assessing the client who is hyperventilating because of acute anxiety, the nurse looks for signs and symptoms of
    1. respiratory acidosis
    2. respiratory alkalosis
    3. metabolic acidosis
    4. metabolic alkalosis

    Nursing Process: Collecting Data
    Client Need: Physiological Integrity

12. When assessing a client for signs and symptoms of hyponatremia, the nurse looks for
    1. weight gain, increased appetite, lethargy
    2. fever, decreased urine output, anxiety
    3. muscle weakness, confusion, restlessness
    4. bradycardia, severe thirst, dry mucous membranes

    Nursing Process: Collecting Data
    Client Need: Physiological Integrity

13. If a client has mild hyponatremia, the nurse can plan to
    1. offer foods high in sodium
    2. offer extra fluids
    3. increase the client's ambulatory activities
    4. keep the client on complete bedrest

    Nursing Process: Planning
    Client Need: Physiological Integrity

14. A client is receiving 500 mL of intravenous normal saline which is to be infused over a period of 8 hours. When entering the room the nurse notes that the intravenous solution infused in 1 hour. The client must now be observed for signs and symptoms of
    1. hypernatremia
    2. hyponatremia
    3. hyperkalemia
    4. respiratory acidosis

    Nursing Process: Collecting Data
    Client Need: Physiological Integrity

15. Ms. Horton has a draining intestinal fistula and has required prolonged gastrointestinal suction. When assessing Ms. Horton, the nurse looks for the signs and symptoms of
    1. hypernatremia
    2. hypokalemia
    3. hyperkalemia
    4. hypomagnesemia

    Nursing Process: Collecting Data
    Client Need: Physiological Integrity

16. A client with a high serum potassium level is closely monitored for

    1. constipation lasting more than 3 days
    2. muscle spasms and paralysis
    3. excessive weight gain
    4. cardiac arrhythmias

    Nursing Process: Collecting Data
    Client Need: Physiological Integrity

17. When developing a plan of care for a client with chronic hypercalcemia and severe loss of calcium from the bones, the nurse includes

    1. limitation of oral fluids
    2. a diet high in calcium
    3. strict bedrest
    4. assistance with ambulatory activities

    Nursing Process: Planning
    Client Need: Safe, Effective Care Environment

18. The client with severe hypocalcemia is frequently assessed for

    1. tetany, seizures, muscle spasms
    2. pain related to kidney stone formation
    3. signs and symptoms of infection
    4. increase in the urine output

    Nursing Process: Collecting Data
    Client Need: Physiological Integrity

19. A client with severe renal disease is closely monitored for signs of hypomagnesemia, which include

    1. flushing
    2. hypotension
    3. neuromuscular irritability
    4. marked weight loss

    Nursing Process: Collecting Data
    Client Need: Physiological Integrity

20. A client with severe hypomagnesemia is given intravenous magnesium sulfate by the physician. While the drug is being administered the client is closely monitored for

    1. a fluid volume excess
    2. a rise in blood pressure and pulse rate
    3. hypocalcemic tetany
    4. a sharp drop in blood pressure

    Nursing Process: Collecting Data
    Client Need: Physiological Integrity

II CRITICAL THINKING EXERCISES

1. Ms. Ash, age 56, is brought to the emergency department by her daughter. She has had severe nausea and vomiting for the past 9 hours. It will be about 10 minutes before she is seen by a physician. What assessments would you make and what questions would you ask her daughter?

2. Mr. Mack has hypocalcemia. What observations would you include in his plan of care?

3. Mr. Border has respiratory acidosis and has difficulty breathing. He has an order for oxygen by nasal catheter for respiratory difficulty. What precautions would you take when giving this client oxygen?

4. Ms. Gordon's serum sodium is 150 mEq/L, indicating that she has mild hypernatremia. This client is 84 years old and often requires assistance with eating as well as her activities of daily living. What actions could the nurse take to correct this mild electrolyte imbalance?

5. A client is to receive 20 mEq of potassium gluconate IV added to 1000 mL of 5% dextrose in water. What special precautions would you take while this drug is being administered?

20/   Caring for Clients in Shock

A serious disorder, *shock* occurs when inadequate peripheral blood flow decreases the amount of oxygen that reaches vital tissues and organs and reduces the removal of the waste products of metabolism.
The following questions deal with the content of Chapter 20.

I. MULTIPLE CHOICE QUESTIONS

Circle the number of the most appropriate answer.

Ms. King is in hypovolemic shock and is being treated with a vasopressor and administration of oxygen.

1. A nurse asks you why Ms. King's 8-hour urinary output is low. The correct answer is that in shock
    1. the bladder capacity is decreased
    2. the renal veins are constricted
    3. there is failure of the right ventricle
    4. there is a reduction of renal blood flow

    Nursing Process: Implementation
    Client Need: Physiological Integrity

2. When evaluating the effectiveness of the treatment of shock, the nurse looks for the minimum essential myocardial perfusion pressure needed to maintain coronary artery blood flow which is a systolic blood pressure of about ____ mm Hg.
    1. 30
    2. 50
    3. 80
    4. 120

    Nursing Process: Evaluation
    Client Need: Physiological Integrity

3. The nurse can relieve Ms. King's restlessness by
    1. oxygen administration
    2. administration of an analgesic or tranquilizer
    3. changing the client's position
    4. encouraging the client to take deep breaths

    Nursing Process: Implementation
    Client Need: Physiological Integrity

4. Unless ordered otherwise, Ms. King is kept supine with the legs elevated 20° to 30°. Keeping Ms. King in this position
    1. decreases pressure in the carotid arteries
    2. increases the workload of the heart
    3. increases blood flow to the brain
    4. enhances urinary output

    Nursing Process: Implementation
    Client Need: Physiological Integrity

5. Ms. King is hypothermic. To correct this problem the nurse can
    1. remove the blanket and cover Ms. King with a sheet
    2. apply light blankets and keep the room warm
    3. apply a warming blanket
    4. use a fan to cool the immediate area

    Nursing Process: Implementation
    Client Need: Physiological Integrity

Individual Questions

6. If a client develops protracted vomiting and diarrhea, the nurse must be alert to the development of

    1. normovolemic shock
    2. hypovolemic shock

    3. neurogenic shock
    4. vasogenic shock

    Nursing Process: Collecting Data
    Client Need: Physiological Integrity

7. Mr. Gold has had a myocardial infarction. The physician states that he has a marked reduction in his cardiac output. Knowing this, the nurse must be alert to signs of

    1. rise in blood pressure and a decrease in pulse
    2. change in the diastolic pressure

    3. widening of the venous pulse pressure
    4. decreased delivery of oxygen to body tissues and organs

    Nursing Process: Collecting Data
    Client Need: Physiological Integrity

8. A client with a spinal cord injury is assessed for the development of neurogenic shock. The most prominent feature of this type of shock is

    1. hypertension
    2. vasodilatation

    3. bradycardia
    4. vasoconstriction

    Nursing Process: Collecting Data
    Client Need: Physiological Integrity

9. When assessing a client who may be in shock, the most critical determinants are

    1. changes in the skin color and increased CVP
    2. an increase in cardiac output

    3. organ blood flow and tissue perfusion
    4. the general appearance of the client

    Nursing Process: Collecting Data
    Client Need: Physiological Integrity

10. To use blood pressure as one criterion for determining whether a client is in shock, the nurse must know the

    1. client's medical history
    2. causes of shock

    3. criteria for shock
    4. client's original blood pressure

    Nursing Process: Collecting Data
    Client Need: Physiological Integrity

11. If a client is in shock, the physician is notified of a urinary output

    1. above 30 mL per hour
    2. below 30 mL per hour

    3. above 100 mL per hour
    4. below 100 mL per hour

    Nursing Process: Implementation
    Client Need: Physiological Integrity

12. To properly evaluate CVP readings, the nurse must first

    1. add dextrose to the CVP line
    2. obtain the client's blood pressure

    3. add saline to the CVP line
    4. obtain a baseline value

    Nursing Process: Implementation
    Client Need: Physiological Integrity

13. To obtain an accurate CVP reading, the zero level of the manometer must be
    1. at the same height in relation to the client's right atrium
    2. below the client's xyphoid process
    3. at the level of the client's hip
    4. at the same height in relation to the client's lower rib cage

    Nursing Process: Implementation
    Client Need: Physiological Integrity

14. If the CVP rapidly rises when the client in shock is receiving intravenous fluids, the
    1. IV administration rate is slowed
    2. intravenous line is discontinued
    3. client is placed in a sitting position
    4. client is placed flat

    Nursing Process: Implementation
    Client Need: Physiological Integrity

II. CRITICAL THINKING EXERCISES

1. Mr. Abrams has had surgery and is now recovering from anesthesia. Describe the changes that may be seen if Mr. Abrams is in actual or impending shock.

2. A nurse assistant asks why she was told not to give morning care to Mr. Rogers. You explain that Mr. Rogers has a severe infection resulting in shock. What rationale would you give for omitting his morning care?

3. You suspect that Mr. Jansen may be in impending shock. What assessments would you make to confirm your suspicions?

21/   Intravenous Therapy

Intravenous (IV) therapy demands skillful administration technique, close observation of the patient, and a number of special nursing considerations. Drugs, solutions (e.g., dextrose, plasma expanders, and amino acids), and whole blood and blood components may be given by the IV route in specific situations.
    The following questions deal with the content of Chapter 21.

I. MULTIPLE CHOICE QUESTIONS

Circle the number of the most appropriate answer.

An inservice program is planned for a surgical unit. All health team members are requested to review and then present the purpose of various types and methods of administering of intravenous solutions.

1. The nurse is correct in stating that the rationale for administration of intravenous fat emulsion is to
   1. prevent electrolyte depletion
   2. prevent and treat fatty acid deficiency
   3. provide carbohydrates
   4. provide calories in the form of proteins

   Nursing Process: Implementation
   Client Need: Safe, Effective Care Environment

2. The nurse is correct in stating that the rationale for administration of amino acid solutions is to
   1. promote carbohydrate synthesis
   2. provide electrolytes
   3. retard wound healing
   4. reduce the rate of protein breakdown

   Nursing Process: Implementation
   Client Need: Safe, Effective Care Environment

3. The nurse is correct in stating that the rationale for administration of plasma expanders is to
   1. maintain the volume of circulating blood
   2. provide white blood cells
   3. maintain protein levels in the blood
   4. provide platelets

   Nursing Process: Implementation
   Client Need: Safe, Effective Care Environment

4. The nurse is correct in stating that the rationale for administration of serum albumin is to
   1. treat severe hypertension
   2. provide a protein fraction of blood
   3. supply erythrocytes
   4. supply essential nutrients

   Nursing Process: Implementation
   Client Need: Safe, Effective Care Environment

5. When a volumetric intravenous electronic controller is used to administer an intravenous solution, the nurse checks the controller to be sure

   1. the intravenous solution is infusing under positive pressure
   2. a pressure infusion sleeve has been added to the IV container

   3. a specific volume is being administered at a specific rate
   4. there is negative pressure in the IV container

   Nursing Process: Evaluation
   Client Need: Physiological Integrity

6. The nurse is correct in stating that the rationale for use of a central venous line is to

   1. administer total parenteral nutrition
   2. monitor serum electrolyte levels

   3. provide short-term intravenous therapy
   4. prevent tissue breakdown

   Nursing Process: Implementation
   Client Need: Safe, Effective Care Environment

7. When charting, the nurse is correct when using the term extravasation to describe the escape of from a blood vessel into surrounding tissues

   1. when the needle or catheter is out of the vein
   2. when the intravenous fluid is administered under pressure

   3. while the needle or catheter is in the vein
   4. when a vasopressor is being administered

   Nursing Process: Implementation
   Client Need: Safe, Effective Care Environment

Mr. Quinn is receiving intravenous therapy for a fluid volume deficit that has occurred as a result of surgery and inability to take oral fluids.

8. While receiving intravenous therapy, Mr. Quinn is observed for signs of fluid overload which include

   1. bradycardia, nonproductive cough, weight loss
   2. hypotension, double vision, paralysis

   3. dyspnea, pulmonary rales, behavioral changes
   4. decreased CVP, increased urine output, anxiety

   Nursing Process: Collecting Data
   Client Need: Physiological Integrity

9. Mr. Quinn is given a blood transfusion to replace some of the blood lost during surgery. While the blood is infusing, Mr. Quinn is assessed for signs and symptoms of a transfusion reaction which include

   1. bradycardia, weight gain, restlessness
   2. oliguria, distended neck veins, anorexia

   3. lumbar pain, urticaria, dyspnea
   4. cough, peripheral edema, headache

   Nursing Process: Collecting Data
   Client Need: Physiological Integrity

10. When monitoring Mr. Quinn's intravenous solution, the nurse plans to add the next solution before the bag or bottle and tubing are empty to prevent

    1. fluid overload
    2. infection

    3. a blood clot forming in the needle
    4. oliguria

    Nursing Process: Planning
    Client Need: Physiological Integrity

11. When developing a plan of care, the nurse includes a change of the dressings over the venipuncture site every

    1. 4 to 8 hours
    2. 48 to 72 hours
    3. 3 to 5 days
    4. week

    Nursing Process: Planning
    Client Need: Safe, Effective Care Environment

12. Mr. Quinn is to receive 40 mEq of potassium gluconate IV. When monitoring the rate of infusion, the nurse calculates that the intravenous solution is not to be infused in less than

    1. 1 hour
    2. 2 hours
    3. 4 to 6 hours
    4. 6 to 12 hours

    Nursing Process: Collecting Data
    Client Need: Physiological Integrity

13. Mr. Quinn's intake and output is measured. The nurse must notify the physician if the

    1. output is above 500 mL/day
    2. intake-output ratio shows a marked change
    3. intake is more than 2000 mL/day
    4. intake is higher than the output

    Nursing Process: Implementation
    Client Need: Physiological Integrity

14. Because of complications following surgery, Mr. Quinn is receiving TPN. When TPN is used to supply nutritional needs, the nurse plans to

    1. check the urine for glucose and ketone bodies q4–6h
    2. adjust the rate of flow according to the urine output
    3. change the TPN catheter weekly
    4. monitor the blood pressure daily

    Nursing Process: Planning
    Client Need: Physiological Integrity

15. Mr. Quinn is to receive a drug by means of a volume-control set. When monitoring the infusion rate, the drug is allowed to infuse over a period of

    1. 1 to 3 minutes
    2. 15 to 30 minutes
    3. 1 hour
    4. 4 hours

    Nursing Process: Implementation
    Client Need: Physiological Integrity

II. CRITICAL THINKING EXERCISES

1. Ms. Corbin is to receive 1000 mL of solution to be administered over 6 hours. The number of drops/milliliter delivered by the macrodrip system selected is 15. When timing the rate of infusion, you determine that the IV is infusing at a rate of 26 drops per minute. What nursing task, if any, would you perform at this time?

2. Mr. Glover is to receive 500 mL of solution to be administered over 8 hours. The number of drops/milliliter delivered by the macrodrip system selected is 20. When timing the rate of infusion, you determine that the IV is infusing at a rate of 40 drops per minute. What nursing task, if any, would you perform at this time?

22/   Caring for Surgical Clients

The performance of a surgical procedure is a common event. Many operations are emergencies because they are performed to correct conditions that are life-threatening (e.g., bowel obstruction and dissecting aortic aneurysm). Other surgical procedures are less urgent and may be performed days after the need for surgery is recognized. Some operations are elective procedures, that is, they are scheduled at the convenience of the physician and client.

The following questions deal with the content of Chapter 22.

I. MULTIPLE CHOICE QUESTIONS

Circle the number of the most appropriate answer.

Ms. Ames, age 31, is scheduled for surgery at 10 a.m. for an open reduction of a fracture of her elbow.

1. When preparing a preoperative medication containing a narcotic and antiemetic, the nurse plans to tell Ms. Ames that drowsiness will occur in about

   1. 5 minutes
   2. 20 minutes

   3. 45 minutes
   4. 1 hour

   Nursing Process: Planning
   Client Need: Safe, Effective Care Environment

2. When explaining the purpose of giving atropine, a cholinergic blocking agent, the nurse tells Ms. Ames that this drug will

   1. help control her blood pressure during surgery
   2. relieve pain and discomfort

   3. cause extreme dryness of the mouth
   4. help in coughing after surgery

   Nursing Process: Implementation
   Client Need: Physiological Integrity

3. When planning preoperative teaching, the nurse must remember that

   1. the surgical procedure must be explained or described in detail
   2. it is best to omit an explanation of the immediate postoperative period

   3. all teaching is best done immediately after giving the preoperative medication
   4. simple, factual explanations, adjusted to the client's ability and need, are essential

   Nursing Process: Planning
   Client Need: Physiological Integrity

4. During the preoperative period the nurse must plan to

1. have Ms. Ames practice deep-breathing and coughing exercises
2. describe what will happen during surgery
3. have Ms. Ames ambulate as much as possible
4. explain postoperative drug therapy to Ms. Ames and her family

Nursing Process: Planning
Client Need: Physiological Integrity

Mr. Hunt is admitted to the postanesthesia recovery room (PARR) following surgery for a bleeding duodenal ulcer and was extubated by the anesthesiologist when he arrived in the PARR.

5. During recovery from anesthesia Mr. Hunt is positioned

1. with the head of the bed elevated 60°
2. with the legs elevated above the level of the heart
3. so that blood flow to the lower extremities is decreased
4. to prevent aspiration of vomitus or secretions

Nursing Process: Implementation
Client Need: Physiological Integrity

6. Mr. Hunt appears to have difficulty breathing. The nurse can insert an oropharyngeal airway to

1. maintain a patent airway
2. prevent excessive postoperative coughing
3. keep secretions in the tracheobronchial tree
4. prevent postoperative hiccups

Nursing Process: Implementation
Client Need: Physiological Integrity

7. To determine if there are any signs of bleeding the nurse inspects the surgical dressing and

1. looks for cyanosis of the nailbeds
2. counts the respiratory rate for 1 full minute
3. places the client on a cardiac monitor
4. the bedding under the client

Nursing Process: Collecting Data
Client Need: Physiological Integrity

Individual Questions

8. Mr. Wagner has had spinal anesthesia and now complains of numbness and a heavy feeling in his legs as the anesthesia wears off. At this time the nurse can tell Mr. Wagner that

1. a medication will be given to relieve the numbness
2. the symptoms will disappear in about 24 hours
3. these symptoms are usual and will subside in a short time
4. if he moves his legs the numbness will be gone by the next day

Nursing Process: Implementation
Client Need: Physiological Integrity

9. Unless ordered otherwise, clients having had spinal anesthesia are kept lying flat in bed for ____ hours.

1. 1 to 3
2. 6 to 12
3. 24
4. 48

Nursing Process: Implementation
Client Need: Physiological Integrity

10. The nurse observes clients for wound dehiscence or evisceration which are most likely to occur between the ____ postoperative days.

1. 1st and 2nd
2. 2nd and 3rd
3. 6th and 8th
4. 10th and 14th

Nursing Process: Collecting Data
Client Need: Physiological Integrity

11. If wound disruption is suspected or has occurred, the client is placed

    1. at complete rest in a position that puts the least strain on the incision
    2. in a lateral recumbent position
    3. supine
    4. prone

    Nursing Process: Implementation
    Client Need: Physiological Integrity

12. The nurse encourages clients to ambulate after surgery because ambulation helps to

    1. decrease the vital capacity
    2. decrease pain
    3. decrease intestinal peristalsis
    4. prevent complications

    Nursing Process: Implementation
    Client Need: Physiological Integrity

13. During the immediate postoperative period, the nurse observes the client for signs and symptoms of a paralytic ileus which may include

    1. rectal bleeding and pain
    2. constipation
    3. abdominal distention and pain
    4. anorexia

    Nursing Process: Collecting Data
    Client Need: Physiological Integrity

14. Ms. Porter has an order for catheterization if she is unable to void after surgery. The nurse performs this procedure if Ms. Porter is unable to void in

    1. 2 to 4 hours
    2. 3 to 6 hours
    3. 8 to 12 hours
    4. 10 to 24 hours

    Nursing Process: Implementation
    Client Need: Physiological Integrity

15. To determine if an infection is developing in or below the surgical incision, the nurse looks for

    1. serosanguinous exudate, blanching of the skin
    2. redness, localized heat, swelling
    3. blood clots, scar tissue, absence of pain
    4. separation of the incision, keloid formation

    Nursing Process: Collecting Data
    Client Need: Safe, Effective Care Environment

16. To remove packing or gauze that has adhered to the skin the nurse can moisten the area with

    1. sterile normal saline
    2. a dilute iodine solution
    3. a dilute saline solution
    4. sterile water

    Nursing Process: Implementation
    Client Need: Physiological Integrity

17. The nurse can help prevent hypostatic pneumonia by

    1. avoiding close client contact
    2. helping the client ambulate
    3. encouraging coughing and deep-breathing
    4. giving antibiotics on time

    Nursing Process: Implementation
    Client Need: Physiological Integrity

II. CRITICAL THINKING EXERCISES

1. Mr. Price's physician tells him that he can have a local or general anesthetic for a skin graft to his ankle. Mr. Price tells you that he does not understand anesthetics. How would you explain these two types of anesthesia to Mr. Price?

2. Ms. Davis is admitted the morning of surgery for a laparoscopic cholecystectomy. She is extremely nervous and frightened. Her vital signs are BP 126/82, pulse 124, respirations 24. What actions would you take?

3. Mr. Williams had a bowel resection 2 days ago. As you enter his room you note that he is pale, his skin is clammy and cool to touch, and he complains of severe pain. You are not familiar with Mr. Williams' past medical and surgical history and postoperative recovery, and you have been off work for 2 days. What information would you obtain and which assessments would you make before contacting his physician?

4. Ms. Jansen, who is extremely obese, had an abdominal hysterectomy. Large retention sutures were used to stabilize the surgical incision. Her surgical dressing and some of the retention sutures were removed by the surgeon. While Ms. Jensen is getting out of bed, she complains of something "giving way" and you note separation of her incision and protrusion of a section of bowel. What actions would you take at this time?

23/   Nursing in Emergencies

Many illnesses are of an emergency nature, both in and out of the hospital. Emergency nursing requires judgment, timing, alertness, and knowledge. An emergency department's primary purpose is to treat the serious, often life-threatening events that require immediate attention.

Many clients seen in an emergency department do not have life-threatening emergencies but still require treatment. Some individuals seeking treatment may have minor injuries or ailments that could be treated in a physician's office, but for various reasons the individual seeks treatment at a hospital.

The following questions deal with the content of Chapter 23.

I. MULTIPLE CHOICE QUESTIONS

Circle the number of the most appropriate answer.

1. Which one of the following assumes the highest priority when administering first aid?

    1. stop the bleeding
    2. obtain vital signs
    3. establish an airway
    4. assess for injuries

    Nursing Process: Implementation
    Client Need: Physiological Integrity

2. In an emergency, most bleeding in an extremity can be stopped by

    1. applying a tight dressing and lowering the affected extremity
    2. application of a loose dressing followed in 10 minutes by application of a tight dressing
    3. pressure on and around the area and elevation of the affected extremity
    4. applying a tourniquet below the bleeding area

    Nursing Process: Implementation
    Client Need: Physiological Integrity

3. The first step in the emergency treatment of respiratory arrest is to

    1. insert an oral airway
    2. administer oxygen
    3. administer a bronchodilator
    4. clear the airway of any mucus, dirt, or other particles

    Nursing Process: Implementation
    Client Need: Physiological Integrity

4. Violent or aggressive clients admitted as psychiatric emergencies

   1. can be left alone as long as they do not threaten others
   2. should be placed in a locked, empty room and left alone until the episode subsides
   3. are protected from harming themselves and others
   4. must be immediately restrained

   Nursing Process: Implementation
   Client Need: Psychosocial Integrity

5. Shock is likely to occur if it has been determined that the client has lost ____ of blood.

   1. 1000 mL or more
   2. 500 to 700 mL
   3. 500 mL
   4. 100 to 400 mL

   Nursing Process: Collecting Data
   Client Need: Physiological Integrity

6. If a victim arrives in the emergency department with an inflatable tourniquet, this device

   1. should not be removed except by a physician
   2. is removed and reapplied every 2 minutes
   3. must remain on the client until a blood pressure is obtained
   4. should never be used outside of the hospital

   Nursing Process: Implementation
   Client Need: Physiological Integrity

7. When assisting with the treatment of shock, which one of the following is done first?

   1. taking an ECG
   2. inserting an intravenous line
   3. placing the client in a sitting position
   4. covering the client with several heavy blankets

   Nursing Process: Implementation
   Client Need: Physiological Integrity

8. The person performing the Heimlich maneuver

   1. stands behind the victim
   2. places the victim flat on a soft surface
   3. places the victim in a sitting position
   4. stands in front of the victim

   Nursing Process: Implementation
   Client Need: Physiological Integrity

9. Vomiting is not induced if a client has ingested

   1. tranquilizers
   2. a strong alkali
   3. antidepressants
   4. birth control pills

   Nursing Process: Implementation
   Client Need: Physiological Integrity

10. When a client seen in the emergency department reports being bitten by a tick, the nurse looks for early symptoms of Lyme disease which include

    1. paralysis, abdominal distention
    2. fatigue, signs of anemia
    3. cyanosis, tachycardia
    4. neck stiffness and pain, headache

    Nursing Process: Collecting Data
    Client Need: Physiological Integrity

11. Following ingestion of a chemical or drug, certain information must be obtained since correct treatment or administration of an antidote depends on

    1. the client's willingness to cooperate
    2. identification of the ingested substance
    3. the age of the client
    4. where the substance came from

    Nursing Process: Collecting Data
    Client Need: Physiological Integrity

12. When doing health teaching the nurse can emphasize that the microorganism causing botulism is found most often in foods that

    1. are left unrefrigerated
    2. are prepared with preservatives
    3. have been improperly canned at home
    4. have been exposed to toxic material such as insecticides

    Nursing Process: Implementation
    Client Need: Health Promotion/Maintenance

13. When teaching a family the importance of keeping ipecac syrup in the household, the nurse can explain that this drug

    1. requires a prescription
    2. is never given to children
    3. may be used to induce vomiting after ingestion of certain substances
    4. is used when certain substances, such as alkalis, are ingested

    Nursing Process: Implementation
    Client Need: Health Promotion/Maintenance

14. When discussing the methods of preventing food poisoning, the nurse can tell clients that

    1. food is best thawed on the kitchen counter
    2. raw food must be cooked at the recommended temperature
    3. cooked food can be allowed to stand until cool before refrigerating
    4. rare meat can be eaten provided it is cooked at the proper temperature

    Nursing Process: Implementation
    Client Need: Health Promotion/Maintenance

15. If carbon monoxide poisoning is suspected, the nurse looks for

    1. muscle rigidity, pallor, nausea, and vomiting
    2. increased respiratory rate, seizures, ataxia
    3. pinpoint pupils, tachycardia, cyanosis
    4. mental confusion, changes in skin color, muscle weakness

    Nursing Process: Collecting Data
    Client Need: Physiological Integrity

16. A victim is brought to the emergency department with heatstroke. The nurse can prepare for treatment of this condition by obtaining

    1. enough cold, wet towels to cover the entire body
    2. warm liquids such as tea or milk
    3. large amounts of cold fluids
    4. a small ice pack to place behind the neck

    Nursing Process: Implementation
    Client Need: Physiological Integrity

17. When teaching those who are subject to frostbite, the nurse can suggest

    1. slow warming of the frostbitten part
    2. massaging the affected part
    3. rubbing ice or snow on the affected part
    4. immersing the part in 150° water

    Nursing Process: Implementation
    Client Need: Health Promotion/Maintenance

II. CRITICAL THINKING EXERCISES

1. Mr. Eden, age 82, is your neighbor. He tells you that his furnace is not working and that he is cold. What medical problem may occur? If the condition is mild, what immediate treatment can be given until he is examined by a physician?

2. While working in the emergency department you receive a telephone call from a mother who asks what she should do because she thinks her child swallowed some pills from the medicine cabinet. What questions would you ask?

3. A client is seen in the emergency department for treatment of a spider bite. The client's condition is stable. What information would you attempt to obtain from the victim?

4. You are standing alone on a street corner. You suddenly hear gunshots and see two youths running from a neighborhood market. They drive away in a car and you cross the street. Inside the market, one man appears dead from a shotgun blast to his face. A woman lying on the floor is bleeding profusely from what appears to be a lower abdominal wound. A teenager is on the floor and appears unconscious or dead. As you pass his body you note a bullet wound in his right temple. What first aid would you give each victim?

V Caring for Clients with Respiratory Disorders

24/ Introduction to the Respiratory System

The upper and lower respiratory airways are subject to many diseases and disorders, some of which are mild, some serious, and some life-threatening. Problems with breathing, the inability to obtain sufficient oxygen, or a disorder resulting in partial or total airway obstruction creates reactions ranging from anxiety to panic.

The following questions deal with the content of Chapter 24.

I. MULTIPLE CHOICE QUESTIONS

Circle the number of the most appropriate answer.

A team conference is scheduled for discussion of respiratory diseases and disorders. All individuals attending the conference are asked to review their inservice notes on the anatomy and physiology of the upper and lower respiratory airway.

1. When asked for the location of the maxillary sinuses, the nurse correctly answers
    1. on either side of the nose
    2. behind the nasal cavity
    3. above the orbital cavities
    4. between the eyes

    Nursing Process: Implementation
    Client Need: Safe, Effective Care Environment

2. When asked for the location of the larynx, the nurse correctly answers between the
    1. pharynx and esophagus
    2. nasopharynx and trachea
    3. cribiform plate and oropharynx
    4. pharynx and trachea

    Nursing Process: Implementation
    Client Need: Safe, Effective Care Environment

3. A nurse assistant asks how speech is produced. The correct answer is by the
    1. larynx and true vocal cords
    2. pharynx, palate, tongue, teeth, lips
    3. larynx, false and true vocal cords
    4. tongue, lips, and larynx

    Nursing Process: Implementation
    Client Need: Safe, Effective Care Environment

4. When asked to describe the glottis, the nurse correctly answers that the glottis is a(n)
   1. opening between the vocal cords
   2. section of tissue that lies immediately below the vocal cords
   3. protective mechanism surrounding the vocal cords
   4. section of tissue immediately above the oropharynx

   Nursing Process: Implementation
   Client Need: Safe, Effective Care Environment

5. When asked to give the function of the epiglottis, the nurse correctly answers that the epiglottis
   1. is part of the lining of the trachea, pharynx, and larynx
   2. opens and closes to direct air or food into the appropriate passages
   3. is the lower section of the larynx
   4. closes when air is expired from the lungs

   Nursing Process: Implementation
   Client Need: Safe, Effective Care Environment

6. A team conference member is asked to name the supporting structures of the trachea. The correct answer is the
   1. oval cartilages
   2. hyaline bone
   3. C-shaped cartilages
   4. osseous bone

   Nursing Process: Implementation
   Client Need: Safe, Effective Care Environment

7. The nurse is asked the name of the entrance of the bronchus into the lung. The correct answer is the
   1. tracheobronchial tree
   2. carina
   3. laryngeal opening
   4. hilus

   Nursing Process: Implementation
   Client Need: Safe, Effective Care Environment

8. The conference leader asks what happens when the carina is stimulated. The correct answer is
   1. more air enters the lungs
   2. coughing and bronchospasm
   3. the respiratory rate decreases
   4. intrathoracic pressure equals atmospheric pressure

   Nursing Process: Implementation
   Client Need: Safe, Effective Care Environment

9. The conference leader asks where the alveoli are located. The correct answer is
   1. at the branching of the secondary bronchi
   2. near the hilum of the lung
   3. near the carina
   4. at the end of the terminal bronchioles

   Nursing Process: Implementation
   Client Need: Safe, Effective Care Environment

10. When asked for a definition of intrapulmonary pressure, the nurse correctly answers that it is the pressure in the
    1. lungs on expiration
    2. thoracic cavity
    3. pleural cavity
    4. trachea, bronchi, and alveoli

    Nursing Process: Implementation
    Client Need: Safe, Effective Care Environment

11. When asked to define the term hypoxemia, the nurse correctly answers
    1. decreased oxygen in the blood
    2. increased oxygen in the blood
    3. increased carbon dioxide in the blood
    4. decreased carbon dioxide in the blood

    Nursing Process: Implementation
    Client Need: Safe, Effective Care Environment

12. The conference leader asks how the pH affects the rate of alveolar ventilation. The correct answer is by a direct action of hydrogen ions on the
    1. higher cerebral centers
    2. respiratory neurons located in the chest wall
    3. respiratory center in the medulla oblongata
    4. lower spinal cord

    Nursing Process: Implementation
    Client Need: Safe, Effective Care Environment

13. The conference leader asks which structures help maintain the normal ratio of carbonic acid to bicarbonate. The correct answer is the
    1. liver and heart
    2. medulla and cerebral cortex
    3. lungs and kidneys
    4. spleen and liver

    Nursing Process: Implementation
    Client Need: Safe, Effective Care Environment

14. A nurse assistant asks, "What is pulse oximetry?" The correct answer is pulse oximetry is a method of
    1. determining whether anemia is present
    2. monitoring the actual oxygen content of hemoglobin
    3. monitoring the carbon dioxide content of the blood
    4. determining blood pH

    Nursing Process: Implementation
    Client Need: Safe, Effective Care Environment

15. The nursing care plan for a client who has had a bronchoscopy under a local anesthetic would include
    1. advising the client to avoid raising sputum
    2. keeping the client lying flat for 6 hours
    3. encouraging fluids for the next 8 hours
    4. keeping the client NPO until the gag reflex returns

    Nursing Process: Planning
    Client Need: Physiological Integrity

Mr. Booth is a client in a medical outpatient clinic. He is scheduled to undergo diagnostic evaluation of his respiratory status.

16. When describing how to obtain a sputum sample, the nurse can tell Mr. Booth to
    1. include some saliva in the sputum sample
    2. raise and discard the first two samples of sputum
    3. save the sputum first expectorated in the morning
    4. rinse his mouth after collecting the sample

    Nursing Process: Implementation
    Client Need: Safe, Effective Care Environment

17. A vital capacity is performed on Mr. Booth. When explaining to another nurse what this test measures, the nurse correctly states that the vital capacity is the
    1. minimum volume of air that can be held in the lungs
    2. maximum volume of air that can be exhaled after maximum inhalation
    3. volume of air remaining in the lungs after expiration
    4. maximum volume of air that can be exhaled with a forced expiratory effort

    Nursing Process: Implementation
    Client Need: Safe, Effective Care Environment

18. Mr. Booth has a direct laryngoscopy. Pain and discomfort after the procedure may be reduced by
    1. applying a heat pack
    2. offering sips of cool fruit juices
    3. applying an ice collar
    4. offering sips of warm water

    Nursing Process: Implementation
    Client Need: Physiological Integrity

II. CRITICAL THINKING EXERCISES

1. Mr. Stone had a mediastinoscopy this morning and has been returned to his room. What special observations or assessments would you perform following this procedure?

2. Ms. Ferris had a thoracentesis 1 hour ago. What observations or assessments would you include in her plan of care for the next 24 hours?

25/ Caring for Clients with Disorders of the Upper Respiratory Airway

Disorders of the upper respiratory airway are common and may be seen in the hospital as well as outpatient setting. Milder problems usually result in unpleasant symptoms and inconvenience, but other problems can be serious and even life-threatening.

The following questions deal with the content of Chapter 25.

I. MULTIPLE CHOICE QUESTIONS

Circle the number of the most appropriate answer.

Mr. Leonard, age 44, developed hoarseness about 8 months ago but did not seek medical advice. After an examination, thorough history, and biopsy of the lesion, the physician had Mr. Leonard admitted to the hospital for a total laryngectomy and radical neck dissection.

1. Mr. Leonard is awake and has returned from the postanesthesia recovery room and is positioned
    1. on his back with the head of the bed elevated 10°
    2. flat with his head turned to the side
    3. in a semi-Fowler's position
    4. in a full Fowler's position

    Nursing Process: Implementation
    Client Need: Physiological Integrity

2. The nurse can tell the difference between a tracheostomy tube and a laryngectomy tube because a laryngectomy tube
    1. is shorter and has a larger diameter
    2. has three separate cannulas
    3. is longer and has a smaller diameter
    4. is metal instead of plastic

    Nursing Process: Collecting Data
    Client Need: Physiological Integrity

3. Mr. Leonard must be checked frequently during the immediate postoperative period. Which one of the following assessments assumes the highest priority? Assessing Mr. Leonard for
    1. pain
    2. signs of respiratory obstruction
    3. evidence of tension on the suture line
    4. evidence of serous drainage on his dressing

    Nursing Process: Collecting Data
    Client Need: Physiological Integrity

4. To prevent extreme movement of Mr. Leonard's head the nurse can
    1. place sandbags on one side of his head
    2. apply a cervical collar when moving or changing his position
    3. support his head when moving or changing his position
    4. place a large pillow behind his shoulders

    Nursing Process: Implementation
    Client Need: Physiological Integrity

5. The nurse can anticipate that Mr. Leonard will have less pain than clients with other types of major surgeries in this area because
   1. there are very few sensory nerves in the neck
   2. they are usually unresponsive the first few days after surgery
   3. of edema around the operative site
   4. sensory nerve endings are severed during surgery

   Nursing Process: Collecting Data
   Client Need: Physiological Integrity

6. During the immediate postoperative period Mr. Leonard will require tracheal suctioning
   1. every hour and as needed
   2. every 4 hours
   3. twice a day
   4. daily

   Nursing Process: Implementation
   Client Need: Physiological Integrity

7. As soon as Mr. Leonard is allowed out of bed the nurse can plan to first teach him how to
   1. speak using an electronic vibrator
   2. change his surgical dressing
   3. suction his oral cavity
   4. insert his laryngectomy tube

   Nursing Process: Planning
   Client Need: Physiological Integrity

8. Oral suctioning is performed gently to
   1. remove all secretions from the nasopharynx
   2. prevent injury to the mucous membranes
   3. keep the oral cavity dry
   4. aid in removing blood from the upper trachea

   Nursing Process: Implementation
   Client Need: Physiological Integrity

9. Mr. Leonard receives nasogastric tube feedings. After the feeding is finished it is followed by insertion of
   1. 50 mL of clean water
   2. 25 mL of tube feeding diluted with 25 mL of water
   3. 25 mL of air
   4. 50 mL of warmed tube feeding

   Nursing Process: Implementation
   Client Need: Physiological Integrity

10. Once oral feedings are started, the nurse remains with Mr. Leonard as he first drinks fluids in case
    1. he needs help in holding a glass
    2. he fails to drink a sufficient quantity of fluids
    3. it is necessary to measure how much he drinks
    4. suctioning is required

    Nursing Process: Implementation
    Client Need: Physiological Integrity

11. A plan for discharge teaching may include
    1. taking a shower rather than a tub bath
    2. a scarf or gauze dressing may be placed over the stoma to keep out dust and dirt
    3. swimming is allowed, provided that the head is kept above water
    4. waiting 1 year before using an electronic vibrator to produce speech

    Nursing Process: Planning
    Client Need: Safe, Effective Care Environment

Ms. Berst had a tracheostomy performed for an upper respiratory tract infection accompanied by severe edema and severe respiratory distress. She has been returned to her room following the procedure.

12. Unless ordered otherwise, the nurse positions the bed
    1. flat
    2. with the head elevated to about 45°
    3. with the feet elevated
    4. with both the head and feet elevated

    Nursing Process: Implementation
    Client Need: Physiological Integrity

13. Ms. Berst has a cuffed tracheostomy tube which requires monitoring the pressure in the cuff which should be between
    1. 10 and 12 mm H_2O
    2. 5 and 10 mm Hg
    3. 20 and 25 mm H_2O
    4. 15 and 25 mm Hg

    Nursing Process: Implementation
    Client Need: Safe, Effective Care Environment

14. If Ms. Berst's tracheostomy tube becomes dislodged and cannot be easily reinserted, the nurse
    1. administers pressurized oxygen
    2. uses a tracheal dilator to keep the stoma open until the physician arrives to reinsert the tube
    3. uses a Venturi mask to inflate the client's lungs and deliver oxygen
    4. administers oxygen by nasal catheter

    Nursing Process: Implementation
    Client Need: Physiological Integrity

15. When performing tracheal suctioning, suction is applied
    1. once the catheter has been passed into the trachea as well as being withdrawn from the trachea
    2. while the catheter is being inserted into the trachea
    3. only when the catheter is being withdrawn from the trachea
    4. when the catheter is in the upper pharynx

    Nursing Process: Implementation
    Client Need: Physiological Integrity

16. Ms. Berst can be encouraged to speak by
    1. taking a breath and briefly covering the tube with a finger
    2. forming words with the mouth while exhaling
    3. exhaling and covering the tube with a finger
    4. forming words with the mouth while inhaling

    Nursing Process: Implementation
    Client Need: Safe, Effective Care Environment

Individual Questions

17. When teaching a client with chronic nasal congestion the nurse recommends avoiding frequent, prolonged use of nose drops since this practice can result in
    1. rebound nasal congestion
    2. physical addiction to the principle ingredient
    3. dilatation of the sinus drainage tracts
    4. shrinkage of the sinus cavities

    Nursing Process: Implementation
    Client Need: Health Promotion/Maintenance

18. Which of the following methods of treatment can be reviewed with the client with chronic sinusitis?

    1. limiting fluid intake, nose drops q4h
    2. high-protein diet, cough suppressants
    3. application of ice packs, analgesics
    4. ample fluid intake, humidification of surrounding air

    Nursing Process: Implementation
    Client Need: Health Promotion/Maintenance

19. Following surgery for nasal polyps the client is

    1. kept flat for 24 hours
    2. kept on the right or left side
    3. placed in a semi-Fowler's position
    4. placed in a head-down position

    Nursing Process: Implementation
    Client Need: Physiological Integrity

20. Following a tonsillectomy clients recovering from anesthesia are

    1. kept flat and on their side
    2. placed in a semi-Fowler's position
    3. kept supine
    4. placed in a prone position

    Nursing Process: Implementation
    Client Need: Physiological Integrity

21. Following surgical drainage of a peritonsilar abscess the client is assessed for signs and symptoms of

    1. lymphadenopathy
    2. respiratory obstruction
    3. pneumonia
    4. gastric bleeding

    Nursing Process: Implementation
    Client Need: Physiological Integrity

22. When a person has a common cold the nurse can advise

    1. eating a low-protein diet
    2. taking an antitussive to decrease coughing
    3. limiting the fluid intake
    4. coughing and deep breathing every 1 to 2 hours

    Nursing Process: Implementation
    Client Need: Health Promotion/Maintenance

23. Discharge teaching of the client having had surgery for tonsillitis or a peritonsilar abscess can include

    1. using ice chips or cold water to relieve throat pain or discomfort
    2. using aspirin to relieve pain
    3. limiting the fluid intake until pain has decreased
    4. using nose drops to relieve nasal congestion

    Nursing Process: Implementation
    Client Need: Health Promotion/Maintenance

24. When preparing materials for treatment of epistaxis, the nurse obtains topical epinephrine because this drug

    1. increases blood flow to the area
    2. helps cauterize superficial blood vessels
    3. results in localized vasoconstriction
    4. reduces blood pressure

    Nursing Process: Implementation
    Client Need: Safe, Effective Care Environment

25. Initial emergency treatment of a minor nosebleed includes
    1. having the client sit with the head tilted back and the mouth closed
    2. applying pressure by holding the soft parts of the nose firmly between the thumb and fore finger
    3. applying pressure with a cold washcloth behind the neck
    4. having the client blow the nose gently to remove accumulated blood

    Nursing Process: Implementation
    Client Need: Physiological Integrity

26. Following insertion of a nasal pack for severe epistaxis the nurse instructs the client to
    1. remove the nasal pack in 24 hours by pulling on the string
    2. avoid drinking fluids for 8 hours
    3. avoid coughing and deep breathing for the next 2 days
    4. breathe through the mouth and spit out any blood

    Nursing Process: Implementation
    Client Need: Safe, Effective Care Environment

27. If aspiration of a foreign body results in total laryngeal obstruction, emergency treatment includes
    1. administration of 100% oxygen
    2. administration of epinephrine
    3. insertion of an endotracheal tube
    4. the use of the Heimlich maneuver

    Nursing Process: Implementation
    Client Need: Physiological Integrity

28. A client with an endotracheal tube is hyperinflated (sighed)
    1. every hour
    2. every 4 hours
    3. every 12 hours
    4. daily

    Nursing Process: Implementation
    Client Need: Physiological Integrity

II. CRITICAL THINKING EXERCISES

1. Mr. Branch had a tracheostomy tube inserted yesterday. While having a bed bath, he suddenly becomes deeply cyanotic and is in obvious severe respiratory distress. You note that his tracheostomy tube appears obstructed. What would you do?

2. Your 16-year-old brother tells you that he has a severe sore throat and fever. He asks you if you know of any medication he can buy that would help relieve his discomfort. What advice would you give him?

3. Ms. Eden had a tracheostomy. What methods can be used to help her communicate with others?

4. You enter Ms. Hunter's room and notice that she is having difficulty breathing. What immediate assessments would you make?

26/ Caring for Clients with Disorders of the Lower Respiratory Airway

Disorders of the lower respiratory airway may be acute or chronic. Some chronic disorders can become acute and some acute disorders can, in turn, become chronic in nature.

When the usual automatic function of breathing enters awareness and becomes a struggle, a vicious cycle ensues. The dyspneic client is anxious because of difficulty in breathing. The anxiety created by difficulty in breathing increases the respiratory rate and depth.

The following questions deal with the content of Chapter 26.

I. MULTIPLE CHOICE QUESTIONS

Circle the number of the most appropriate answer.

A team conference is held to discuss the nursing management of clients with lower respiratory airway disorders.

1. The nurse is ask to define bronchiectasis. The correct response is that this disorder is a chronic infectious disease in which there is (are)
   1. changes in the parenchyma of the lung
   2. structural changes in the walls of the bronchi and bronchioles
   3. a marked decrease in sputum production
   4. an increase in the vital capacity and forced expiratory volume

   Nursing Process: Implementation
   Client Need: Safe, Effective Care Environment

2. The nurse is ask to define pleurisy. The correct response is pleurisy is a(n)
   1. collection of fluid between the visceral and parietal pleura
   2. inflammation of the alveoli
   3. infection of the surface of the lung
   4. inflammation of the visceral and parietal pleura

   Nursing Process: Implementation
   Client Need: Safe, Effective Care Environment

3. The nurse is asked to name three signs and symptoms of pneumonia. The most correct answer is
   1. nonproductive cough, nausea, weight loss
   2. bradycardia, anorexia, chills
   3. chest pain, fever, shallow respirations
   4. diarrhea, chest pain, hypothermia

   Nursing Process: Implementation
   Client Need: Safe, Effective Care Environment

4. The nurse is asked to define thoracic empyema. The most correct answer is
   1. pus or infected fluid within the pleural cavity
   2. air or fluid in the lungs
   3. rupture of the alveoli
   4. trauma to the chest followed by entrance of air

   Nursing Process: Implementation
   Client Need: Safe, Effective Care Environment

5. A nurse assistant asks, "What causes the flu?" The correct answer is that influenza is caused by
   1. *Streptococcus viridans*
   2. a virus
   3. *Staphlococcus aureus*
   4. a fungus

   Nursing Process: Implementation
   Client Need: Safe, Effective Care Environment

6. When discussing the incidence of tuberculosis, the conference leader asks, "What segment of the population has the highest incidence of tuberculosis?" The most correct answer is

    1. the elderly, school-aged children
    2. sexually promiscuous teenagers, factory workers

    3. the mentally retarded, middle-aged adults
    4. alcoholics, those with AIDS

    Nursing Process: Implementation
    Client Need: Safe, Effective Care Environment

Mr. Bauer has tuberculosis and is admitted for treatment of malnutrition, advanced tuberculosis, and pneumonia.

7. Mr. Bauer is encouraged to

    1. take shallow breaths when the pain is severe
    2. cough and deep breathe every 2 hours while awake

    3. lie on his affected side
    4. change his position at least twice a day

    Nursing Process: Implementation
    Client Need: Physiological Integrity

8. If Mr. Bauer has pain on coughing, the nurse may

    1. administer the prescribed narcotic analgesic before the client coughs
    2. support the chest with both hands and use firm pressure to splint the chest wall

    3. have the client sit upright when it is necessary to cough
    4. have the client lie on the unaffected side when it is necessary to cough

    Nursing Process: Implementation
    Client Need: Physiological Integrity

9. Mr. Bauer takes oral fluids poorly. When determining the total daily urine output, the nurse notifies the physician if the output is less than

    1. 1500 mL/day
    2. 500 mL/8 hours

    3. 250 mL/8 hours
    4. 500 mL/day

    Nursing Process: Implementation
    Client Need: Physiological Integrity

10. Mr. Bauer has a fever and is given an antipyretic. Following oral administration Mr. Bauer's temperature is taken in

    1. 15 minutes
    2. 30 minutes

    3. 1 hour
    4. 2 hours

    Nursing Process: Implementation
    Client Need: Physiological Integrity

11. When teaching Mr. Bauer, the nurse emphasizes the importance of

    1. taking antitubercular drugs for a long period of time
    2. eating a low-protein, high-caloric diet

    3. adhering to the short-term drug regimen
    4. avoiding all contact with family members and friends

    Nursing Process: Implementation
    Client Need: Health Promotion/Maintenance

Ms. Garner has pulmonary emphysema and was seen in the respiratory clinic for evaluation and treatment. She is admitted to the hospital with marked respiratory distress and possible pneumonia.

12. A history of symptoms is obtained from Ms. Garner. One of the first symptoms that she may have noticed is
    1. pain on coughing
    2. rust-colored sputum
    3. hypotension
    4. exertional dyspnea

    Nursing Process: Collecting Data
    Client Need: Physiological Integrity

13. It is determined that Ms. Garner has advanced pulmonary emphysema. During assessment the nurse may note that Ms. Garner has
    1. a distended abdomen
    2. a chronic productive cough
    3. a ruddy complexion
    4. distended neck veins during inspiration

    Nursing Process: Collecting Data
    Client Need: Physiological Integrity

14. If Ms. Garner requires oxygen, the safest method of administration is a flow rate set at
    1. 6–7 L/min
    2. 1 L/min
    3. no more than 2–3 L/min
    4. 3–6 L/min

    Nursing Process: Implementation
    Client Need: Physiological Integrity

15. Oxygen administration to Ms. Garner is discontinued if
    1. her level of consciousness decreases
    2. she appears restless
    3. her color remains cyanotic
    4. her respiratory rate increase

    Nursing Process: Implementation
    Client Need: Physiological Integrity

16. The nurse can teach Ms. Garner to use therapeutic breathing exercises which
    1. use thoracic muscles to breathe
    2. relieve the burden on muscles of the upper thorax
    3. increase the respiratory rate
    4. decrease the respiratory rate

    Nursing Process: Implementation
    Client Need: Health Promotion/Maintenance

17. Ms. Garner can be taught pursed-lip breathing which helps control the respiratory rate and depth and
    1. slows expiration
    2. slows inspiration
    3. increases inspiration
    4. increases expiration

    Nursing Process: Implementation
    Client Need: Health Promotion/Maintenance

Individual Questions

18. When developing a plan of nursing management for the client with acute bronchitis, the nurse includes
    1. monitoring vital signs daily
    2. limiting fluids until coughing and chest pain decreases
    3. encouraging coughing and deep breathing q2h while awake
    4. keeping room air warm and dry

    Nursing Process: Planning
    Client Need: Physiological Integrity

19. When teaching the client with chronic bronchitis, the nurse encourages the client to

    1. avoid exposure to sunlight and wind
    2. drink extra fluids to loosen bronchial secretions
    3. avoid exposure to hot, humid air during the summer months
    4. stay indoors as much as possible during the winter months

    Nursing Process: Implementation
    Client Need: Health Promotion/Maintenance

20. Placing the client with a disorder of the lower respiratory airway in a semi-Fowler's position

    1. takes the strain off the lower back muscles
    2. increases the amount of blood going to the lungs
    3. decreases circulation to the legs
    4. increases the amount of air taken with each breath

    Nursing Process: Implementation
    Client Need: Physiological Integrity

21. A lung abscess can sometimes be prevented in the unconscious client by

    1. changing the client's position every 4 hours
    2. avoiding the aspiration of secretions
    3. suctioning the oral cavity daily
    4. keeping the bed flat

    Nursing Process: Implementation
    Client Need: Safe, Effective Care Environment

22. When assessing the client with bronchial asthma, the nurse may expect to note

    1. dyspnea, wheezing, cough
    2. anorexia, anxiety, decreased mucus production
    3. fear, marked weight loss, fever
    4. copious sputum, cyanosis, periods of apnea

    Nursing Process: Collecting Data
    Client Need: Physiological Integrity

23. When teaching the client having frequent attacks of bronchial asthma, the nurse may recommend

    1. decreasing the fluid intake during an attack
    2. increasing food intake between attacks
    3. avoiding exposure to sunlight
    4. humidification of inspired air

    Nursing Process: Implementation
    Client Need: Health Promotion/Maintenance

24. When teaching the client who works in an area where dust is present in high concentrations, the nurse can recommend

    1. drinking extra fluids during working hours
    2. wearing a mask capable of filtering dust particles
    3. avoiding the area when dust is present
    4. using saline nose drops to remove dust particles

    Nursing Process: Implementation
    Client Need: Health Promotion/Maintenance

25. When giving care to the client with pulmonary hypertension, the nurse can reduce the body's need for oxygen by

    1. preventing fatigue
    2. having the client ambulate at frequent intervals
    3. increasing the fluid intake
    4. encouraging a well-balanced diet

    Nursing Process: Implementation
    Client Need: Safe, Effective Care Environment

26. When assessing the client with a possible small pulmonary embolus, the nurse looks for
    1. cough, tachycardia, dyspnea
    2. hypothermia, cyanosis, apnea
    3. hypertension, restlessness, petechiae
    4. bradycardia, hyperthermia, anorexia

    Nursing Process: Collecting Data
    Client Need: Physiological Integrity

27. When a pulmonary embolism occurs, an intravenous infusion is started as soon as possible to
    1. administer 5% dextrose to treat shock
    2. monitor the central venous pressure
    3. establish a patent vein before shock occurs
    4. obtain blood gas samples

    Nursing Process: Implementation
    Client Need: Physiological Integrity

28. The nurse can help prevent atelectasis by encouraging
    1. frequent ambulation
    2. extra fluids during waking hours
    3. eating a well-balanced diet
    4. coughing and deep breathing at frequent intervals

    Nursing Process: Implementation
    Client Need: Physiological Integrity

29. Acute respiratory failure requires immediate recognition of symptoms which include
    1. severe hypertension
    2. use of the accessory muscles of respiration
    3. a pulse rate below 60/min
    4. prolonged periods of apnea

    Nursing Process: Collecting Data
    Client Need: Physiological Integrity

30. Which one of the following clients is a candidate for adult respiratory distress syndrome (ARDS) and therefore requires close observation? The client with a recent history of
    1. diarrhea
    2. anorexia
    3. marked weight loss
    4. drug overdose

    Nursing Process: Collecting Data
    Client Need: Physiological Integrity

31. Which of the following may indicate the development of ARDS and require contacting the physician immediately?
    1. cyanosis; shallow, labored breathing
    2. bradycardia; hypertension
    3. pale, clammy skin; abdominal distention
    4. restlessness; hypovolemia

    Nursing Process: Collecting Data
    Client Need: Physiological Integrity

32. When caring for the client with decreased lower respiratory function,
    1. vital signs are monitored daily
    2. fluids are restricted
    3. the airway must be kept patent at all times
    4. position changes are avoided

    Nursing Process: Implementation
    Client Need: Physiological Integrity

33. Clients requiring mechanical ventilation must
    1. have the lungs auscultated daily
    2. receive frequent oral care
    3. never be suctioned
    4. have the endotracheal tube removed daily

    Nursing Process: Implementation
    Client Need: Physiological Integrity

34. Which one of the following can be included when doing health teaching for the client with decreased function of the lower airway?

    1. avoid respiratory irritants; take frequent rest periods
    2. limit fluids; avoid dry, heated areas
    3. exercise for 1 hour each day; avoid foods high in protein
    4. keep the living area cool; avoid exposure to sunlight

    Nursing Process: Implementation
    Client Need: Health Promotion/Maintenance

35. At a team conference the nurse presents the fact that lung cancer

    1. produces early symptoms
    2. cannot be cured
    3. often has few early symptoms
    4. is easily detected by chest radiograph

    Nursing Process: Implementation
    Client Need: Safe, Effective Care Environment

36. When developing a long-term plan of care for Mr. Ward, who has a malignant mediastinal tumor, the nurse must be aware of the fact that these tumors are

    1. easily treated with surgery and chemotherapy
    2. almost always can be removed surgically
    3. almost always inoperable
    4. usually cured with chemotherapy

    Nursing Process: Planning
    Client Need: Physiological Integrity

37. When describing the use of heparin in the treatment of a pulmonary embolus to another nurse, the most correct explanation is that heparin

    1. dissolves the thrombus
    2. prevents extension of the thrombus and development of additional thrombi
    3. shortens the bleeding and clotting time and thins the blood
    4. corrects a blood clotting deficiency

    Nursing Process: Implementation
    Client Need: Safe, Effective Care Environment

38. At a team conference a nurse asks why acute asthma may be treated with an adrenergic agent. The most correct response is that an adrenergic agent reduces bronchospasm by

    1. acting on the respiratory center in the medulla
    2. sedating the client and reducing anxiety
    3. stimulating nerve fibers in the lung
    4. relaxation of smooth muscle lining the bronchi and larger bronchioles

    Nursing Process: Implementation
    Client Need: Safe, Effective Care Environment

39. If a client is receiving anticoagulant therapy for a pulmonary embolism, the nurse should

    1. give all drugs orally
    2. monitor the plasma pH and platelet count
    3. keep the client on the left or right side
    4. place prolonged pressure on intramuscular injection sites

    Nursing Process: Implementation
    Client Need: Physiological Integrity

II. CRITICAL THINKING EXERCISES

1. Ms. Keller, a 60-year-old widow, has severe emphysema. She had to take early retirement from her job as a secretary and apply for disability. She is now concerned that she will be unable to perform household tasks such as cleaning, laundry, and cooking, tasks that she was able to pay to have done in the past. What advice could you give Ms. Keller?

2. Mr. Eubanks is receiving oxygen by nasal catheter for severe emphysema. You walk into his room and note that his wife is sitting near him and that his respiratory rate is lower than normal. What is the first thing you would check after you have timed his respiratory rate?

3. You are working in an outpatient clinic. Mr. Cole comes to the clinic for an initial visit, complaining of a chronic cough with copious amounts of dark-colored sputum. When giving an initial history to you, he tells you that he is from West Virginia and that he is now retired. What questions would you ask? Would a work history be relevant?

4. Mrs. Pierce developed intrinsic asthma at age 30. What advice can the nurse give for possibly reducing the frequency and severity of asthma attacks? What facts should be known before planning a teaching program?

27/ Caring for Clients Undergoing Thoracic Surgery

Thoracic surgery may be performed for a variety of conditions. Surgery on structures of the chest such as the lungs and heart requires opening the thoracic cavity. After most thoracic surgeries, chest tubes and a closed drainage system are used.

The following questions deal with the content of Chapter 27.

I. MULTIPLE CHOICE QUESTIONS

Circle the number of the most appropriate answer.

1. When inspecting chest tubes connected to an underwater seal system, the nurse makes sure the system is kept
    1. at the level of the bed
    2. 6 inches higher than the level of the bed
    3. close to the bedside stand
    4. below the level of the bed

    Nursing Process: Collecting Data
    Client Need: Physiological Integrity

2. When inspecting a one- or two-bottle closed drainage system, the nurse makes sure that the end of the drainage tube coming from the client and going to the drainage bottle
    1. is kept underwater at all times
    2. must be placed at least 1 inch above the water level
    3. is kept at the same level as the tube going to the client
    4. is connected to suction by means of a Y-connector

    Nursing Process: Collecting Data
    Client Need: Physiological Integrity

3. At a team conference, when explaining the use of chest tubes, the nurse is most correct in saying that it is usually necessary to drain secretions, air, and blood from the thoracic cavity in order to
    1. create positive pressure within the chest cavity
    2. collapse the lung on the operative side in order to encourage healing
    3. equalize alveolar pressure
    4. reexpand the lung

    Nursing Process: Implementation
    Client Need: Safe, Effective Care Environment

4. Chest tubes are inspected at frequent intervals since any break in the system could
   1. decrease thoracic pressure
   2. increase the amount of drainage from the chest
   3. allow air to be drawn into the pleural space
   4. decrease abdominal pressure

   Nursing Process: Implementation
   Client Need: Safe, Effective Care Environment

5. When answering a family's question about when the chest tubes will be removed, the nurse is most correct in saying that they are usually not removed until
   1. all drainage ceases
   2. bubbling in the drainage system ceases
   3. the lung has fully expanded
   4. water begins rising in the drainage tube

   Nursing Process: Implementation
   Client Need: Safe, Effective Care Environment

6. If any break or major leak in the underwater seal system occurs, the nurse
   1. turns the client on his unoperative side
   2. immediately clamps the chest tube
   3. administers oxygen at 2 L/min
   4. begins tracheal suctioning

   Nursing Process: Implementation
   Client Need: Physiological Integrity

7. In the beginning, the nurse knows that an underwater seal drainage system is functioning correctly when
   1. fluid in the water-seal chamber fluctuates with each respiration
   2. fluid in the drainage chamber is absent
   3. air is not present in the water-seal chamber
   4. fluid is not present in the water-seal chamber

   Nursing Process: Evaluation
   Client Need: Physiological Integrity

8. Subcutaneous emphysema can be detected when
   1. crackling sounds are heard on auscultation of the lungs
   2. a crackling sensation is felt on palpation
   3. the skin appears ecchymotic
   4. the client complains of pain

   Nursing Process: Collecting Data
   Client Need: Physiological Integrity

9. Following chest surgery the client is placed in a semi-Fowler's position to
   1. move drainage to the upper apex
   2. prevent a paralytic ileus
   3. prevent nausea and vomiting
   4. improve lung capacity

   Nursing Process: Implementation
   Client Need: Physiological Integrity

10. Encouraging the client to cough and deep breathe after chest surgery
    1. helps ventilate and expand the lung
    2. helps secretions to move into the lower chest cavity
    3. prevents excessive bleeding
    4. encourages exercise of the chest muscles and thus reduce pain

    Nursing Process: Implementation
    Client Need: Physiologic Integrity

11. When explaining the purpose of an incentive spirometer to another nurse, the nurse correctly states that this device

    1. measures the amount of air that is inhaled
    2. measures lung expansion
    3. measures drainage from the chest tubes
    4. helps ventilation

Nursing Process: Implementation
Client Need: Safe, Effective Care Environment

II. CRITICAL THINKING EXERCISES

1. Mr. Ward had a right upper lobe lobectomy for lung cancer. He returns from surgery with anterior and posterior chest tubes. He refuses to cough because of pain. What nursing measures can be taken to help Mr. Ward cough and deep breathe?

2. Four days after chest surgery Ms. Parsons' chest tubes are removed. What specific nursing measures can be taken to prevent ankylosis of the shoulder and muscle atrophy on the operative side?

VI Caring for Clients with Cardiovascular Disorders

28/ Introduction to the Cardiovascular System

Heart disease is the leading cause of death for adults in the United States. Preserving or duplicating the pumping action of the heart does not come easily once the heart is damaged. Although a human heart transplant and the temporary use of an artificial heart are available, preserving the natural heart by preventing heart disease or treating cardiac disorders early is more preferable.

The following questions deal with the content of Chapter 28.

I. MULTIPLE CHOICE QUESTIONS

Circle the number of the most appropriate answer.

A student nurse is scheduled for clinical experience on a nursing unit where clients with cardiac problems are hospitalized.

1. The student uses a medical-surgical nursing reference text to review the care of clients with cardiovascular disorders. The nursing student looks for the term that refers to the ability of the heart to initiate its own electrical impulse. The term the student is looking for is

   1. excitability
   2. conductivity

   3. automaticity
   4. rhythmicity

   Nursing Process: Implementation
   Client Need: Safe, Effective Care Environment

2. The student reads in a client's past health history that the client was born with an opening in the wall between the right and left chambers of the heart. The student nurse would be most correct in identifying this structure as the

   1. atria
   2. ventricle
   3. aorta
   4. septum

   Nursing Process: Implementation
   Client Need: Safe, Effective Care Environment

3. A client's medical record indicates that the client has a condition that causes great difficulty pumping blood to and through the lungs. When reviewing the client's diagnostic tests, the student nurse is most likely to find the heart chambers that are most impaired are the

   1. right and left atria
   2. right and left ventricle
   3. right atria and ventricle
   4. left atria and ventricle

   Nursing Process: Assessment
   Client Need: Safe, Effective Care Environment

4. The student nurse plans to count the client's heart rate by auscultating over the heart's apex. If the procedure is done correctly, the nurse will place the stethoscope

   1. on the left side of the chest below the nipple
   2. on the left side of the chest above the nipple
   3. on the right side of the chest below the nipple
   4. on the right side of the chest above the nipple

   Nursing Process: Implementation
   Client Need: Safe, Effective Care Environment

5. A client with a heart disorder asks the student nurse to explain why his physician told him he has a greater risk for infection. The student nurse would be most correct in explaining that microorganisms that are present in blood are most likely to infect that layer with which it is in direct contact, which is the

   1. myocardium
   2. epicardium
   3. endocardium
   4. pericardium

   Nursing Process: Implementation
   Client Need: Health Promotion/Maintenance

6. A client tells the student nurse that his brother had the valve between the left atria and ventricle replaced. He asks what that valve is called. The nurse would be most correct in telling the client it is the

   1. aortic valve, which is a semilunar valve
   2. mitral valve, which is a bicuspid valve
   3. pulmonic valve, which is a semilunar valve
   4. tricuspid valve, which has three leaflets

   Nursing Process: Implementation
   Client Need: Health Promotion/Maintenance

7. As the client describes his brother's valvular problem, which one of the following explanations should the nurse confirm is correct? "The doctor said my brother's blood

   1. left the heart too soon"
   2. seeped back into an upper chamber"
   3. plugged up the circulatory pathway"
   4. was too thin to even clot"

   Nursing Process: Implementation
   Client Need: Health Promotion/Maintenance

8. A client asks the student, "What did my physician mean when he said I had good capillary blood flow?" The nurse would be most correct in explaining that the capillaries are divisions of the vascular system which connect

   1. chordae tendinae and papillary muscles
   2. the tunica media and tunica intima
   3. two heart chambers
   4. arterioles and venules

   Nursing Process: Implementation
   Client Need: Safe, Effective Care Environment

Individual Questions

9. A client has a venous catheter in his heart through which fluids are being administered. If the client asks the nurse through which vessel the catheter was threaded to reach the right atria of his heart, the most correct answer would be

   1. the aorta
   2. the vena cava

   3. the pulmonary artery
   4. a pulmonary vein

   Nursing Process: Implementation
   Client Need: Safe, Effective Care Environment

10. In order to help a client understand cardiac circulation, the nurse would be most correct in explaining that the vessels that actually supply the heart with oxygenated blood are the

    1. pulmonary veins
    2. coronary arteries

    3. carotid arteries
    4. vena cavae

    Nursing Process: Implementation
    Client Need: Health Promotion/Maintenance

11. A student nurse uses an anatomy text to find how venous blood from coronary circulation returns to the heart. The most accurate information is that the coronary veins empty into an opening in the right side of the heart referred to as the

    1. subclavian vein
    2. jugular vein

    3. coronary sinus
    4. transverse sinus

    Nursing Process: Implementation
    Client Need: Safe, Effective Care Environment

12. A client says, "I know that when my heart beats, it causes a pulsation. What is happening between each beat?" The best response from the nurse is that during the pause

    1. no one knows what is happening
    2. cardiac activity is at a standstill

    3. the atria are filling with blood
    4. the ventricles are filling with blood

    Nursing Process: Implementation
    Client Need: Safe, Effective Care Environment

13. A client's electrical cardiac activity is being observed with a cardiac monitor. If the client asks what structure initiates the electrical impulse that keeps the heart beating, the most correct answer from the nurse is the specialized tissue known as the

    1. bundle of His
    2. atrioventricular node

    3. Purkinje fibers
    4. sinoatrial node

    Nursing Process: Implementation
    Client Need: Safe, Effective Care Environment

14. The nurse goes on to explain that the area of the heart that normally initiates each impulse is often referred to as the

    1. trendsetter
    2. pacemaker

    3. governor
    4. commander

    Nursing Process: Implementation
    Client Need: Health Promotion/Maintenance

15. Because of its potential for altering normal cardiac conduction, which one of the following electrolyte values would be most appropriate for the nurse to report immediately if it were elevated?

    1. potassium
    2. chloride

    3. sodium
    4. bicarbonate

    Nursing Process: Implementation
    Client Need: Physiological Integrity

16. A nurse administers a prescribed drug that blocks the calcium channels in the cell membranes of cardiac tissue. When planning this client's care, based upon the nurse's knowledge concerning the role of calcium in cardiac function, which assessment would be most essential to determine the drug's effectiveness?

    1. auscultation of heart sounds
    2. palpation of the pulse rate
    3. percussion of the heart border
    4. inspection of the chest size

    Nursing Process: Planning
    Client Need: Physiological Integrity

17. The nurse measures the cardiac output on four hospitalized clients. Which one is most likely to have a cardiac output that is greater than all the others?

    1. Ms. Foreman, who is 35 years old
    2. Mr. Riley, who is 6' 2" tall
    3. Mr. Al-Amed, who is Iranian
    4. Ms. Simpson, who is an asthmatic

    Nursing Process: Assessment
    Client Need: Health Promotion/Maintenance

18. To calculate a client's cardiac output, the nurse must multiply the volume of blood ejected during ventricular contraction times the client's

    1. heart rate
    2. present age
    3. systolic pressure
    4. diastolic pressure

    Nursing Process: Implementation
    Client Need: Safe, Effective Care Environment

19. A client with a cardiac disorder will be undergoing several diagnostic tests. The nurse makes the physician and staff aware that this client is allergic to seafood. The nurse's action is

    1. inappropriate since he will be restricted from eating
    2. inappropriate since the client will be discharged immediately afterwards
    3. appropriate because the client may have a reaction to iodine based dyes
    4. appropriate because many dyes are made from fish derivatives

    Nursing Process: Implementation
    Client Need: Safe, Effective Care Environment

20. When a client reveals he is experiencing chest pain, besides asking the client to describe the pain, the nurse should obtain which other essential data at this time?

    1. his family history
    2. his drug allergies
    3. whether the pain radiates
    4. any history of similar pain

    Nursing Process: Assessment
    Client Need: Physiological Integrity

21. A nurse plans to determine whether a client has a pulse deficit. To do this the nurse must count the radial pulse rate while

    1. evaluating the palpated volume
    2. another nurse counts the apical rate
    3. noting if there are similar pauses between each beat
    4. feeling the pulsations just below the left nipple

    Nursing Process: Assessment
    Client Need: Safe, Effective Care Environment

22. A nurse charts the following admission note: B.P. 150/78 in R arm while lying, 146/74 in L arm while sitting, and 142/74 while standing. The best analysis of this nurse's documentation is that it is

    1. appropriate if the client is not acutely ill
    2. appropriate if the client has chest pain
    3. inappropriate since it did not reveal significant changes
    4. inappropriate since only one measurement is necessary

    Nursing Process: Evaluation
    Client Need: Safe, Effective Care Environment

23. To determine whether the data displayed and recorded by a cardiac monitor are correct, which one of the following nursing actions is most appropriate? The nurse

    1. measures the client's blood pressure
    2. palpates the client's pulse rate
    3. requests a chest radiography
    4. uses a pulse oximeter machine

    Nursing Process: Assessment
    Client Need: Safe, Effective Care Environment

24. A nurse auscultates the chest to assess the client's heart sounds. When listening for the S2 (second heart sound), or "dub," which placement of the chestpiece indicates that the nurse is performing this assessment accurately? The nurse listens

    1. at the 4th intercostal space to the left of the sternum
    2. at the 5th intercostal space in the midclavicular line
    3. at the 2nd intercostal space to the left of the sternum
    4. at the 2nd intercostal space to the right of the sternum

    Nursing Process: Assessment
    Client Need: Safe, Effective Care Environment

25. Checking a client's popliteal pulse is an order on the nursing care plan. If this assessment is performed correctly, the nurse will palpate

    1. on top of the foot
    2. behind the knee
    3. in the groin
    4. at the inner ankle

    Nursing Process: Assessment
    Client Need: Safe, Effective Care Environment

26. While assessing a client's skin, which other finding suggests that the client has poor peripheral circulation?

    1. The hair growth is sparse over the legs.
    2. The leg muscles are small and weak.
    3. The skin feels warm and moist.
    4. The toenails are thin and rough.

    Nursing Process: Assessment
    Client Need: Physiological Integrity

27. A nurse reads in the medical record that a client has +4 pitting edema. This means that the examiner found the amount of fluid in the tissue to be

    1. slight
    2. moderate
    3. serious
    4. severe

    Nursing Process: Assessment
    Client Need: Physiological Integrity

28. A nurse observes a colleague assessing a client for jugular vein distention. Which one of the following indicates that the nurse is performing this assessment accurately? The nurse places the client in a sitting position at a

    1. 30° angle of head elevation
    2. 45° angle of head elevation
    3. 60° angle of head elevation
    4. 90° angle of head elevation

    Nursing Process: Evaluation
    Client Need: Safe, Effective Care Environment

29. Which one of the following assessment findings would support the practical nurse's suspicion that a client is experiencing pulmonary edema? The

    1. client refuses to lay flat
    2. client's feet are swollen
    3. client's skin is flushed
    4. client's abdomen is distended

    Nursing Process: Assessment
    Client Need: Physiological Integrity

30. A nursing student reviews the results of laboratory tests performed at the time of the client's admission. Which one of the following is most suggestive of heart disease? The client's

    1. urine contains ketones
    2. cholesterol is elevated
    3. blood contains platelets
    4. hemoglobin is low

    Nursing Process: Assessment
    Client Need: Safe, Effective Care Environment

31. If a client asks the nurse to explain what the physician meant when stating, "Your enzymes are elevated," the best response is that it is

    1. a normal finding associated with tissue healing
    2. an abnormal finding associated with cell damage
    3. a normal finding associated with the aging process
    4. an abnormal finding associated with an infection

    Nursing Process: Implementation
    Client Need: Health Promotion/Maintenance

32. The laboratory report of creatine kinase isoenzymes is transmitted to the nursing unit. An elevation in which one of the following should be reported since it indicates cardiac muscle damage?

    1. CK-MM
    2. CK-BB
    3. CK-MB
    4. CK-CM

    Nursing Process: Implementation
    Client Need: Physiological Integrity

33. A client with cardiovascular disease asks the nurse to explain why he is scheduled to have a chest radiograph. The best explanation is that this diagnostic procedure is being done to

    1. analyze circulation
    2. diagnose pneumonia
    3. identify lung tumors
    4. determine heart size

    Nursing Process: Implementation
    Client Need: Safe, Effective Care Environment

34. A client asks the nurse to explain the reason a stress test has been ordered. The best explanation is that this test demonstrates

    1. the effectiveness of blood circulation
    2. how the heart responds to exercise
    3. the manner in which emotions affect the heart
    4. which structures within the heart are impaired

    Nursing Process: Implementation
    Client Need: Safe, Effective Care Environment

35. Which information would best prepare the client on what may be experienced during the cardiac catheterization?

    1. "You will be given a general anesthetic."
    2. "You may experience a slight headache."
    3. "You will hear repetitive clicks and noises."
    4. "You may feel fluttering in your chest."

    Nursing Process: Implementation
    Client Need: Health Promotion/Maintenance

36. The best evidence that a client has understood the explanation concerning the use of dye during a cardiac catheterization is that the client says, "When the dye is instilled, I will feel

    1. a fluttering feeling in my chest"
    2. a warm sensation over my body"
    3. like I need to cough"
    4. lightheaded and dizzy"

    Nursing Process: Evaluation
    Client Need: Safe, Effective Care Environment

37. Which one of the following is most important for the nurse to assess following a coronary arteriogram?

    1. bleeding from the catheter insertion site
    2. fluid accumulation in the lung fields
    3. edema in both of the lower extremities
    4. numbness and tingling in the fingertips

    Nursing Process: Assessment
    Client Need: Physiological Integrity

38. After a coronary arteriogram, the nurse should intervene if a nursing assistant places the client in a

    1. Fowler's position
    2. supine position
    3. Trendelenburg position
    4. prone position

    Nursing Process: Implementation
    Client Need: Safe, Effective Care Environment

39. The nurse plans to measure a client's central venous pressure. Before filling the manometer with fluid, it is essential that the nurse place the zero mark at the level of the client's

    1. jugular vein
    2. iliac crest
    3. xiphoid process
    4. right atrium

    Nursing Process: Planning
    Client Need: Safe, Effective Care Environment

40. During a diagnostic test, a client experiences chest pain. Which one of the following actions should the nurse perform first?

    1. administer a precordial thump
    2. have the client stop and rest
    3. finish testing the client
    4. give a prescribed narcotic

    Nursing Process: Implementation
    Client Need: Physiological Integrity

II. CRITICAL THINKING EXERCISES

1. Mr. Samuel Shapiro is admitted to the coronary care unit. What questions are important to ask as part of the initial data base?

2. You are the nurse who schedules Mr. Frederick Jenkins for a stress electrocardiogram. What teaching would be appropriate to help the client understand why and how the test will be performed?

3. Alva Montgomery has just been returned to the nursing unit following a cardiac catheterization. Discuss the nursing care that would be appropriate at this time.

4. The nurse observes that a client who has just arrived in the outpatient department for a diagnostic test is quite anxious. What nursing actions would help to reduce the client's anxiety?

5. A client who supposedly has no known allergies has a significant change in his condition immediately after radiopaque dye is instilled. What assessment findings would support that the client is experiencing an allergic reaction to the dye?

29/ Caring for Clients with Infectious and Inflammatory Disorders of the Heart and Blood Vessels

Clients with infectious or inflammatory disorders of the heart and blood vessels often require treatment extending over a long period of time. The treatment of these disorders is often slow and tedious, with the client requiring long-term medical management and nursing care. As a result, it may become necessary for some clients to change their occupation, modify their lifestyle, and adjust their role and family responsibilities.

The following questions deal with the content of Chapter 29.

I. MULTIPLE CHOICE QUESTIONS

Circle the number of the most appropriate answer.

1. A nurse reads the medical record of a client who has infective endocarditis. If this client is typical of most others with this disorder, the nurse is most likely to find that the client has had

   1. rheumatic fever
   2. infectious mononucleosis
   3. pulmonary tuberculosis
   4. hepatitis B

   Nursing Process: Assessment
   Client Need: Physiological Integrity

2. The physician orders all of the following laboratory tests for a client who is suspected of having rheumatic heart disease. Which one is the nurse most correct in identifying for the client as being used to detect structural changes in the heart valves?

   1. cardiac catheterization
   2. coronary arteriography
   3. echocardiogram
   4. aortogram

   Nursing Process: Implementation
   Client Need: Safe, Effective Care Environment

3. A client is admitted with possible infective endocarditis. If all of the following occurred in the client's recent past history, which one is most likely related to the client's current condition? The client reports having

   1. diarrhea for 3 days
   2. wisdom teeth extracted
   3. traveled to Canada
   4. changed occupations

   Nursing Process: Assessment
   Client Need: Safe, Effective Care Environment

4. A client with infective endocarditis asks the nurse to explain what the physician meant by the term vegetations. The best answer is that they are

   1. collections of tissue and inflammatory products
   2. the consequence of inadequate exercise
   3. microscopic plants that grow in unwashed skin
   4. the growths that appear in tissue cultures

   Nursing Process: Implementation
   Client Need: Health Promotion/Maintenance

5. A client experiences all of the following signs and symptoms. Which one is most likely due to a complication associated with infective endocarditis?

   1. frequent vomiting
   2. increased urination

   3. epigastric burning
   4. labored breathing

   Nursing Process: Assessment
   Client Need: Physiological Integrity

6. A client with infective endocarditis asks how long he will need to take his prescribed drug therapy. The best answer is

   1. for one or two doses now and again in 6 weeks
   2. every day for the rest of a lifetime

   3. continuously for the next month and a half
   4. for several weeks now and periodically throughout life

   Nursing Process: Implementation
   Client Need: Health Promotion/Maintenance

7. A physician writes the following order for antibiotic therapy to treat a client during an acute stage of infective endocarditis: nafcillin sodium (Unipen) 1 g q4h. The nurse checks with the physician concerning the route for administration; at this stage of the disease, it is most common that this drug will be given

   1. orally
   2. intramuscularly

   3. subcutaneously
   4. intravenously

   Nursing Process: Implementation
   Client Need: Physiological Integrity

8. A physician orders carbenicillin indanyl disodium (Geocillin) 764 mg PO qid for a client with infective endocarditis. Using military time, which one of the following scheduling routines would be most appropriate for achieving the best therapeutic effect?

   1. 1000, 1400, 1800, 2200
   2. 0800, 1200, 1600, 2000

   3. 0900, 1300, 1700, 2100
   4. 0600, 1200, 1800, 0000

   Nursing Process: Implementation
   Client Need: Physiological Integrity

9. A client tells the nurse that the physician has informed him of the possible complications associated with myocarditis and asks which one is most serious. The best answer is

   1. activity intolerance
   2. irregular heart rate

   3. cardiomyopathy
   4. tachycardia

   Nursing Process: Implementation
   Client Need: Health Promotion/Maintenance

10. A client with myocarditis asks the nurse the outcome that would result if he acquired cardiomyopathy. The best response is that the condition often

   1. reduces cardiac output
   2. elevates blood pressure

   3. decreases heart size
   4. slows heart conduction

   Nursing Process: Implementation
   Client Need: Health Promotion/Maintenance

11. When caring for a client with myocarditis, which position should the nurse plan to use to promote the most comfort and relief from symptoms?

   1. dorsal recumbent
   2. left lateral

   3. high Fowler's
   4. reverse Trendelenburg

   Nursing Process: Planning
   Client Need: Physiological Integrity

12. The physician prescribes all of the following interventions for the treatment of a client with myocarditis. Which one of the following should the nurse explain is used to reduce the volume of blood the heart must circulate?

    1. antibiotic therapy
    2. complete bedrest

    3. sodium-restricted diet
    4. oxygen per nasal cannula

    Nursing Process: Implementation
    Client Need: Safe, Effective Care Environment

13. When caring for a client with myocarditis, which one of the following should the nurse plan to use to assess the client's oxygenation status?

    1. cardiac monitor
    2. pulse oximeter

    3. incentive spirometer
    4. tympanic thermometer

    Nursing Process: Planning
    Client Need: Safe, Effective Care Environment

14. Digoxin (Lanoxin) is prescribed for a client with complications associated with myocarditis. Which one of the following would be essential to report before administering the medication?

    1. The client is constipated.
    2. The client is restless.

    3. The client's heart rate is 54 bpm.
    4. The client's temperature is 97.6°F.

    Nursing Process: Implementation
    Client Need: Physiological Integrity

15. When assessing the client with pericarditis, the signs and symptoms are most likely to mimic a

    1. gallbladder attack
    2. collapsed lung

    3. myocardial infarction
    4. ruptured appendix

    Nursing Process: Assessment
    Client Need: Safe, Effective Care Environment

16. When the nurse auscultates the chest of a client with pericarditis, which one of the following abnormal sounds is most likely to be heard?

    1. gurgles
    2. murmur

    3. friction rub
    4. inspiratory wheeze

    Nursing Process: Assessment
    Client Need: Physiological Integrity

17. A nurse notes that when auscultating a client's blood pressure, there is a span of 10 mm Hg when the Korotkoff sounds occur during both expiration and inspiration. The nurse would be most correct in identifying this phenomenon as

    1. pulse deficit
    2. pulse pressure

    3. pulsus paradoxus
    4. pulsus bigeminus

    Nursing Process: Assessment
    Client Need: Physiological Integrity

18. A client with pericarditis experiences precordial pain. Which one of the following nursing measures would be best for relieving the client's discomfort?

    1. have the client ambulate about the room
    2. temporarily withhold all food and fluids

    3. instruct the client to take a deep breath and bear down
    4. instruct the client to sit up and lean forward

    Nursing Process: Implementation
    Client Need: Physiological Integrity

19. Which one of the following assessments would be most indicative to the nurse that the client with pericarditis is developing cardiac tamponade? The client develops
    1. severe hypotension
    2. a loud S_1 heart sound
    3. flushed, warm skin
    4. sudden bradycardia

    Nursing Process: Assessment
    Client Need: Physiological Integrity

20. Which one of the following is the best evidence that the client's condition has improved following pericardiocentesis?
    1. urine output increases
    2. Homans' sign is negative
    3. blood pressure is reduced
    4. peripheral edema is absent

    Nursing Process: Evaluation
    Client Need: Physiological Integrity

21. A client with pericarditis develops respiratory difficulty while sleeping. What alternative plan would be best at this time to resolve the client's sleep disturbance and improve breathing?
    1. give a prescribed sleeping medication each night
    2. use a reclining chair for sleep instead of the bed
    3. restrict oral fluids after the evening meal
    4. avoid allowing naps during daytime hours

    Nursing Process: Planning
    Client Need: Physiological Integrity

22. A client with an infectious and inflammatory disorder of the heart is depressed because he becomes fatigued and cannot complete all of his hygiene. The nurse could best improve the client's self-esteem by
    1. distributing the activity between periods of rest
    2. eliminating hygiene activities for the time being
    3. asking the client's wife to assist with his hygiene
    4. telling him that his endurance will improve soon

    Nursing Process: Planning
    Client Need: Psychosocial Integrity

23. A client with an infectious and inflammatory disorder of the heart must restrict his intake of oral fluids. Which one of the following measures would be most appropriate to add to the plan for care?
    1. offer reconstituted fruit juices
    2. suggest sucking on hard, sour candy
    3. substitute carbonated drinks for water
    4. have the client sip fluid through a straw

    Nursing Process: Planning
    Client Need: Physiological Integrity

24. Before discharging the client with an infectious or inflammatory disorder of the heart, which one of the following is the most important point for the nurse to stress about the drug regimen?
    1. wearing a Medic-Alert tag or bracelet
    2. taking the full dose for the full time
    3. the drug's mechanism of action
    4. how to request a generic form

    Nursing Process: Implementation
    Client Need: Health Promotion/Maintenance

25. Which one of the following techniques would be best for evaluating whether the client has understood the nurse's discharge instructions?
    1. have the client repeat the instructions
    2. ask the client if he or she has any questions
    3. call the client at home following discharge
    4. request that the client sign the instructions

    Nursing Process: Evaluation
    Client Need: Health Promotion/Maintenance

26. Which one of the following signs is most important to report to the physician since it indicates a suggestive sign of thrombophlebitis in a lower extremity?

    1. bright, flushed skin over the lower leg
    2. tiny, reddish hemorrhagic spots on the foot
    3. leg fatigue following periods of activity
    4. calf pain on dorsiflexion of the foot

    Nursing Process: Assessment
    Client Need: Physiological Integrity

27. Which one of the following should the nurse plan to explain while preparing a client for an impedence plethysmography?

    1. A cardiac monitor will be used to assess heart rhythm.
    2. A blood pressure cuff will be applied to the leg.
    3. A pulse oximeter will be attached to one finger.
    4. A light anesthetic will be administered intravenously.

    Nursing Process: Planning
    Client Need: Safe, Effective Care Environment

28. A nurse observes all of the following as a nursing assistant provides care for a client with a thrombophlebitis of the left lower leg. For which one is it essential to intervene? The nursing assistant

    1. applies a warm compress to the calf
    2. rubs lotion into the skin on the legs
    3. supports the knee and ankle during position changes
    4. provides a variety of oral fluids for the client

    Nursing Process: Implementation
    Client Need: Safe, Effective Care Environment

29. When caring for an inactive client, which one of the following would be most important to add to the plan for care in order to prevent a thrombophlebitis?

    1. perform isometric leg exercises q2h while awake
    2. dangle the legs over the bedside q4h while awake
    3. seat client in a chair for 2 hours daily
    4. provide 2000 mL of oral fluids per day

    Nursing Process: Planning
    Client Need: Physiological Integrity

30. Which one of the following laboratory test results would be the best resource for determining the effectiveness of heparin sodium (Liquaemin) prescribed for the treatment of thrombophlebitis?

    1. platelet count
    2. partial thromboplastin time (PTT)
    3. prothrombin time (PT)
    4. plasmin level

    Nursing Process: Evaluation
    Client Need: Physiological Integrity

31. Which one of the following assessments must be reported to the physician when a client is receiving warfarin sodium (Coumadin)?

    1. swollen ankles
    2. red skin rash
    3. jaundiced sclera
    4. bleeding gums

    Nursing Process: Implementation
    Client Need: Physiological Integrity

32. All of the following are important for health promotion. For clients with thromboangiitis obliterans, which one of the following would be especially important for the nurse to stress during discharge instructions?

    1. maintain normal weight
    2. consume less dietary fat
    3. avoid smoking cigarettes
    4. increase daily exercise

    Nursing Process: Implementation
    Client Need: Health Promotion/Maintenance

33. Which one of the following should the nurse instruct the client with thromboangiitis obliterans to report to the physician immediately?

    1. black skin areas
    2. redness of the feet
    3. burning leg pain
    4. thickened toenails

    Nursing Process: Implementation
    Client Need: Health Promotion/Maintenance

34. A nursing colleague obtains all of the following data after assessing a client with thromboangiitis obliterans. Which one is most important to report to the physician?

    1. There are crackles in the bases of the client's lungs.
    2. The blood pressure is 138/88 in the left arm while sitting.
    3. The dorsalis pedis pulses in both feet are not palpable.
    4. The skin temperature over both lower extremities is cool.

    Nursing Process: Implementation
    Client Need: Physiological Integrity

II. CRITICAL THINKING EXERCISES

1. How could the nurse respond to a client, subsequently diagnosed as having pericarditis, who asks why he was treated as though he had had a myocardial infarction immediately after being assessed in the emergency department.

2. A nurse is caring for all four of the following clients: Mr. Sands, who is scheduled for an echocardiogram; Ms. King, who had an abdominal hysterectomy; Mr. Goetz, who has bronchopneumonia; and Ms. Poindexter, who has gallstones. Which one is at highest risk for developing thrombophlebitis and why?

3. Mr. Carl Edwards will be taking oral anticoagulants on a daily basis to prevent a reoccurrence of thrombophlebitis. What teaching should the nurse plan to provide?

4. Mr. Harold Teeter has thromboangiitis obliterans. Explain how you would instruct him to perform Buerger-Allen exercises.

30/ Caring for Clients with Valvular Disorders of the Heart

Valvular disorders of the heart range from mild to potentially life-threatening. Valvular disorders may respond to conservative treatment or require major heart surgery. The client with a valvular disorder may be faced with many decisions as well as changes in lifestyle and personal commitments.

The following questions deal with the content of Chapter 30.

I. MULTIPLE CHOICE QUESTIONS

Circle the letter of the most appropriate answer.

1. An older client asks the nurse how he acquired aortic stenosis since it was not diagnosed until he was 75 years old. The best explanation that the nurse could provide is that

   1. calcium precipitates within valvular cells with age
   2. the heart muscle begins to get overstretched with age
   3. collagen is not formed as abundantly as individuals age
   4. pericardial adhesions constriction the heart with age

   Nursing Process: Implementation
   Client Need: Health Promotion/Maintenance

2. A client with aortic stenosis experiences dizziness. Which one of the following aspects of nursing care is the most important?

    1. attending to hygiene
    2. preventing injury

    3. monitoring vital signs
    4. orienting the client

    Nursing Process: Planning
    Client Need: Safe, Effective Care Environment

3. When assessing a client with aortic stenosis, the best location on the chest for hearing the sound made by the aortic valve closing is

    1. at the 2nd intercostal space in the left midaxillary line
    2. at the 5th intercostal space in the left midclavicular line

    3. below the left nipple at the 5th intercostal space
    4. to the right of the sternum at the 2nd intercostal space

    Nursing Process: Assessment
    Client Need: Physiological Integrity

4. A client with aortic stenosis is placed on a low sodium diet. Which one of the following would be most appropriate to tell the client to avoid?

    1. dried beans
    2. ripe bananas

    3. canned soup
    4. fresh fish

    Nursing Process: Implementation
    Client Need: Health Promotion/Maintenance

5. After being examined by a physician, a client with aortic stenosis asks the nurse to re-explain a treatment referred to as balloon valvuloplasty. The nurse would be most accurate in explaining that this procedure involves

    1. compressing plaque in an artery
    2. stretching the narrowed valve

    3. replacing the valve with a balloon
    4. grafting a section of new tissue

    Nursing Process: Implementation
    Client Need: Health Promotion/Maintenance

6. When the nurse assesses the radial pulse of a client with aortic insufficiency, which one of the following findings is most characteristic? The pulse is apt to feel strong

    1. with slow, regular beats
    2. with slow, irregular beats

    3. with fast, thready beats
    4. with quick, sharp beats

    Nursing Process: Assessment
    Client Need: Physiological Integrity

7. When taking the blood pressure of a client with aortic insufficiency, which one of the following is most typical? There is a

    1. wide pulse pressure
    2. large pulse deficit

    3. high diastolic pressure
    4. low systolic pressure

    Nursing Process: Assessment
    Client Need: Physiological Integrity

8. When giving report on a postoperative client who underwent a surgical repair of the aortic valve, the nurse would be most correct in explaining that a vascular graft was required because

    1. the aorta was also diseased
    2. the valve could not be replaced

    3. the prosthetic valve did not fit securely
    4. the left ventricle pumped too much blood

    Nursing Process: Implementation
    Client Need: Safe, Effective Care Environment

9. A client with mitral stenosis tells the nurse that she is going to have a root canal performed on one of her molars next week. Which of the following would be the most appropriate health teaching the nurse could provide?

   1. remind the client of a need to resume taking an antibiotic
   2. identify the advantages for regular brushing and flossing
   3. suggest that the client have a complete blood count beforehand
   4. recommend that the dentist monitor the client's heart rate

   Nursing Process: Implementation
   Client Need: Health Promotion/Maintenance

10. The pathology report on a client who underwent a mitral valve replacement says that the tissue showed evidence of commissures. The best explanation the nurse could provide is that the natural valve was narrowed by

    1. extra valve cusps
    2. stationary clots
    3. tumorous growths
    4. thick, rigid scars

    Nursing Process: Implementation
    Client Need: Health Promotion/Maintenance

11. Which one of the following assessment findings is the best evidence that the right ventricle of a client with mitral stenosis is failing as an effective pump?

    1. The client's skin is quite pale.
    2. The client's legs are edematous.
    3. The client has lost weight.
    4. The client is very thirsty.

    Nursing Process: Assessment
    Client Need: Physiological Integrity

12. The nurse examines the sputum of a client with pulmonary complications associated with mitral stenosis. If this client is typical of others, the sputum is likely to appear

    1. green and thick
    2. pink and frothy
    3. clear and sticky
    4. white and curdlike

    Nursing Process: Assessment
    Client Need: Physiological Integrity

13. The nurse hears a murmur when auscultating the chest of a client with mitral stenosis, which, if typical of most with this disorder, is best described as sounding like a

    1. rumbling train
    2. distant whistle
    3. steaming teakettle
    4. chirping bird

    Nursing Process: Assessment
    Client Need: Physiological Integrity

14. The physician recommends cardioversion to correct an arrhythmia called atrial fibrillation. The nurse would be most correct in explaining that during cardioversion

    1. the heart is stopped briefly to restore proper conduction
    2. a battery-charged electrode is placed in the right atria
    3. a catheter is inserted in the heart and blood is removed
    4. the blood is circulated and oxygenated outside the body

    Nursing Process: Implementation
    Client Need: Health Promotion/Maintenance

15. When caring for a client with mitral valve insufficiency, which one of the following findings would suggest that the client's stroke volume is low? The client develops

    1. tachycardia
    2. bradycardia

    3. a fever
    4. petechiae

    Nursing Process: Assessment
    Client Need: Physiological Integrity

16. When reviewing the data of a client with chest pain, which one of the following findings would be most suggestive that the pain is caused by a prolapsed mitral valve rather than angina? The chest pain

    1. occurs with exertion
    2. is not relieved by rest

    3. is of short duration
    4. radiates up the neck

    Nursing Process: Assessment
    Client Need: Physiological Integrity

17. The client with mitral valve prolapse asks the nurse why the physician recommended taking a single aspirin every day. The best response is that aspirin reduces the potential for

    1. experiencing anxiety
    2. producing scar tissue

    3. developing a fever
    4. forming blood clots

    Nursing Process: Implementation
    Client Need: Health Promotion/Maintenance

18. The best evidence that a client with mitral valve prolapse has understood the dietary recommendations provided by the nurse is if the client says it is best to avoid

    1. products that contain lactose
    2. staples containing preservatives

    3. beverages that contain caffeine
    4. grains that contain gluten

    Nursing Process: Evaluation
    Client Need: Health Promotion/Maintenance

19. Which one of the following nursing measures would be appropriate to add to the plan of care for a client with aortic stenosis to prevent the Valsalva maneuver?

    1. dangle the legs over the bedside before walking
    2. encourage the selection of foods high in fiber

    3. have the client inhale deeply and cough while exhaling
    4. have the client rise slowly from a sitting position

    Nursing Process: Planning
    Client Need: Physiological Integrity

20. A nursing assistant with a sore throat has been assigned to care for a client with mitral stenosis. Which one of the following is most appropriate?

    1. reassign the client's care to another person
    2. have the nursing assistant wear a face mask

    3. ask the physician to prescribe an antibiotic
    4. transfer the client to another nursing unit

    Nursing Process: Implementation
    Client Need: Safe, Effective Care Environment

II. CRITICAL THINKING EXERCISES

1. A client has had a prosthetic valve inserted to replace an incompetent mitral valve. Describe the assessment findings that would suggest that the valve has ruptured or become displaced.

2. A client has a prolapsed mitral valve. What information could the nurse provide about why people with this disorder experience physical symptoms that mimic severe anxiety?

3. What instructions could be given to a client to relieve the chest pain associated with mitral valve prolapse?

31/ Caring for Clients with Occlusive Disorders of Coronary and Peripheral Blood Vessels

Clients with heart disease may be chronically or critically ill. The chronically ill client probably has been ill for many years, is seen by a physician frequently, has taken many different types of medications, and has probably been told to follow a special diet. Both critically and chronically ill clients require skilled nursing management—one needing the skills required in an emergency, the other needing the patience and understanding required for the management of the chronically ill.

The following questions deal with the content of Chapter 31.

I. MULTIPLE CHOICE QUESTIONS

Circle the number of the most appropriate answer.

Mr. Harris, age 57, is an insurance salesman. He has a history of coronary artery disease (CAD) and hypertension, and he has seen a physician at regular intervals. While at work he experienced symptoms and was immediately taken to the hospital by a co-worker. While Mr. Harris is in the emergency department, the physician makes a tentative diagnosis of myocardial infarction, and Mr. Harris is admitted to the coronary care unit.

1. If Mr. Harris understands the etiology of his medical problem, he will be able to explain to the nurse that his

   1. heart is enlarged and does not pump efficiently
   2. arteries are hard and narrowed by fatty deposits
   3. heart valves are narrowed with residual scar tissue
   4. conduction system does not relay impulses correctly

   Nursing Process: Evaluation
   Client Need: Health Promotion/Maintenance

2. Mr. Harris has a prescription for nitroglycerin tablets which he takes sublingually when necessary. If Mr. Harris has a correct understanding of the drug's mechanism of action, he will tell the nurse that this medication

   1. lowers his blood cholesterol
   2. clears the arteries of plaque
   3. keeps blood from clotting
   4. dilates blood vessels

   Nursing Process: Evaluation
   Client Need: Health Promotion/Maintenance

3. During the assessment interview, based upon the fact that Mr. Harris has CAD, the nurse is most likely to find that the client's chief complaint at this time is severe

   1. headache
   2. dyspnea
   3. chest pain
   4. heart palpitations

   Nursing Process: Assessment
   Client Need: Safe, Effective Care Environment

4. Which of the following assessments most supports the presumption that Mr. Harris is presently having a myocardial infarction? He is

   1. nauseated and diaphoretic
   2. flushed and lethargic
   3. cyanotic and hypertensive
   4. pale and breathing slowly

   Nursing Process: Assessment
   Client Need: Physiological Integrity

5. While awaiting a definitive diagnosis, the nurse would be most correct in telling Mr. Harris that the viability of myocardial tissue is related to

    1. restoring adequate arterial circulation
    2. maintaining adequate pumping function
    3. reducing his arterial blood pressure
    4. changing his future lifestyle habits

    Nursing Process: Implementation
    Client Need: Health Promotion/Maintenance

6. The nurse reviews the rhythm strip from the cardiac monitor several days after Mr. Harris has been admitted to the coronary care unit. The wave changes that are most characteristic of a myocardial infarction include

    1. prolonged PR interval, wide QRS complex, depressed ST segment
    2. a definite Q wave, ST segment elevation, T wave inversion
    3. nonuniform P waves, normal QRS complex, tall peaked T waves
    4. a tall P wave, short PR interval, appearance of a U wave

    Nursing Process: Assessment
    Client Need: Physiological Integrity

7. During and after administering streptokinase, a thrombolytic agent, it would be essential for the nurse to monitor Mr. Harris for

    1. hypertension
    2. bleeding
    3. nausea
    4. diarrhea

    Nursing Process: Implementation
    Client Need: Safe, Effective Care Environment

Individual Questions

8. A client who has been diagnosed as having atherosclerosis asks the nurse what possible consequences might occur with this disease. The most correct answer is that atheroslcerosis can lead to

    1. lung damage, kidney failure, and strokes
    2. valvular disorders, diabetes, and strokes
    3. heart attacks, kidney failure, and strokes
    4. anemia, liver damage, and heart attacks

    Nursing Process: Implementation
    Client Need: Health Promotion/Maintenance

9. A client asks the nurse why blood vessels like his become hard and inelastic. The best answer the nurse could give is that arteriosclerosis results from

    1. eating too much saturated fat
    2. ineffective stress management
    3. calcium deposits within arterial walls
    4. acquiring an inherited genetic defect

    Nursing Process: Implementation
    Client Need: Health Promotion/Maintenance

10. A nurse reviews the data from the medical record of a client with coronary artery disease. If this client is typical of others with this disorder, the nurse will most likely find that the client

    1. is a thin male who is less than 35 years old
    2. does not smoke cigarettes or drink alcohol
    3. reacts passively to emotional stressors
    4. has relatives who died of heart disease

    Nursing Process: Assessment
    Client Need: Physiological Integrity

11. A client with CAD disease asks the nurse to explain the difference between angina and a myocardial infarction. The nurse would be most correct in telling the client that both result from ischemia, but with angina

    1. the arteries are dilated
    2. the pain is more severe

    3. the pain does not radiate
    4. heart muscle does not die

    Nursing Process: Implementation
    Client Need: Health Promotion/Maintenance

12. When the nurse performs a head-to-toe assessment on a client, which finding would support the possibility that the client has hyperlipidemia?

    1. The client's toenails are thick.
    2. The client has jaundiced sclera.

    3. There are yellow skin lesions about the eyelids.
    4. There is only sparse hair growth on the extremities.

    Nursing Process: Assessment
    Client Need: Physiological Integrity

13. When the laboratory blood test results are returned on a client with CAD, which one of the following is the nurse most likely to find?

    1. The total cholesterol is elevated.
    2. The red blood cell count is low.

    3. The prothrombin time is prolonged.
    4. The serum calcium level is high.

    Nursing Process: Assessment
    Client Need: Physiological Integrity

14. A client with CAD is placed on a low-fat diet. Which one of the following laboratory results would indicate to the nurse that the client has been compliant? The client's

    1. LDL (low density lipoprotein) level is reduced
    2. HDL (high density lipoprotein) level is reduced

    3. blood urea nitrogen level is reduced
    4. serum potassium level is reduced

    Nursing Process: Evaluation
    Client Need: Health Promotion/Maintenance

15. A nurse is assigned to the following four clients. Which one should the nurse plan to explain is at risk for developing CAD?

    1. Mr. Grant, who has bronchial asthma
    2. Mr. Joyner, who has diabetes mellitus

    3. Ms. Davis, who has a duodenal ulcer
    4. Ms. Engler, who has uterine fibroid tumors

    Nursing Process: Planning
    Client Need: Health Promotion/Maintenance

16. Which one of the following could the nurse recommend to healthy adults who want to promote the development of collateral arteries throughout the myocardium?

    1. maintaining normal weight
    2. taking 1 aspirin daily

    3. performing regular aerobic exercise
    4. utilizing stress management techniques

    Nursing Process: Implementation
    Client Need: Health Promotion/Maintenance

17. A client demonstrates accurate information if he refers to which one of the following as a procedure in which a balloon-tipped catheter is inserted into a diseased coronary artery?

    1. balloon valvuloplasty
    2. percutaneous transluminal coronary angioplasty (PTCA)

    3. coronary artery bypass graft (CABG)
    4. carotid endarterectomy

    Nursing Process: Evaluation
    Client Need: Safe, Effective Care Environment

18. The nurse assesses a client after a coronary arteriography. Which one of the following is the best evidence that there is a clot at the vascular access site?

    1. The client has chest pain.
    2. Distal leg pulses are absent.

    3. Petechiae are present on the chest.
    4. The dressing appears bloody.

    Nursing Process: Assessment
    Client Need: Physiological Integrity

19. A nurse restricts the physical activity of a client who has had a severe myocardial infarction from the 4th to the 7th postrecovery days. The nurse's action is

    1. appropriate since this is when the infarcted area is in its softest state
    2. appropriate since this is when the client is most prone to an arrhythmia

    3. inappropriate because sufficient scar tissue has formed by this time
    4. inappropriate since complications are more likely to occur about 8 to 10 days later

    Nursing Process: Evaluation
    Client Need: Safe, Effective Care Environment

20. A client who has had a myocardial infarction asks the nurse why the physician has prescribed a diuretic. The best answer the nurse could give is that, in this case, the drug is given to

    1. prevent kidney damage
    2. reduce blood volume

    3. excrete toxic wastes
    4. regulate fluid balance

    Nursing Process: Implementation
    Client Need: Safe, Effective Care Environment

21. A client who is being monitored with a pulmonary artery catheter asks the nurse why the measurements are being taken. The best response is that the data provide an early indication of a complication called

    1. ventricular rupture
    2. atrial fibrillation

    3. aortic insufficiency
    4. cardiogenic shock

    Nursing Process: Implementation
    Client Need: Safe, Effective Care Environment

22. Which one of the following nursing measures would be most appropriate to add to the care plan of a client with a myocardial infarction to reduce the potential for developing venous thrombosis?

    1. apply antiembolism stockings and remove q8h for 20 minutes
    2. limit fluid intake to 1500 mL during each 24 hour period

    3. supervise deep-breathing exercises q4h while awake
    4. discourage straining while having a bowel movement

    Nursing Process: Planning
    Client Need: Safe, Effective Care Environment

23. The best evidence that the heart is pumping effectively following a myocardial infarction is that the

    1. client is oriented
    2. heart rate is regular

    3. urine output is ≥ 100 mL/hr
    4. mucous membranes are moist

    Nursing Process: Evaluation
    Client Need: Physiological Integrity

24. Following a myocardial infarction, the nurse is likely to observe the client manifest which one of the following as a mechanism for coping with the fear and anxiety of the diagnosis?

    1. regression
    2. repression

    3. undoing
    4. denial

    Nursing Process: Assessment
    Client Need: Psychological Integrity

25. Which one of the following nursing approaches would most help the family of the client with a myocardial infarction cope with the client's change in health status?

    1. contact a psychotherapist
    2. keep the family informed

    3. avoid discussing medical issues
    4. have them keep their visits brief

    Nursing Process: Implementation
    Client Need: Psychosocial Integrity

26. The best plan for helping a client restore his sense of control following a myocardial infarction would be to

    1. let the client make decisions affecting his care
    2. screen emotionally upsetting news from the client

    3. defer discussions about his condition to the physician
    4. let the client see business associates on a limited basis

    Nursing Process: Planning
    Client Need: Psychosocial Integrity

27. When assessing the client with Raynaud's disease, it is especially important for the nurse to monitor the color of the client's

    1. urine
    2. skin

    3. sclera
    4. nailbeds

    Nursing Process: Assessment
    Client Need: Physiological Integrity

28. Which one of the following measures could the nurse plan to teach a client with Raynaud's disease in order to help him or her abort an attack of symptoms?

    1. take an aspirin daily
    2. imagine a warm activity

    3. drink a cold beverage
    4. elevate the legs

    Nursing Process: Planning
    Client Need: Health Promotion/Maintenance

29. It would be most appropriate for the nurse to instruct a client with Raynaud's disease to avoid

    1. smoking cigarettes and cold temperatures
    2. drinking alcohol and physical exercise

    3. inadequate sleep and emotional stress
    4. weight gain and bowel irregularity

    Nursing Process: Implementation
    Client Need: Health Promotion/Maintenance

30. The best evidence that a peripheral artery in an extremity is totally occluded is that the arm or leg will be

    1. withered, weak, and numb
    2. white, cold, and painful

    3. flushed, swollen, and warm
    4. mottled, puffy, and throb

    Nursing Process: Assessment
    Client Need: Physiological Integrity

31. If all of the following actions are observed when a nursing colleague administers an injection of heparin subcutaneously, for which one should the nurse intervene? The nurse

    1. selects the abdomen as the site for injection
    2. aspirates a bubble of air within the syringe

    3. swabs the site with an alcohol pledget
    4. rubs the site after withdrawing the needle

    Nursing Process: Evaluation
    Client Need: Safe, Effective Care Environment

32. In the event that the client's clotting mechanisms are extremely prolonged while undergoing heparin therapy, the nurse should plan to have which one of the following drugs on hand?

    1. vitamin K
    2. vitamin C
    3. protamine sulfate
    4. atropine sulfate

    Nursing Process: Planning
    Client Need: Safe, Effective Care Environment

33. When developing a teaching plan for a client with peripheral vascular disease, one of the best measures to include to prevent future complications is

    1. appropriate foot care
    2. simple aerobic exercises
    3. weight reduction techniques
    4. therapeutic positioning

    Nursing Process: Planning
    Client Need: Health Promotion/Maintenance

34. After a client has a sympathectomy, which one of the following is the nurse most likely to find associated with the procedure? The client's

    1. emotions are dulled
    2. appetite is reduced
    3. skin is extremely dry
    4. taste is diminished

    Nursing Process: Assessment
    Client Need: Physiological Integrity

35. Which one of the following should the nurse advise a client with varicose veins to avoid?

    1. leg elevation
    2. prolonged standing
    3. forced coughing
    4. active exercise

    Nursing Process: Implementation
    Client Need: Health Promotion/Maintenance

36. Which one of the following assessments should be reported to the physician because it is an indication that the client may have an aneurysm in the descending aorta?

    1. sudden abdominal distention
    2. a pounding temporal headache
    3. a pulsating abdominal mass
    4. twisted, ropelike leg veins

    Nursing Process: Implementation
    Client Need: Safe, Effective Care Environment

37. Which one of the following would be a priority when planning the nursing care for a client with an aortic aneurysm? Controlling

    1. heart rhythm
    2. bowel elimination
    3. blood pressure
    4. dietary intake

    Nursing Process: Planning
    Client Need: Physiological Integrity

II. CRITICAL THINKING EXERCISES

1. A client who is experiencing chest pain is brought to the emergency department. What assessments are important to perform at this time?

2. A 70-year-old client has had a massive myocardial infarction and may not survive. His wife, four children, and grandchildren fill the hall outside the coronary care unit. How might the nurse provide support for the client's family?

3. The wife of a 38-year-old client who has had a myocardial infarction confides to the nurse that she is fearful that her husband might die if they have sexual intercourse. What health teaching would be important to provide?

4. What information would be essential to provide before discharging a client with Raynaud's disease?

32/ Caring for Clients with Cardiac Arrhythmias

To pump blood, the heart must alternately contract and relax, allowing blood to enter its chambers during the relaxation phase and exit during the contraction phase. The alternate contraction and relaxation are provided by an inherent rhythmicity of cardiac muscle. In disease, the pacemaker of the heart can be too fast or too slow. The myocardial cells can become overexcitable or develop a shortened refractory period; the Purkinje system can be damaged, or blocks can develop in the conduction system.

The following questions deal with the content of Chapter 32

I. MULTIPLE CHOICE QUESTIONS

Circle the number of the most appropriate answer.

1. A nursing assistant asks the nurse to explain what the term arrhythmia means. The nurse would be most correct in explaining that arrhythmia means that the client has a disturbance in

    1. heart rhythm or rate, or both
    2. heart filling or emptying, or both
    3. venous or arterial circulation, or both
    4. central or peripheral blood flow, or both

    Nursing Process: Implementation
    Client Need: Safe, Effective Care Environment

2. When a client asks the nurse to clarify what the physician meant when he was told he had sinus brady-cardia, the best explanation is that

    1. the heart rate is more than 60 bpm and regular
    2. the heart rate is less than 60 bpm and regular
    3. the heart rate is more than 60 bpm and irregular
    4. the heart rate is less than 60 bpm and irregular

    Nursing Process: Implementation
    Client Need: Health Promotion/Maintenance

3. When assessing a client, the nurse finds that the client's heart rate is 54 beats per minute (bpm). For which one of the following clients might this finding be considered acceptable?

    1. Ms. Davis, 22 years old, who is 6 months pregnant
    2. Mr. O'Rourke, 56 years old, who is a strict vegetarian
    3. Mr. Snyder, 20 years old, who jogs 5 miles daily
    4. Ms. Cone, 38 years old, who had heart surgery as an infant

    Nursing Process: Assessment
    Client Need: Safe, Effective, Care Environment

4. A nurse observes the ECG rhythm of her assigned client on a cardiac monitor. If the client bears down and strains while having a bowel movement, which one of the following is most likely to occur?

    1. The heart rate may speed up.
    2. The heart rate may slow down.
    3. The impulse conduction may be incomplete.
    4. The impulse conduction may be accelerated.

    Nursing Process: Assessment
    Client Need: Physiological Integrity

5. A nurse finds that a client's heart rate is 48 bpm. Which medication should be withheld until the nurse consults with the physician?

   1. cimetidine (Tagamet)
   2. meperidine (Demerol)
   3. digoxin (Lanoxin)
   4. prednisolone (Delta-Cortef)

   Nursing Process: Implementation
   Client Need: Physiological Integrity

6. Which one of the following drugs should the nurse plan to have on hand for the treatment of a slow heart rate?

   1. digoxin (Lanoxin)
   2. propranolol (Inderal)
   3. atropine sulfate
   4. morphine sulfate

   Nursing Process: Planning
   Client Need: Physiological Integrity

7. A nurse reviews a client's medical record. Which one of the findings below best supports the documented statement that the client has sinus tachycardia? The client's heart rate is regular and is beating at a rate

   1. between 60 and 100 bpm
   2. between 75 and 90 bpm
   3. between 100 and 150 bpm
   4. between 150 and 200 bpm

   Nursing Process: Evaluation
   Client Need: Safe, Effective Care Environment

8. A nurse is assigned the following four clients. Which one is the most likely to manifest sinus tachycardia?

   1. Ms. Jones, who has hyperthyroidism
   2. Ms. Dunn, who had a hysterectomy
   3. Mr. Higgins, who has a fractured hip
   4. Mr. Wallace, who had a hernia repaired

   Nursing Process: Assessment
   Client Need: Safe, Effective Care Environment

9. A physician orders all of the following drugs. Which one would the nurse be most correct in explaining may slow a rapid heart rate?

   1. warfarin sodium (Coumadin), an anticoagulant
   2. acetaminophen (Tylenol), a nonsalicylate
   3. verapamil (Calan), a calcium channel blocker
   4. furosemide (Lasix), a loop diuretic

   Nursing Process: Implementation
   Client Need: Safe, Effective Care Environment

10. A nurse would be most correct in explaining to a client who has just experienced atrial fibrillation that during this arrhythmia the atria

    1. are totally inactive
    2. quiver rapidly
    3. contract forcefully
    4. are electrically unresponsive

    Nursing Process: Implementation
    Client Need: Health Promotion/Maintenance

11. When discharging a client with atrial fibrillation, which of the following information would be most accurate to share with the client? "Your arrhythmia may cause clots to form within your heart so the physician has recommended that you take

    1. acetylsalicylic acid (aspirin)"
    2. ketorolac (Toradol)"
    3. vitamin K (Synkayvite)"
    4. labetolol (Normodyne)"

    Nursing Process: Implementation
    Client Need: Health Promotion/Maintenance

12. A client is admitted and found to have a complete heart block. When explaining the condition to the family, the nurse would be most correct in saying that in heart block there is a problem in transmitting the electrical conduction through the

    1. SA node
    2. internodal pathways
    3. intraatrial pathways
    4. AV node

    Nursing Process: Implementation
    Client Need: Health Promotion/Maintenance

13. The physician tells a client with complete heart block that if the condition does not improve by adjusting the drug therapy, some other form of treatment may be used. The client asks the nurse to what the physician may have been referring. The nurse would be most correct in saying that with this type of arrhythmia, a more normal heart rhythm may be restored by

    1. inserting a pacemaker
    2. performing cardioversion
    3. massaging the carotid arteries
    4. doing a heart transplant

    Nursing Process: Implementation
    Client Need: Safe, Effective Care Environment

14. A nurse is caring for four clients who are being monitored by cardiac telemetry. Which one of them is most likely to manifest an occasional PVC (premature ventricular contraction)?

    1. Ms. White, who has been vomiting
    2. Mr. Keegan, who drinks a lot of fruit juice
    3. Mr. Loren, who is restricted from eating
    4. Ms. Dayton, who is anxious about discharge

    Nursing Process: Assessment
    Client Need: Safe, Effective Care Environment

15. Which one of the following statements is most indicative of the feeling that some clients experience with a premature ventricular contraction? The client says,

    1. "My heart occasionally goes 'flip-flop'"
    2. "I get this squeezed feeling in my chest"
    3. "There's discomfort radiating to my neck"
    4. "It feels like I have acid indigestion"

    Nursing Process: Assessment
    Client Need: Safe, Effective Care Environment

16. A nurse is watching the cardiac monitors that are being used in the care of four clients. All of the clients are having PVCs. Which one of the following is the most dangerous and requires reporting?

    1. Client A has had three PVCs in the last 3 hours.
    2. Client B has just had a run of six PVCs in a row.
    3. Client C has had six PVCs in the last hour that look alike.
    4. Client D has had three PVCs about 6 minutes apart.

    Nursing Process: Implementation
    Client Need: Physiological Integrity

17. If a client is experiencing dangerous forms of PVCs, it would be most appropriate for the nurse to check the emergency drug box to make sure that there is a supply of

    1. digoxin (lanoxin)
    2. verapamil (Calan)
    3. nitroglycerin (Nitrol IV)
    4. lidocaine (Xylocaine)

    Nursing Process: Implementation
    Client Need: Safe, Effective Care Environment

18. While monitoring the cardiac rhythm of a client, which one of the following assessments is most suggestive of ventricular fibrillation?

    1. There is a chaotic, undulating line on the monitor.
    2. There is a straight line across the monitor screen.
    3. There are wide, bizarre-looking QRS complexes.
    4. There are several saw-toothed waves before each QRS complex.

    Nursing Process: Assessment
    Client Need: Physiological Integrity

19. A client collapses while ambulating and is unresponsive to shaking and shouting. After yelling for assistance, the nurse should take the next step which is to

    1. seal the client's nose
    2. check the carotid pulse
    3. give two quick breaths
    4. open the client's airway

    Nursing Process: Implementation
    Client Need: Physiological Integrity

20. When no pulse is felt, the nurse prepares to administer cardiac compressions. The most correct placement for the nurse's hands is over the lower half of the sternum

    1. even with the tip of the xiphoid process
    2. about 1 ½ inches to the left of the xiphoid process
    3. about 1 ½ inches above the tip of the xiphoid process
    4. about 1 ½ inches below the tip of the xiphoid process

    Nursing Process: Implementation
    Client Need: Physiological Integrity

21. A nurse prepares to administer cardiopulmonary resuscitation. If all of the following measures are performed in sequence, which one indicates that the nurse needs additional practice? The nurse

    1. opens the airway by lifting the neck
    2. gives breaths that last 1 ½ seconds
    3. gives two breaths after 15 compressions
    4. maintains a compression rate of 88 per minute

    Nursing Process: Evaluation
    Client Need: Physiological Integrity

22. Which one of the following is the best indication that cardiopulmonary resuscitation can be discontinued?

    1. the client's pupils are small and fixed
    2. the client is breathing and has a pulse
    3. the client's color no longer appears pale
    4. the client begins to vomit and choke

    Nursing Process: Evaluation
    Client Need: Physiological Integrity

23. A client is scheduled to have a permanent pacemaker implanted. Where can the nurse tell the client the battery will be located?

    1. above the xiphoid process
    2. below the left nipple
    3. below the right clavicle
    4. underneath the sternum

    Nursing Process: Implementation
    Client Need: Safe, Effective Care Environment

24. After a client undergoes elective cardioversion, which of the following is most important to add to the plan for care?

    1. monitor the vital signs q15min × 2 hours
    2. offer full liquids when alert and oriented
    3. ambulate in the hall with assistance
    4. record intake and output each shift

    Nursing Process: Planning
    Client Need: Safe, Effective Care Environment

25. Before applying defibrillator paddles to the client's chest, it would be most appropriate for the nurse to

    1. shave the hair above and below the nipple line
    2. protect the skin with saline pads or gel
    3. count the client's apical heart rate
    4. explain the procedure to the client

    Nursing Process: Implementation
    Client Need: Safe, Effective Care Environment

26. Which one of the following should the nurse inform a client may cause his or her pacemaker to malfunction?

    1. high tension wires
    2. cellular phones
    3. electronic pagers
    4. personal computers

    Nursing Process: Implementation
    Client Need: Health Promotion/Maintenance

II. CRITICAL THINKING EXERCISES

1. A nurse finds that a client who was just assessed a few minutes ago now appears to be dead. What actions would be appropriate for the nurse to take at this time?

2. Ms. Moudry, who had a permanent pacemaker inserted, will be discharged in 2 days. What health teaching would be important to provide?

3. When receiving a report, you are asked by the nurse working the next shift to explain the difference between a pacemaker that is set at a fixed rate and one that is set on demand. What response would you make?

4. A client is receiving an antiarrhythmic drug. What assessments are important to document?

33/ Caring for Clients with Hypertension

Blood pressure reflects the ability of the arteries to stretch and fill with blood, the efficiency of the heart as a pump, and the volume of circulating blood. Studies of healthy persons show that blood pressure can fluctuate within a wide range and still be normal. The term *hypertension* refers to a disease entity characterized by sustained elevation of arterial pressure.

The following questions deal with the content of Chapter 33.

I. MULTIPLE CHOICE QUESTIONS

Circle the number of the most appropriate answer.

Mrs. Kibler, age 44, is diagnosed as having essential hypertension during a routine physical examination. She will be followed in the physician's office.

1. When Ms. Kibler asks the nurse to explain what hypertension means, the best answer is that a person is considered to be hypertensive when the systolic blood pressure is equal to or exceeds 140 mm Hg and the diastolic is equal to or exceeds

    1. 85 mm Hg
    2. 90 mm Hg

    3. 95 mm Hg
    4. 100 mm Hg

    Nursing Process: Implementation
    Client Need: Health Promotion/Maintenance

2. The nurse would also be correct in explaining to Ms. Kibler that when the physician referred to her type of disorder as essential hypertension, it means that

   1. it is due to aging
   2. the cause is unknown

   3. the cause must be determined
   4. it is due to another illness

   Nursing Process: Implementation
   Client Need: Health Promotion/Maintenance

3. Ms. Kibler admits to all of the following. If she agrees to make one lifestyle change to help control her hypertension, which one would be most important for the nurse to recommend? Eliminate

   1. drinking carbonated beverages
   2. consuming dairy products

   3. smoking cigarettes
   4. eating dried beans

   Nursing Process: Planning
   Client Need: Health Promotion/Maintenance

4. Besides restricting dietary sodium, it would be appropriate for the nurse to tell Ms. Kibler that new research indicates that it may be beneficial to

   1. increase sources of calcium, like milk
   2. increase sources of potassium, like bananas

   3. decrease sources of magnesium, like nuts
   4. decrease sources of zinc, like wheat germ

   Nursing Process: Implementation
   Client Need: Health Promotion/Maintenance

Individual Questions

5. Which one of the following assessment findings is most likely to be correlated with hypertension?

   1. frequent urination
   2. unusual thirst

   3. spontaneous nosebleeds
   4. chronic constipation

   Nursing Process: Assessment
   Client Need: Physiological Integrity

6. When the nurse obtains a general appraisal of a client with hypertension, one of the most striking observations is that these clients tend to have

   1. a flushed face
   2. constricted pupils

   3. protruding eyes
   4. difficulty thinking

   Nursing Process: Assessment
   Client Need: Safe, Effective Care Environment

7. A nurse reviews the laboratory test results on a client diagnosed with hypertension. Which one of the following best supports the possibility that atherosclerosis is a contributing cause? The client's

   1. erythrocyte count is low
   2. leukocyte count is high

   3. hemoglobin is decreased
   4. cholesterol is elevated

   Nursing Process: Assessment
   Client Need: Physiological Integrity

8. Which one of the following is the best evidence that the hypertensive client understands how he will be tested while undergoing a fluorescein angiography test? The client says,

   1. "An instrument will be placed on my cornea"
   2. "Dye will be injected into my vein"

   3. "The physician will look into my eyes"
   4. "I will have to read an eye chart"

   Nursing Process: Evaluation
   Client Need: Safe, Effective Care Environment

9. A newly diagnosed hypertensive client asks the nurse how the physician will most likely treat his disorder. The nurse would be most correct in stating that the last measure that may be used would be

   1. dietary modifications
   2. weight reduction
   3. increasing exercise
   4. medication therapy

   Nursing Process: Implementation
   Client Need: Safe, Effective Care Environment

10. The physician prescribes the calcium channel blocker dilitazem (Cardizem) for the treatment of a client's hypertension. When explaining the mechanism of action, the nurse states most accurately that this type of drug

    1. reduces the reabsorption of sodium
    2. blocks the effects of catecholamines
    3. dilates arteries and arterioles
    4. interferes with forming angiotensin I

    Nursing Process: Implementation
    Client Need: Safe, Effective Care Environment

11. A nurse obtains a client's blood pressure measurement and finds that it is 210/115 mm Hg in the left arm while lying down. The most appropriate action to take is to recommend

    1. rechecking the blood pressure within 2 years
    2. remeasuring the blood pressure within 1 year
    3. evaluating the measurement again in 2 weeks
    4. referring the client for prompt medical assessment

    Nursing Process: Planning
    Client Need: Physiological Integrity

12. The nurse uses a reference to determine what characteristics distinguish accelerated hypertension from other findings associated with this disorder. The nurse is most likely to find that the sign that is most unique to accelerated hypertension is

    1. hemorrhages and exudates in the eye
    2. a pounding headache in the frontal region
    3. numbness and tingling in all extremities
    4. loss of the central field of vision

    Nursing Process: Implementation
    Client Need: Safe, Effective Care Environment

13. A client is admitted with malignant hypertension. Which one of the following assessment findings suggests that the client is developing renal failure?

    1. The client experiences pain during urination.
    2. The urine is extremely clear, resembling water.
    3. The client excretes less than 30 mL of urine.
    4. The bladder is distended above the umbilicus.

    Nursing Process: Assessment
    Client Need: Physiological Integrity

14. When caring for a client with a blood pressure of 220/110 at rest, which one of the following is the highest priority for nursing care?

    1. protecting the client's safety
    2. providing adequate nutrition
    3. assisting with hygiene measures
    4. ensuring sufficient sleep

    Nursing Process: Planning
    Client Need: Physiological Integrity

15. If a client with hypertension requested all of the following beverages, which one would be most appropriate to provide?

    1. cola
    2. coffee
    3. orange juice
    4. iced tea

    Nursing Process: Implementation
    Client Need: Physiological Integrity

16. If a client being treated for hypertension says he often feels as though he will faint, it would be best to recommend that he

    1. eat less salt
    2. drink more fluids
    3. take deep breaths
    4. promptly lie down

    Nursing Process: Implementation
    Client Need: Health Promotion/Maintenance

17. While awaiting a return phone call from the physician in response to a hypertensive client who is having chest pain, the nurse's most appropriate action would be to

    1. administer oxygen
    2. obtain a urine specimen
    3. monitor respirations
    4. elevate the legs

    Nursing Process: Implementation
    Client Need: Physiological Integrity

18. After the nurse has observed signs that a hypertensive client is anxious, which one of the following comments would be most therapeutic?

    1. "You have nothing to be frightened about."
    2. "Many individuals have high blood pressure."
    3. "You seem worried; I'll stay with you a while."
    4. "The hospital is the best place when you're ill."

    Nursing Process: Implementation
    Client Need: Psychosocial Integrity

19. A nurse observes that when a client's brother visits for an extended period of time, the client becomes restless, tachycardic, and his blood pressure rises even higher than his usual hypertensive levels. Which one of the following actions is most appropriate? Tell the brother

    1. his visits disturb the client
    2. he may visit for up to 15 minutes
    3. his presence endangers the client
    4. to call before visiting the client

    Nursing Process: Implementation
    Client Need: Psychosocial Integrity

20. When developing the teaching plan for a hypertensive client, it would be most correct to tell the client that hypertension is a chronic condition that requires

    1. drug therapy
    2. lifelong attention
    3. early retirement
    4. great expense

    Nursing Process: Planning
    Client Need: Health Promotion/Maintenance

21. If a hypertensive client reports all of the following, which one indicates that additional teaching is needed?

    1. "I have kept a daily log of my blood pressure measurements."
    2. "I have begun walking a mile each morning and afternoon."
    3. "I take an extra dose of medication when I feel tense."
    4. "I don't eat pastries, snacks, or fried foods anymore."

    Nursing Process: Evaluation
    Client Need: Health Promotion/Maintenance

II. CRITICAL THINKING EXERCISES

1. A nurse has been asked to discuss factors that contribute to hypertension. What topics would be most appropriate to include?

2. A client who attends the nurse's presentation tells the group that the cause of his hypertension is athero-sclerosis. What other diseases are also likely to elevate the blood pressure?

3. When collecting data on a new client, what would be the most thorough approach for the nurse to take in assessing the client's blood pressure?

4. When caring for clients with accelerated or malignant hypertension, what complications might the nurse detect?

34/ Caring for Clients with Heart Failure

The pumping action of the heart circulates blood in a loop from the venous circulation to the lungs and then into the arterial circulation. This provides a continuous supply of oxygen and nutrients for cellular energy and a mechanism for eliminating carbon dioxide and metabolic wastes. Disturbances in one part of the heart, if they are severe enough or last long enough, eventually affect the entire circulation.

The following questions deal with the content of Chapter 34.

I. MULTIPLE CHOICE QUESTIONS

Circle the number of the most appropriate answer.

Mr. Katz, age 67, is admitted to the hospital with a diagnosis of possible heart failure.

1. Mr. Katz's wife asks the nurse to explain what the physician meant by the term congestive in relation to her husband's condition. The most correct response is that when the heart fails as an efficient pump, it causes

   1. an accumulation of blood and fluids in organs and tissues
   2. an excessive burden on the kidneys to excrete body fluids
   3. the bone marrow to produce additional blood cells
   4. the spleen to enlarge from absorbing uncirculated blood cells

   Nursing Process: Implementation
   Client Need: Health Promotion/Maintenance

2. It would be accurate for the nurse to further explain that if the pumping function on the left side of the heart fails, Mr. Katz will experience symptoms primarily affecting his

   1. intestine and elimination
   2. liver and clotting
   3. lungs and breathing
   4. extremities and mobility

   Nursing Process: Implementation
   Client Need: Health Promotion/Maintenance

3. When explaining the pathophysiology of heart failure to Mrs. Katz, it would be accurate for the nurse to tell her that of the four heart chambers, the one whose function is most likely to become impaired first in most individuals is the

   1. right atrium
   2. left atrium
   3. right ventricle
   4. left ventricle

   Nursing Process: Implementation
   Client Need: Health Promotion/Maintenance

4. In regard to the medical record of Mr. Katz, if he is typical of other individuals who develop heart failure, his past health history will most likely indicate that he has had

   1. chronic hypertension
   2. rheumatoid arthritis
   3. hypothyroidism
   4. diabetes mellitus

   Nursing Process: Assessment
   Client Need: Safe, Effective Care Environment

5. The nurse performs a head-to-toe physical assessment of Mr. Katz. If Mr. Katz has left-sided heart failure, the nurse would most likely hear ____ when auscultating his lungs.

   1. loud bronchial wheezes
   2. moist basilar crackles

   3. soft tracheal sounds
   4. clear alveolar sounds

   Nursing Process: Assessment
   Client Need: Physiological Integrity

6. Mr. Katz is breathing rapidly and shallowly. When the arterial blood gas results are returned, the nurse is most likely to find that his blood pH is more than 7.45 due to

   1. respiratory acidosis
   2. respiratory alkalosis

   3. metabolic acidosis
   4. metabolic alkalosis

   Nursing Process: Assessment
   Client Need: Physiological Integrity

7. A colleague asks the nurse caring for Mr. Katz to explain what the drug reference on digoxin (Lanoxin) refers to as inotropic action. The nurse would be most correct in explaining that an inotropic action is one that affects

   1. heart rate
   2. heart contraction

   3. blood pressure
   4. renal output

   Nursing Process: Implementation
   Client Need: Safe, Effective Care Environment

Mrs. O'Leary, age 59, has been hospitalized for 2 days for treatment of right-sided heart failure. She has been experiencing symptoms for 2 months before seeing her physician.

8. If Mrs. O'Leary is typical of most individuals with right-sided heart failure, which one of the following conditions is she most likely to have?

   1. cancer
   2. emphysema

   3. arthritis
   4. pharyngitis

   Nursing Process: Assessment
   Client Need: Safe, Effective Care Environment

9. In an examination of Mrs. O'Leary, which one of the following would most likely be in evidence?

   1. dyspnea when lying flat
   2. blood-streaked sputum

   3. slow, irregular pulse
   4. pitting, pedal edema

   Nursing Process: Assessment
   Client Need: Physiological Integrity

10. If Mrs. O'Leary is typical of others with right-sided heart failure, during the examination of her abdomen the nurse is most likely to find that

    1. bowel sounds are hypoactive
    2. her skin appears jaundiced

    3. her abdomen is quite large
    4. there is generalized tenderness

    Nursing Process: Assessment
    Client Need: Physiological Integrity

11. The best evidence that the oxygen which has been prescribed for Mrs. O'Leary is beneficial is that her

    1. heart rate is reduced
    2. lungs sound clear

    3. abdomen is soft
    4. urine output rises

    Nursing Process: Evaluation
    Client Need: Physiological Integrity

Individual Questions

12. When renin is produced as a consequence of heart failure, the nurse is most likely to note a change in the client's

   1. blood pressure
   2. heart rate

   3. heart rhythm
   4. pulse quality

   Nursing Process: Assessment
   Client Need: Physiological Integrity

13. It would be most appropriate for the nurse who administers digoxin (Lanoxin) to provide food sources that are rich in

   1. sodium
   2. calcium

   3. potassium
   4. zinc

   Nursing Process: Implementation
   Client Need: Physiological Integrity

14. When collecting subjective data, the nurse could expect that a client who is developing left-sided congestive heart failure would describe having

   1. to sleep in a reclining chair
   2. intolerance for fatty foods

   3. tight-fitting shoes
   4. to urinate frequently

   Nursing Process: Assessment
   Client Need: Safe, Effective Care Environment

15. When performing a data-base assessment, a client with right-sided heart failure is most likely to describe

   1. being constantly thirsty and voiding excessive amounts of urine
   2. having swollen feet and ankles, particularly at the end of each day

   3. having to lie flat in bed to improve breathing
   4. losing weight despite the usual consumption of food

   Nursing Process: Assessment
   Client Need: Safe, Effective Care Environment

16. If a client requires treatment for acute pulmonary edema, which item in the list that follows can the nurse most expect to use for monitoring and evaluating the client's response?

   1. pulmonary artery catheter
   2. mechanical ventilator

   3. pulse oximeter
   4. ECG heart monitor

   Nursing Process: Planning
   Client Need: Physiological Integrity

17. When a client's heart is forced to pump against elevated pressure in the pulmonary vascular system, the client is most likely to develop signs of

   1. right ventricular hypertrophy
   2. left ventricular hypertrophy

   3. right ventricular atrophy
   4. left ventricular atrophy

   Nursing Process: Assessment
   Client Need: Physiological Integrity

18. When monitoring the client with heart failure, which daily assessment would be appropriate to add to the plan for care?

   1. weight
   2. appetite

   3. sleep pattern
   4. stool color

   Nursing Process: Planning
   Client Need: Physiological Integrity

19. If a client with left-sided heart failure experiences paroxysmal nocturnal dyspnea, which one of the following would be most appropriate to add to the plan for care?

   1. place the client on an alternating pressure mattress
   2. use several pillows to support the head and thorax
   3. administer oxygen per nasal cannula before bedtime
   4. cough forcefully to expectorate accumulated secretions

   Nursing Process: Planning
   Client Need: Safe, Effective Care Environment

20. The laboratory test result that would most likely reveal if renal perfusion has been affected by congestive heart failure is

   1. urinary hemoglobin
   2. urinary bilirubin
   3. C-reactive protein (CRP)
   4. blood urea nitrogen (BUN)

   Nursing Process: Assessment
   Client Need: Physiological Integrity

21. If a client with heart failure ate all of the following foods regularly prior to his acute episode, which one should the nurse instruct the client to avoid after being discharged?

   1. ripe bananas
   2. orange juice
   3. frankfurters
   4. apple sauce

   Nursing Process: Implementation
   Client Need: Health Promotion/Maintenance

22. For which one of the following reasons would the nurse be most correct in explaining why a client with pulmonary edema is given morphine sulfate?

   1. to relieve chest pain
   2. to reduce anxiety
   3. to slow the heart rate
   4. to improve heart contraction

   Nursing Process: Implementation
   Client Need: Safe, Effective Care Environment

23. What nursing action is most appropriate when planning the care of a client who is receiving digoxin (Lanoxin), a cardiac glycoside?

   1. monitor the pulse rate
   2. measure urinary output
   3. limit oral fluid intake
   4. assist with hygiene

   Nursing Process: Planning
   Client Need: Safe, Effective Care Environment

24. Besides measuring the urinary output of a client receiving furosemide (Lasix), a loop diuretic, it would be most appropriate to monitor the client's

   1. serum potassium level
   2. apical heart rate
   3. level of consciousness
   4. tolerance of activity

   Nursing Process: Assessment
   Client Need: Physiological Integrity

25. If a client is prescribed a calcium channel blocker, such as verapamil (Calan), the best evidence that its action is producing a therapeutic effect is that

   1. the client's blood pressure is reduced
   2. the client's skin is warm and dry
   3. the client does not have palpitations
   4. the client experiences less dizziness

   Nursing Process: Evaluation
   Client Need: Physiological Integrity

26. An intraaortic balloon pump (IABP) is being used to treat a client in heart failure who has developed cardiogenic shock. The nurse would be most correct in explaining to the client's spouse that the balloon inflates

    1. during the ventricles' resting phase
    2. at the time of ventricular contraction
    3. when the client takes a deep breath
    4. simultaneously with each pulse beat

    Nursing Process: Implementation
    Client Need: Health Promotion/Maintenance

27. The best evidence that an intraaortic balloon pump is achieving a therapeutic effect is that

    1. urine output increases
    2. heart rhythm is regular
    3. peripheral pulses are strong
    4. pupils are widely dilated

    Nursing Process: Evaluation
    Client Need: Physiological Integrity

28. A client receiving digoxin (Lanoxin) reports all of the following. Which one suggests digitalis toxicity?

    1. insomnia
    2. anorexia
    3. thirst
    4. dizziness

    Nursing Process: Evaluation
    Client Need: Physiological Integrity

29. When examining a client, the nurse finds which one of the following assessment findings as being most suggestive that the client's symptoms may be due to right-sided heart failure? In a sitting position, the client's

    1. jugular veins are distended
    2. heart sounds are not audible
    3. respirations are rapid and deep
    4. systolic blood pressure is low

    Nursing Process: Assessment
    Client Need: Physiological Integrity

30. A client is anxious about his impaired respirations. Which one of the following nursing actions would be inappropriate?

    1. coaching the client to breathe slowly
    2. curtailing current activities
    3. sitting the client upright
    4. pulling the privacy curtains

    Nursing Process: Implementation
    Client Need: Psychosocial Integrity

31. A client with heart failure is to receive a diuretic daily. At what time of day would it be best to administer this drug?

    1. early in the morning
    2. with the noon meal
    3. during mid-afternoon
    4. just before bedtime

    Nursing Process: Implementation
    Client Need: Physiological Integrity

32. If rotating tourniquets are used to treat pulmonary edema, each extremity will have a tourniquet applied for ____ minutes.

    1. 15
    2. 30
    3. 45
    4. 60

    Nursing Process: Intervention
    Client Need: Safe, Effective Care Environment

II. CRITICAL THINKING EXERCISES

1. Mr. Henry Ratcliff has been admitted with left-sided congestive heart failure and Mr. Carl Allen has right-sighted congestive heart failure. What assessment findings will be unique in each of these two clients?

2. Mr. George Hass is receiving digoxin (Lanoxin), a cardiac glycoside. How does this drug relieve heart failure?

3. Several clients with heart failure are awaiting a heart transplant. What treatment approaches may be used to support the function of their natural hearts until a donor heart may be found.

4. Before the time of discharge, what health teaching would be important to provide a client with heart failure?

5. How should rotating tourniquets be removed when a client's condition has been stabilized with *dry phlebotomy*?

35/ Caring for Clients Undergoing Cardiovascular Surgery

The individual who decides to have surgery performed on his or her heart is taking a calculated risk for a longer and healthier life. Clients enter the hospital with varying degrees of emotional readiness. The preoperative period is very important because it helps the client feel secure in the hospital situation, understand the procedures required before and after surgery, and develop confidence in the surgical team.

The following questions deal with the content of Chapter 35.

I. MULTIPLE CHOICE QUESTIONS

Circle the number of the most appropriate answer.

1. A client who is scheduled for cardiac surgery asks the nurse how his blood will be circulated and oxygenated when his heart is stopped during the operation. The best answer is that
   1. the blood remains stationary when the heart is stopped
   2. a mechanical ventilator provides oxygen for the blood
   3. a special machine substitutes for the heart and lungs
   4. the heart is stopped so briefly that nothing else is needed

   Nursing Process: Implementation
   Client Need: Safe, Effective Care Environment

2. A client asks the nurse to re-explain what the physician meant when he recommended a procedure called a *comissurotomy*. The most accurate answer is that this procedure widens a narrowed valve by
   1. stretching its opening with a finger
   2. inflating a ballooned catheter
   3. replacing it with an animal's valve
   4. substituting a mechanical valve

   Nursing Process: Implementation
   Client Need: Safe, Effective Care Environment

3. The best evidence that a client understands what will be done during a coronary artery bypass graft (CABG) procedure is when he describes that the surgeon will use one of his own blood vessels to
   1. re-route blood around a narrowed section of a coronary artery
   2. totally replace one or more diseased coronary arteries
   3. shunt blood from a coronary vein into a coronary artery
   4. provide drainage channels to remove blood from the myocardium

   Nursing Process: Evaluation
   Client Need: Safe, Effective Care Environment

4. If the surgeon plans to use the saphenous vein for a coronary artery bypass graft (CABG), the nurse would be most correct to scrub the skin preoperatively in the

   1. arm
   2. abdomen
   3. neck
   4. leg

   Nursing Process: Implementation
   Client Need: Safe, Effective Care Environment

5. A client with a ventricular aneurysm understands the health risks associated with this condition if he indicates that which two of the following complications may occur?

   1. infection and occlusion
   2. infarct and hypertension
   3. thrombi and hemorrhage
   4. pericarditis and emboli

   Nursing Process: Evaluation
   Client Need: Health Promotion/Maintenance

6. A client with a myocardial infarction complicated by the formation of a ventricular aneurysm asks the nurse why the physician has recommended waiting 4 to 8 weeks to repair it. The most accurate answer is that there is a better outcome

   1. following a period of weight loss
   2. if the heart is allowed to rest
   3. when blood flow has increased
   4. after scar tissue has formed

   Nursing Process: Implementation
   Client Need: Safe, Effective Care Environment

7. A client who will have a heart tumor removed has accurate information if he states that the type of tumor that has the best prognosis is one that

   1. extends from a pedicle or stem
   2. is located within the septum
   3. has invaded transmural tissue
   4. occurs in the heart's apex

   Nursing Process: Evaluation
   Client Need: Health Promotion/Maintenance

8. If the nurse suspects that a trauma victim's heart may be bleeding into the pericardium, the best plan would be to

   1. auscultate heart sounds hourly
   2. inspect the chest for bruises
   3. keep the client on bedrest
   4. administer oxygen per mask

   Nursing Process: Planning
   Client Need: Physiological Integrity

9. A client with cardiomyopathy asks the nurse how a donor heart is obtained for heart transplantation. The most accurate answer is that

   1. organs are harvested and preserved in a tissue bank
   2. donor hearts are frozen and thawed when one is needed
   3. each hospital obtains and stores a supply of donated organs
   4. after death, the donor heart is matched with a recipient

   Nursing Process: Implementation
   Client Need: Safe, Effective Care Environment

10. The nurse would be most correct in explaining to a potential heart transplant client that the most serious long-term problem associated with this procedure is

    1. myocardial infarction
    2. organ rejection
    3. infective endocarditis
    4. congestive heart failure

    Nursing Process: Implementation
    Client Need: Safe, Effective Care Environment

11. When monitoring a client following a heart transplant, which one of the following would be most suggestive that the client is experiencing organ rejection? The client

1. has chest pain
2. bleeds easily
3. has an elevated white blood cell count
4. has a decreased red blood cell count

Nursing Process: Assessment
Client Need: Physiological Integrity

12. A nurse finds a client crying the evening before surgery. Which one of the following statements would be most therapeutic at this time?

1. "It's quite normal to feel distraught."
2. "You'll feel relieved after the surgery."
3. "Don't cry. You're just upsetting yourself."
4. "You're under the care of the best surgeon."

Nursing Process: Implementation
Client Need: Psychosocial Integrity

13. When assessing a cardiac surgery client on a mechanical ventilator with an endotracheal tube in place, the nurse should immediately report which finding?

1. The client's respiratory rate is 22 per minute.
2. Breath sounds are heard on one side below the bronchi.
3. The pilot balloon on the endotracheal tube is inflated.
4. The client is not able to communicate by speaking.

Nursing Process: Implementation
Client Need: Physiological Integrity

14. Which one of the following would be the maximum volume of drainage the nurse could expect in 1 hour from a chest tube following cardiac surgery?

1. 30 mL
2. 50 mL
3. 75 mL
4. 100 mL

Nursing Process: Assessment
Client Need: Safe, Effective Care Environment

15. Which one of the following assessments is most indicative of hypoxia when monitoring a postoperative cardiac surgery client? The client is

1. hungry
2. shivering
3. restless
4. in pain

Nursing Process: Assessment
Client Need: Physiological Integrity

16. Which one of the following is the best evidence that the client is adequately oxygenated after cardiac surgery?

1. Peripheral pulses are strong.
2. The client's skin is warm and dry.
3. Arterial blood gases are normal.
4. Urine output is ≥ 30 mL/hour.

Nursing Process: Evaluation
Client Need: Physiological Integrity

17. A client asks the nurse why he must have a nasogastric tube following cardiac surgery. The best answer is that this tube

1. will be used to provide liquid nourishment postoperatively
2. removes gas that might otherwise restrict ventilation
3. provides a route for administering oral medications
4. enables measuring the pH of gastric secretions

Nursing Process: Implementation
Client Need: Safe, Effective Care Environment

18. A femoral artery catheter has just been removed from a client recovering from cardiac surgery. Which one of the following positions would be contraindicated?

    1. dorsal recumbent
    2. semi-Fowler's
    3. Trendelenburg
    4. lateral oblique

    Nursing Process: Planning
    Client Need: Physiological Integrity

19. An arterial line within the radial artery is being used to directly monitor a postoperative client's blood pressure. Which one of the following assessments would be most important to report? In the arm with the arterial catheter,

    1. the client's fingers are pale and cold
    2. the client's capillary refill is ≤ 3 seconds
    3. heparinized saline clears the line of blood
    4. the brachial artery is strongly palpable

    Nursing Process: Assessment
    Client Need: Physiological Integrity

20. The physician explains to the spouse of a postoperative client that the client is temporarily disoriented and confused due to postcoronary psychosis. The nurse would be correct in explaining that a major cause for this is

    1. alcohol withdrawal
    2. sensory overload
    3. drug reactions
    4. low blood volume

    Nursing Process: Implementation
    Client Need: Health Promotion/Maintenance

21. A client is hoarse following removal of an endotracheal tube. It would be most appropriate for the nurse to recommend that the client

    1. rest his voice
    2. whisper his words
    3. talk in a lower pitch
    4. speak as usual

    Nursing Process: Implementation
    Client Need: Safe, Effective Care Environment

22. A client is scheduled for an endarterectomy. If this client is typical of most who have this surgery, which condition is most likely to be a concurrent health problem?

    1. arrhythmias
    2. hypotension
    3. atherosclerosis
    4. endocarditis

    Nursing Process: Assessment
    Client Need: Safe, Effective Care Environment

23. If an endarterectomy was performed on the carotid artery, which one of the following would be most important to assess?

    1. ability to swallow
    2. ability to talk
    3. pupil size and response
    4. time of capillary refill

    Nursing Process: Planning
    Client Need: Physiological Integrity

24. Which of the following is the best evidence that a client understands how to care for an extremity from which a vascular graft was taken? The client says he should

    1. apply moist heat or use an electric heating pad
    2. sit as much as possible and avoid walking
    3. wear warm stockings and shoes with hard soles
    4. avoid driving a car or flying in an airplane

    Nursing Process: Evaluation
    Client Need: Health Promotion/Maintenance

II. CRITICAL THINKING EXERCISES

1. Besides the usual postoperative risks, what other potential problems are associated with a heart transplant procedure?

2. Mr. Otto Yablonski has indicated he is extremely anxious and fearful about undergoing cardiac surgery in the morning. What nursing interventions would help to relieve this client's insecurity?

3. A recovery room nurse calls to inform the nursing unit that a client has reacted from anesthesia following cardiac surgery and is awaiting transfer to the surgical nursing unit. What further information would be important to obtain prior to the transfer?

4. Darrell Upton is recovering from vascular surgery in a lower extremity. What nursing interventions would promote tissue perfusion in the operative leg?

VII Caring for Clients with Hematopoietic and Lymphatic Disorders

36/ Introduction to the Hematopoietic and Lymphatic Systems

Blood is a viscous (thick) fluid that transports vital substances to every part of the body and removes the waste products of cellular metabolism. The heart circulates blood throughout the body by means of a vast network of arteries, arterioles, capillaries, veins, and venules. The lymphatic system is a network of lymph nodes connected by ducts.

The following questions deal with the content of Chapter 36.

I. MULTIPLE CHOICE QUESTIONS

Circle the number of the most appropriate answer.

Eight rooms of a medical unit have been set aside for the care of clients with hematologic disorders. In preparation for the admission of clients to the unit, the charge nurse has scheduled team conferences for a review of the anatomy and physiology of the hematopoietic and lymphatic systems. The nurses on the unit will be presenting various parts of the team conference.

1. When presenting basic information about blood, the nurse is most correct in stating that the average individual has approximately
    1. 3.5 quarts of blood
    2. 5 liters of blood
    3. 8 quarts of blood
    4. 9 liters of blood

    Nursing Process: Implementation
    Client Need: Safe, Effective Care Environment

2. When describing how lymph circulates through the lymph nodes and connected ducts, the nurse is most correct in saying that lymph moves by
   1. changes in the gradient pressure in veins
   2. action of arteries on nearby lymph vessels
   3. means of contraction of skeletal muscles
   4. gravity

   Nursing Process: Implementation
   Client Need: Safe, Effective Care Environment

3. When defining the term *erythroblast,* the nurse is most correct in stating that an erythroblast is a(n)
   1. immature erythrocyte
   2. type of nucleated, immature white blood cell
   3. red blood cell produced by yellow bone marrow
   4. mature erythrocyte

   Nursing Process: Implementation
   Client Need: Safe, Effective Care Environment

4. When describing a decrease below the normal number of leukocytes, the nurse correctly uses the term
   1. leukocytosis
   2. leukosis
   3. leukopenia
   4. leukomiosis

   Nursing Process: Implementation
   Client Need: Safe, Effective Care Environment

5. When discussing the number one defense against bacterial infection, the nurse correctly names
   1. granulocytes
   2. basophils
   3. eosinophils
   4. neutrophils

   Nursing Process: Implementation
   Client Need: Safe, Effective Care Environment

6. When giving the alternative term for platelets, the nurse is correct in using the term
   1. thrombocytes
   2. erythrocytes
   3. leukocytes
   4. neutrophils

   Nursing Process: Implementation
   Client Need: Safe, Effective Care Environment

7. When giving the alternative term for gamma globulins, the nurse is correct in using the term
   1. protein globulins
   2. immunoglobulins
   3. amino acid globulins
   4. plasma globulins

   Nursing Process: Implementation
   Client Need: Safe, Effective Care Environment

8. When discussing blood types, the nurse is correct in saying that universal donors have type ____ blood.
   1. A
   2. O
   3. B
   4. AB

   Nursing Process: Implementation
   Client Need: Safe, Effective Care Environment

9. When defining the term *positive Rh factor,* the nurse is correct in saying that this factor is a(n)
   1. antigen present in blood plasma
   2. antibody found in red blood cells
   3. immunoglobulin present in plasma
   4. protein substance found on the red blood cell membrane

   Nursing Process: Implementation
   Client Need: Safe, Effective Care Environment

10. When describing the site where a bone marrow aspiration may be performed, the nurse is most correct in stating the
    1. femur or ulna
    2. sternum or iliac crest
    3. radius or sternum
    4. iliac arch or pubic bone

    Nursing Process: Implementation
    Client Need: Safe, Effective Care Environment

II. CRITICAL THINKING EXERCISES

1. Ms. Randall is seen in the clinic because she has experienced bruises that appear to develop even though she has not had any injury. What questions would you ask and what topics would you cover when obtaining an initial history from Ms. Randall?

37/ Caring for Clients with Disorders of the Hematopoietic System

The term *blood dyscrasia* (blood disease) describes a large group of disorders that affect the blood. Although blood dyscrasias affect the blood in some way, the disorders themselves are manifestations of many different pathologic processes.

The following questions deal with the content of Chapter 37.

I. MULTIPLE CHOICE QUESTIONS

Circle the number of the most appropriate answer.

Mr. Weaver, age 19, is admitted to the hospital with a tentative diagnosis of sickle cell anemia.

1. When reviewing Mr. Weaver's laboratory reports, the nurse knows that sickle cell anemia is present when
   1. the hemoglobin is below 9.0 gms.
   2. the sickle cell screening test is positive for hemoglobin S
   3. a urine sample is positive for sickle cell anemia
   4. the white blood count is elevated

   Nursing Process: Collecting Data
   Client Need: Safe, Effective Care Environment

2. Mr. Weaver is in sickle cell crisis. When developing a plan of care, the nurse must know that the crisis form of this disorder results from the
   1. release of hemoglobin R from red blood cells
   2. increase in the production of erythrocytes
   3. blockage of small blood vessels
   4. decrease in the production of thrombocytes

   Nursing Process: Planning
   Client Need: Safe, Effective Care Environment

3. When assessing Mr. Weaver, the nurse looks for
   1. signs of tissue anoxia in the extremities
   2. an increase in the force of peripheral pulses
   3. distention of the carotid arteries
   4. a sudden increase in his blood pressure

   Nursing Process: Collecting Data
   Client Need: Physiological Integrity

Ms. Stewart has pernicious anemia and is receiving vitamin B$_{12}$.

4. When giving a report to the nurses on the next shift, a nurse asks, "What causes pernicious anemia?" The most correct answer is that pernicious anemia is due to a
   1. lack of the intrinsic factor in gastric secretions
   2. lack of the extrinsic factor in the liver
   3. formation of immature leukocytes
   4. formation of erythroblasts

   Nursing Process: Implementation
   Client Need: Safe, Effective Care Environment

5. The nurse also asks why Ms. Stewart is receiving vitamin B$_{12}$. The most correct response is that this vitamin is necessary for the
   1. production of white cells
   2. normal maturation of red blood cells
   3. production of platelets
   4. destruction of stem cells

   Nursing Process: Implementation
   Client Need: Safe, Effective Care Environment

6. The nurse asks what would happen if Ms. Stewart were not treated promptly. The most correct answer is
   1. a decrease in her production of the extrinsic factor
   2. degenerative changes in her nervous system
   3. a decrease in her white blood cell count
   4. degenerative changes in her liver

   Nursing Process: Implementation
   Client Need: Safe, Effective Care Environment

Ms. Larson, age 68, has had fatigue and weakness for the past year. After performing a physical examination and routine blood work, her physician admits her to the hospital with the diagnosis of possible chronic lymphocytic leukemia (CLL).

7. A nurse assistant asks questions about Ms. Larson's diagnosis and the meaning of the term *leukemia*. The most correct answer is that leukemia is characterized by a
   1. marked anemia and loss of bone marrow stem cells
   2. sudden increase in lymphocytes and thrombocytes
   3. rampant, unregulated proliferation of immature leukocytes
   4. marked increase in platelets and mature leukocytes

   Nursing Process: Implementation
   Client Need: Safe, Effective Care Environment

8. When planning for preparing Ms. Larson for diagnostic tests, the nurse is aware of the fact that the diagnosis of leukemia may be confirmed by
   1. radioisotope studies
   2. CT scan
   3. examination of peripheral blood and bone marrow
   4. radiographic studies

   Nursing Process: Planning
   Client Need: Safe, Effective Care Environment

9. During treatment, Mrs. Larson develops thrombocytopenia. The nurse must assess Ms. Larson for signs of
   1. an overwhelming infection
   2. alopecia
   3. extreme fatigue and dyspnea
   4. easy bruising and excessive bleeding

   Nursing Process: Collecting Data
   Client Need: Physiological Integrity

10. Ms. Larson is discharged and receives outpatient chemotherapy. When working in the hematology clinic, the nurse notes that there is an increase in the serum uric acid level. To effectively plan client teaching, the nurse knows that this increase is most probably due to
    1. massive cell destruction during chemotherapy
    2. the effect of corticosteroids on the kidney
    3. erythroblastosis
    4. leukocytosis

    Nursing Process: Planning
    Client Need: Physiological Integrity

11. Because of the elevated serum uric acid level, Mrs. Larson is encouraged to
    1. walk more frequently
    2. drink extra fluids
    3. eat foods high in protein
    4. limit her fluid intake

    Nursing Process: Implementation
    Client Need: Physiological Integrity

12. Ms. Larson also has thrombocytopenia. The nurse can advise Ms. Larson to
    1. eat a soft, bland diet
    2. avoid other people who have an infection
    3. take precautions to avoid physical injury
    4. increase her protein and iron intake

    Nursing Process: Implementation
    Client Need: Health Promotion/Maintenance

Mr. Young is admitted with a diagnosis of multiple myeloma. A team conference is scheduled to discuss a plan of care for this client.

13. When developing a care plan for Mr. Young, the nurse must know that multiple myeloma is a malignant disease of
    1. plasma cells
    2. erythrocytes
    3. leukocytes
    4. thrombocytes

    Nursing Process: Planning
    Client Need: Safe, Effective Care Environment

14. When planning nursing management, the nurse must be aware of the fact that in multiple myeloma single or multiple osteolytic tumors are found in the
    1. urine
    2. blood
    3. bone
    4. lungs

    Nursing Process: Planning
    Client Need: Safe, Effective Care Environment

15. When performing an initial physical assessment on Mr. Young, the nurse must be aware of the fact that prominent symptoms of multiple myeloma include
    1. fatigue
    2. generalized edema
    3. dyspnea
    4. severe, localized bone pain

    Nursing Process: Collecting Data
    Client Need: Physiological Integrity

16. Mr. Young is encouraged to increase his fluid intake to
    1. help remove tumor cells from his urine
    2. prevent renal damage from hypercalcemia
    3. prevent congestive heart failure
    4. increase his serum uric acid levels

    Nursing Process: Implementation
    Client Need: Physiological Integrity

17. Mr. Young is encouraged to ambulate because immobilization can
    1. increase calcium loss from the bone
    2. decrease the loss of calcium in the urine
    3. increase the concentration of potassium in the blood
    4. decrease serum uric acid levels

    Nursing Process: Implementation
    Client Need: Physiological Integrity

18. When developing a plan of discharge teaching, the nurse includes the importance of avoiding injuries because Mr. Young is subject to
    1. bladder stones
    2. pathological fractures
    3. cardiac arrhythmias
    4. stasis ulcers

    Nursing Process: Implementation
    Client Need: Health Promotion/Maintenance

Individual Questions

19. To reduce the signs and symptoms of chronic anemia, the nurse can plan to advise the client to
    1. take frequent rest periods and to space activities
    2. take multivitamins daily
    3. sleep at least 10 hours per night
    4. eat a diet low in iron and high in vitamin C

    Nursing Process: Planning
    Client Need: Health Promotion/Maintenance

20. When developing a care plan for the client with polycythemia vera, the nurse must be aware of the fact that these clients have a tendency to develop
    1. thrombi
    2. excessive bleeding tendencies
    3. anemia
    4. leukopenia

    Nursing Process: Planning
    Client Need: Safe, Effective Care Environment

21. The term *leukocytosis* is noted on a client's chart. When checking a dictionary the nurse finds that this term is defined as a(n)
    1. increase in the number of leukocytes
    2. destruction of leukocytes
    3. absorption of leukocytes by the bone marrow
    4. decrease in the number of leukocytes

    Nursing Process: Implementation
    Client Need: Safe, Effective Care Environment

22. When assessing the client with agranulocytosis, the nurse looks for
    1. fever, chills, ulcers on the mucous membranes
    2. hypertension, stasis ulcers, tachycardia
    3. diarrhea, headache, peripheral erythema
    4. anorexia, hypotension, double vision

    Nursing Process: Collecting Data
    Client Need: Physiological Integrity

23. When developing a plan of care for the client with agranulocytosis, the nurse includes
    1. encouraging a high-protein diet
    2. limiting fluids to prevent congestive heart failure
    3. use of alcohol mouth rinses to control mouth infections
    4. careful aseptic technique to prevent infection

    Nursing Process: Planning
    Client Need: Safe, Effective Care Environment

24. When assessing the client with thrombocytopenia, the nurse looks for
    1. small hemorrhages in the skin, mucous membranes, or subcutaneous tissues
    2. distended neck veins
    3. discoloration of the nails and sclera
    4. thrombus formation in the extremities

    Nursing Process: Collecting Data
    Client Need: Physiological Integrity

25. When defining hemophilia at a team conference, the nurse is correct in stating that hemophilia is a hereditary
    1. clotting factor deficiency
    2. increase in the antihemophilic factor
    3. decrease in the number of erythrocytes
    4. an increase in the number of white blood cells

    Nursing Process: Implementation
    Client Need: Safe, Effective Care Environment

26. Clients with hemophilia are observed for early warning signs of internal bleeding which include
    1. hypotension, bradycardia
    2. absence of urine output, headache
    3. tachycardia, increased pain in an area
    4. constipation, anorexia

    Nursing Process: Collecting Data
    Client Need: Physiological Integrity

27. When a client has hemophilia, gastrointestinal bleeding may be evidenced by
    1. anorexia
    2. coffee-ground emesis
    3. constipation
    4. clay-colored stools

    Nursing Process: Collecting Data
    Client Need: Physiological Integrity

28. When developing a care plan for the client with aplastic anemia, the nurse must be aware of the fact that this blood dyscrasia is manifested by a(n)
    1. increase in the number of thrombocytes
    2. depression of bone marrow activity
    3. increase in plasma volume
    4. decrease in the number of leukocytes

    Nursing Process: Planning
    Client Need: Safe, Effective Care Environment

29. A nursing care plan for the client with aplastic anemia includes
    1. limitation of the fluid intake
    2. taking the temperature rectally
    3. prevention of infection
    4. having the client ambulate at frequent intervals

    Nursing Process: Planning
    Client Need: Safe, Effective Care Environment

II. CRITICAL THINKING EXERCISES

1. Mr. Shields has leukemia. The laboratory reports his hemoglobin as 5.8 grams and platelet count as 66,000. His physician has been notified. What two major problems are associated with these two laboratory results?

2. Ms. Day has leukemia and is scheduled for chemotherapy. She tells you that she has heard that anyone receiving chemotherapy will lose their hair. What would you tell her?

3. Mr. Green has aplastic anemia. His white blood cell count (WBC) is 1800. What precautions are taken when the WBC is this low? Why?

38/ Caring for Clients with Disorders of the Lymphatics

Disorders affecting the lymphatics are those that are infectious, inflammatory, occlusive, and malignant. Lymphatic malignancies are the most serious problem affecting the lymphatics because they can be life-threatening.
The following questions deal with the content of Chapter 38.

I. MULTIPLE CHOICE QUESTIONS

Circle the number of the most appropriate answer.

Lymphatic disorders are to be discussed at a scheduled refresher conference for all members of a medical unit. All those attending the conference are asked to review anatomy and physiology of the lymphatic system as well as the more common lymphatic disorders.

1. When asked for the composition of lymph, the nurse correctly answers that lymph is similar in composition to
   1. whole blood
   2. serosanguinous fluid
   3. gastric juices
   4. tissue fluid and plasma

   Nursing Process: Implementation
   Client Need: Safe, Effective Care Environment

2. When asked for the effects of lymphedema, the nurse correctly answers that lymphedema results in
   1. swelling of the affected lymph node
   2. deformity and poor tissue nutrition
   3. a collection of plasma in tissues
   4. enlarged, reddened areas

   Nursing Process: Implementation
   Client Need: Safe, Effective Care Environment

3. When asked to describe a prominent symptom of lymphangitis, the nurse correctly replies
   1. swelling of the lymph nodes
   2. blanching of the affected area
   3. red streaks that follow the course of the lymph channels
   4. cyanosis distal to the affected part

   Nursing Process: Implementation
   Client Need: Safe, Effective Care Environment

4. When asked for the cause of infectious mononucleosis, the nurse correctly answers
   1. *Staphylococcus aureus*
   2. the protozoa *Toxoplasma*
   3. the Epstein-Barr virus
   4. the cytomegalovirus

   Nursing Process: Implementation
   Client Need: Safe, Effective Care Environment

5. When the nurse is asked to give the reason why clients with a lymphoma have a decreased resistance to infection, the most correct reply is the
   1. rapid proliferation of abnormal lymphocytes
   2. increase in abnormal thrombocytes
   3. decrease in leukocytes
   4. decrease in erythrocytes

   Nursing Process: Implementation
   Client Need: Safe, Effective Care Environment

Individual Questions

6. The nurse can help relieve lymphedema by
   1. elevating the affected part
   2. having the client ambulate at frequent intervals
   3. encouraging the client to drink 8 or more glasses of fluid per day
   4. keeping the client flat in bed 16 or more hours per day

   Nursing Process: Implementation
   Client Need: Safe, Effective Care Environment

7. When performing a physical assessment on the client with non-Hodgkin's lymphoma, the nurse looks for
   1. painful, red lymph nodes
   2. enlarged cervical, axillary, and inguinal lymph nodes
   3. abdominal distention
   4. peripheral edema

   Nursing Process: Collecting Data
   Client Need: Physiological Integrity

8. Which of the following can the nurse offer to the client experiencing nausea and vomiting following radiation therapy?
   1. a diet high in carbohydrates
   2. crackers and fruit juices
   3. clear liquids such as carbonated beverages, popsicles
   4. a soft diet

   Nursing Process: Implementation
   Client Need: Physiological Integrity

II. CRITICAL THINKING EXERCISES

1. What suggestions for disguising the condition could you give a client who has lymphedema of the legs?

2. Ms. Foss developed oral ulcerations while undergoing outpatient chemotherapy for Hodgkin's disease. What suggestions regarding her dietary and fluid can you give to this client?

VIII Caring for Clients with Immune Disorders

39/ Introduction to the Immune System

The immune system functions as the word implies—it provides *immunity*. Immunity is a vital protective mechanism that enables the body to destroy invading foreign agents and microorganisms.

The following questions deal with the content of Chapter 39.

I. MULTIPLE CHOICE QUESTIONS

Circle the number of the most appropriate answer.

A new addition to the hospital contains units that specialize in allergies, disorders of the immune system, and organ transplantation. All nurses are required to attend conferences providing information about these new areas as well as a review of various body systems. Today, the conference focuses on the immune system. All nurses are expected to actively participate in the conference.

1. When asked for the basic components of the immune system, the nurse correctly answers
   1. thrombocytes and white blood cells
   2. the liver, spleen, and bone marrow
   3. erythrocytes, the liver, and leukocytes
   4. specialized lymphoid tissues and white blood cells

   Nursing Process: Implementation
   Client Need: Safe, Effective Care Environment

2. When asked to describe the role of the thymus gland after birth, the nurse correctly answers the
   1. production of leukocytes and thrombocytes
   2. programming of T-lymphocytes to become regulator or effector cells
   3. destruction of erythrocytes and thrombocytes
   4. manufacture of B-lymphocytes

   Nursing Process: Implementation
   Client Need: Safe, Effective Care Environment

3. When asked which cells recognize foreign antigens and stimulate B-lymphocytes, the nurse correctly answers
   1. helper T cells (T4 cells)
   2. suppressor T cells (T8 cells)
   3. effector T cells
   4. cytotoxic cells

   Nursing Process: Implementation
   Client Need: Safe, Effective Care Environment

4. When asked for the name of the cells formed after exposure to an antigen, the nurse correctly answers
   1. lymphokines
   2. B-lymphocytes memory cells
   3. effector T cells
   4. regulator T cells

   Nursing Process: Implementation
   Client Need: Safe, Effective Care Environment

5. When asked for a definition of an autoimmune disorder, the nurse defines the disorder as one in which the body
   1. produces its own antigens
   2. is unable to produce T-lymphocytes
   3. recognizes some of its own cells as foreign cells
   4. manufactures protein markers

   Nursing Process: Implementation
   Client Need: Safe, Effective Care Environment

6. When asked for another term for antibodies, the nurse correctly replies
   1. antigens
   2. immunoglobulins
   3. alpha globulins
   4. plasma proteins

   Nursing Process: Implementation
   Client Need: Safe, Effective Care Environment

7. When asked about the formation of antibodies following an invasion by a microorganism, the nurse correctly replies that this response is negotiated by
   1. B-lymphocytes
   2. T-lymphocytes
   3. lymphokines
   4. immunoglobulins

   Nursing Process: Implementation
   Client Need: Safe, Effective Care Environment

8. When asked to name the type of immunity resulting from a previous invasion by a specific microorganism, the nurse correctly replies a
   1. naturally acquired active immunity
   2. passive immunity
   3. artificially acquired active immunity
   4. naturally acquired active immunity

   Nursing Process: Implementation
   Client Need: Safe, Effective Care Environment

9. When asked to name the type of immunity resulting from a injection of an antitoxin, the nurse correctly replies
   1. naturally acquired active immunity
   2. passive immunity
   3. artificially acquired active immunity
   4. naturally acquired active immunity

   Nursing Process: Implementation
   Client Need: Safe, Effective Care Environment

10. When asked to explain the importance of a thorough drug history during the initial assessment of the client with an immune disorder, the nurse correctly replies that
    1. many drugs interfere with the formation of immunoglobulins
    2. some drugs prevent the formation of antibodies
    3. certain drugs may affect the immune system
    4. certain drugs interfere with passive immunity

    Nursing Process: Implementation
    Client Need: Safe, Effective Care Environment

II. CRITICAL THINKING EXERCISES

1. Mr. Decker is seen by a physician for vague symptoms he has had over the past 7 months. The physician asks you to obtain a history and perform a general physical assessment. What areas would you cover in a history and physical assessment?

40/ Caring for Clients with Allergic and Autoimmune Disorders

Allergy refers to a state of *altered* immunologic reactivity whereby the body is injured in the course of its immune response against a substance that is recognized as something foreign. An allergic reaction may affect various organs and structures such as the skin, nasal mucosa, and gastrointestinal tract. Autoimmune disorders are those due to an immune response to oneself.

The following questions deal with the content of Chapter 40.

I. MULTIPLE CHOICE QUESTIONS

Circle the number of the most appropriate answer.

Ms. Graf has a history of possible allergies. Her physician has advised her to be seen as an outpatient in the allergy clinic of the hospital.

1. Ms. Graf states that the physician used the term *allergen* and asks what this word means. The nurse tells Ms. Graf that an allergen is a(n)

   1. hypersensitivity reaction in mucous membranes
   2. substance capable of causing an allergic response
   3. substance produced in response to an antibody
   4. microorganism capable of causing the production of immunogens

   Nursing Process: Implementation
   Client Need: Health Promotion/Maintenance

2. Ms. Graf asks about the more common symptoms of an allergy. The nurse tells Ms. Graf
   1. sneezing, nasal congestion, excessive nasal discharge
   2. anorexia, chest pain, indigestion
   3. constipation, vomiting, weight loss
   4. heart palpitations, coughing, headache

   Nursing Process: Implementation
   Client Need: Health Promotion/Maintenance

3. Ms. Graf asks how the physician will be able to tell if she has allergies. The nurse answers that the physician will
    1. take a detailed drug history
    2. prescribe a drug to see if it relieves symptoms
    3. skin test her with extracts of various substances
    4. apply skin patches containing an antihistamine

    Nursing Process: Implementation
    Client Need: Health Promotion/Maintenance

4. Ms. Graf asks why her physician prescribed an antihistamine. The nurse tells Ms. Graf that the antihistamine
    1. prevents more allergies from developing
    2. cures the allergy
    3. relieves the symptoms of the allergy
    4. prevents the allergies from becoming worse

    Nursing Process: Implementation
    Client Need: Health Promotion/Maintenance

5. Ms. Graf states that her physician ordered an expectorant and asks why she needs this drug. The nurse tells her that an expectorant
    1. prevents excessive coughing
    2. dries secretions in the nose and throat
    3. relieves the symptoms of an allergy
    4. thins secretions and helps to raise sputum

    Nursing Process: Implementation
    Client Need: Health Promotion/Maintenance

Individual Questions

6. Which one of the following might alert the nurse that the client has developed a dermatitis medicamentosa?
    1. sudden appearance of a generalized skin rash
    2. severe sneezing and coughing
    3. sudden onset of diarrhea
    4. symptoms of asthma

    Nursing Process: Evaluation
    Client Need: Physiological Integrity

7. When asked at a team conference what can be done for a persistent food allergy, the nurse correctly replies institution of a(n)
    1. low-fat diet until symptoms are relieved
    2. rice and tea diet
    3. elimination diet
    4. course of corticosteroid therapy

    Nursing Process: Implementation
    Client Need: Safe, Effective Care Environment

8. During a report to the next shift the nurse is asked why epinephrine was given IM to a client with allergies. The nurse correctly replies that epinephrine is used in the treatment of
    1. serious allergic reactions
    2. skin rashes due to allergies
    3. contact dermatitis
    4. excessive nasal congestion and sneezing

    Nursing Process: Implementation
    Client Need: Safe, Effective Care Environment

9. When asked by a client how immunotherapy appears to help in the treatment of allergies, the nurse correctly replies that these injections appear to
    1. prevent the offending allergens from entering the body
    2. stimulate antibody formation against the offending allergens
    3. prevent the development of new allergies
    4. stimulate masts cells to produce antibodies

    Nursing Process: Implementation
    Client Need: Physiological Integrity

10. If angioedema occurs following administration of a drug, the physician is contacted immediately and the nurse
    1. asks a nurse assistant to stay with the client
    2. closely monitors the blood pressure and respiratory status
    3. connects the client to a cardiac monitor
    4. administers oxygen at 1 L/min

    Nursing Process: Implementation
    Client Need: Physiological Integrity

11. At a team conference the conference leader asks how the body is able to recognize foreign cells and its own cells. The nurse correctly replies by means of
    1. antibodies present in the serum
    2. antigens located in the cell nucleus
    3. autoantibodies present in the bone marrow
    4. individual cell surface antigens coded by genes

    Nursing Process: Implementation
    Client Need: Safe, Effective Care Environment

II. CRITICAL THINKING EXERCISES

1. Ms. Hunt has severe allergic rhinitis and has been found to be allergic to grasses, trees, and weeds. What recommendations could you make to help Ms. Hunt avoid these allergens?

2. Mr. Blake has developed a severe contact dermatitis on various areas of his body, including his hands, arms, face, and neck. Which specific questions would you ask Mr. Blake when taking a history of exposure to substances that may be causing his contact dermatitis?

3. Ms. Curtis received oxacillin IM 20 minutes ago. When entering her room you note that she is slightly cyanotic and is having difficulty breathing. You immediately notify the physician, stating that you believe she may be having a serious allergic reaction to the drug. What specific observations and tasks are performed until Ms. Curtis is seen by the physician?

41/   Caring for Clients with AIDS

AIDS stands for *acquired immunodeficiency syndrome.* AIDS can be described as the end result of an infection with HIV (human immunodeficiency virus). In the United States AIDS was first recognized as a disease about early 1981. At that time the infection was primarily found in homosexual and a few bisexual men. Shortly thereafter, it was detected in male and female intravenous drug abusers who shared needles. Although the highest incidence of the disease is in men, the incidence in women is rising at a rapid rate.

The following questions deal with the content of Chapter 41.

I. MULTIPLE CHOICE QUESTIONS

Circle the number of the most appropriate answer.

Mr. Norris has been diagnosed as having AIDS. Presently, he is not acutely ill and is being seen in the clinic as an outpatient.

1. The physician states that Mr. Norris is immunocompromised. When developing a teaching plan, the nurse must be aware of the fact that Mr. Norris is
   1. subject to polycythemia
   2. a candidate for bone marrow transplantation
   3. going to receive many blood transfusions
   4. unable to fight infection

   Nursing Process: Planning
   Client Need: Physiological Integrity

2. When performing an initial physical assessment on Mr. Norris, the nurse questions him about his symptoms which may include
   1. constipation, anorexia, edema of the extremities
   2. weight gain, cardiac arrhythmias, headache
   3. fever, pronounced weight loss, diarrhea
   4. nasal stuffiness, dry mouth, nausea

   Nursing Process: Collecting Data
   Client Need: Physiological Integrity

3. Mr. Norris asks how his physician determines when he is ready to take zidovudine (Retrovir). The nurse correctly answers that the physician will monitor his
   1. T4 cell count
   2. hemoglobin and hematocrit
   3. ELISA test
   4. T8 cell count

   Nursing Process: Implementation
   Client Need: Safe, Effective Care Environment

Individual Questions

4. A client asks the nurse about the screening tests for the AIDS virus. The nurse correctly replies that a screening test is positive when the
   1. client has been infected with the AIDS virus
   2. client has produced antibodies against the AIDS virus
   3. AIDS virus has begun to replicate
   4. AIDS virus becomes an immunogen

   Nursing Process: Implementation
   Client Need: Health Promotion/Maintenance

5. If a PEG tube is inserted for feeding, the nurse must closely observe the client for
   1. difficulty breathing
   2. localized skin infection
   3. Kaposi's sarcoma
   4. evidence of weight gain

   Nursing Process: Collecting Data
   Client Need: Safe, Effective Care Environment

6. If a T4 cell count is 180 cells/mm^3 the client is closely observed for
   1. adverse drug effects
   2. Kaposi's sarcoma
   3. signs and symptoms of infection
   4. orthopnea and dyspnea

   Nursing Process: Collecting Data
   Client Need: Safe, Effective Care Environment

7. The client with CNS involvement can be helped with activities of daily living by
   1. making tasks as simple as possible
   2. having all ADL performed early in the morning
   3. keeping the client awake during the morning hours
   4. doing the more complicated tasks first

   Nursing Process: Implementation
   Client Need: Safe, Effective Care Environment

8. At a team conference a nurse asks what happens after an infection with the human immunodeficiency virus (HIV). The nurse correctly replies
   1. the virus appears to damage T4 lymphocytes
   2. CD4 surface markers are destroyed by the HIV
   3. the virus invades T8 lymphocytes
   4. autoantibodies are formed

   Nursing Process: Implementation
   Client Need: Safe, Effective Care Environment

9. A nurse asks what AIDS-related complex (ARC) is. The nurse correctly replies that ARC is a group of signs and symptoms present from the time HIV enters the body to the
   1. time the antibody test becomes positive
   2. development of an immune system response
   3. development of opportunistic infections
   4. time when the T4 cell count is above 500

   Nursing Process: Implementation
   Client Need: Safe, Effective Care Environment

10. Which of the following might be noted during a physical assessment or obtained during a history of the client with ARC?
    1. abdominal tenderness, pronounced bradycardia
    2. lymph node enlargement, night sweats
    3. weight gain, edema of the extremities
    4. constipation, anorexia

    Nursing Process: Collecting Data
    Client Need: Physiological Integrity

II. CRITICAL THINKING EXERCISES

1. You work in surgery and have learned that one of your co-workers, a scrub nurse, is HIV-positive. No one else is aware of this fact. Do you think this nurse should be allowed to scrub in surgery when needles and sharp instruments can and do pierce sterile gloves, resulting in a possible transmission of the virus to the surgical client or other co-workers? Give one or more reasons for your answer.

2. John has AIDS and is dissatisfied with the medical care he has been receiving. He tells you that he has heard of a physician in another country who has helped many of those with AIDS—some of whom are said to be cured of the disease. What warnings would you give John regarding seeking treatment from this physician?

3. One of your friends is getting married. She suspects that her fiance has had sexual partners prior to their decision to get married. She asks your advice regarding having her fiance tested for AIDS, even though he has no symptoms of any illness. What advice would you give her and what reason would you give for your advice?

4. Besides observing universal precautions, what other safety measures should the nurse observe when handling needles and sharp instruments?

IX Caring for Clients with Neurological Disorders

42/ Introduction to the Nervous System

The nervous system consists of the brain, spinal cord, and peripheral nerves. It is responsible for coordinating many body functions and responding to changes in or stimuli from the internal and external environment.

The following questions deal with the content of Chapter 42.

I. MULTIPLE CHOICE QUESTIONS

Circle the number of the most appropriate answer.

The nurses on a clinical unit are asked to give conferences on neurological diseases. The first conference is scheduled to cover the anatomy and physiology of the nervous system. Each nurse is encouraged to actively participate in the conferences and review the scheduled topic before the conference.

1. When asked to give the name of the membranes covering the brain, the nurse answers
   1. ventricles
   2. meninges
   3. neurilemma
   4. myelin

   Nursing Process: Implementation
   Client Need: Safe, Effective Care Environment

2. When asked to give the function of the ventricles of the brain, the nurse states that the ventricles
   1. act as passageways for motor neurons
   2. protect the spinal cord
   3. contain the hypothalamus and associated structures
   4. manufacture and absorb cerebrospinal fluid

   Nursing Process: Implementation
   Client Need: Safe, Effective Care Environment

3. When asked by the conference leader for the name of the structure that connects the two hemispheres of the cerebrum, the nurse answers the
   1. hypothalamus
   2. basal ganglia
   3. corpus callosum
   4. thalamus

   Nursing Process: Implementation
   Client Need: Safe, Effective Care Environment

4. When asked to give the function of the cerebellum, the nurse answers that the cerebellum
   1. supports the thalamus
   2. controls and coordinates muscle movement
   3. is a passageway for the sympathetic nervous system
   4. receives impulses from sensory neurons

   Nursing Process: Implementation
   Client Need: Safe, Effective Care Environment

5. When asked to name two neurohormones of the sympathetic nervous system, the nurse answers
   1. acetylcholine and acetylcholinesterase
   2. choline and paracholine
   3. dopamine and choline
   4. epinephrine and norepinephrine

   Nursing Process: Implementation
   Client Need: Safe, Effective Care Environment

6. When asked to name the area where the spinal cord ends, the nurse answers between the
   1. 1st and 2nd lumbar vertebrae
   2. 2nd and 3rd lumbar vertebrae
   3. 4th and 5th thoracic vertebrae
   4. 5th and 6th sacral vertebrae

   Nursing Process: Implementation
   Client Need: Safe, Effective Care Environment

7. When asked the purpose of an electroencephalogram, the nurse answers to
   1. determine blood flow through the cerebral arteries
   2. study the changes in the electrical potential of muscles
   3. determine brain size and activity
   4. obtain a record of the electrical activity of the brain

   Nursing Process: Implementation
   Client Need: Safe, Effective Care Environment

Mr. Breck is admitted with the diagnosis of a possible CVA (cerebrovascular accident).

8. When performing a physical assessment, normal or abnormal function of the 8th cranial nerve can be determined by testing Mr. Breck's
   1. visual acuity and gag reflex
   2. ability to distinguish odors and colors
   3. eye movements and pupil size
   4. hearing and equilibrium

   Nursing Process: Collecting Data
   Client Need: Physiological Integrity

9. When performing a physical assessment, which of the following responses may indicate somnolence or lethargy? Mr. Breck is
   1. aroused only by vigorous and continuous stimulation
   2. drowsy or sleepy at inappropriate times but can be aroused
   3. unresponsive to all but painful stimuli
   4. unable to answer questions

   Nursing Process: Evaluation
   Client Need: Physiological Integrity

10. Which of the following could the nurse use to evaluate Mr. Breck's motor function?
    1. finger-to-nose test with the eyes closed
    2. ability to identify common objects
    3. eliciting a gag reflex
    4. eliciting sensations of pressure and pain

    Nursing Process: Evaluation
    Client Need: Physiological Integrity

11. To evaluate Mr. Breck's 3rd cranial nerve, the nurse tests the
    1. movements of his facial muscles as he frowns and smiles
    2. ability to stand upright with the eyes closed
    3. size and equality of the pupils and their reaction to light
    4. ability to identify substances placed on the anterior tongue

    Nursing Process: Evaluation
    Client Need: Physiological Integrity

12. Mr. Breck is to have a lumbar puncture. Unless directed otherwise, Mr. Breck is placed ____ immediately prior to the procedure.
    1. prone with his head turned to the left
    2. on his side with the head and knees flexed
    3. on his side with the head and knees extended
    4. supine with his head and knees flexed

    Nursing Process: Implementation
    Client Need: Safe, Effective Care Environment

13. When the lumbar puncture is performed, the physician states that Mr. Breck's spinal fluid pressure is 300 mm H_2O. Normal spinal fluid pressure is _____ mm H_2O.
    1. 40 to 80
    2. 80 to 180
    3. 100 to 300
    4. over 300

    Nursing Process: Evaluation
    Client Need: Physiological Integrity

14. Following the lumbar puncture, the nurse
    1. raises the head of the bed 45°
    2. places Mr. Breck in a full Fowler's position
    3. keeps Mr. Breck flat for 3 hours
    4. places Mr. Breck in a prone position

    Nursing Process: Implementation
    Client Need: Safe, Effective Care Environment

15. Mr. Breck is scheduled for a cerebral angiogram. Mr. Breck's family can be told that this test
    1. calculates the speed of blood flow to the brain
    2. determines the size of the brain
    3. measures the depth of the motor cortex
    4. detects distortion of the arteries of the brain

    Nursing Process: Implementation
    Client Need: Safe, Effective Care Environment

16. Prior to a cerebral angiogram the nurse asks if the family if Mr. Breck
    1. is allergic to iodine or seafood
    2. has ever had a chest radiograph
    3. is cooperative
    4. can tolerate some pain or discomfort

    Nursing Process: Implementation
    Client Need: Safe, Effective Care Environment

II. CRITICAL THINKING EXERCISES

1. Ms. Campbell is scheduled for a myelogram. What specific questions are asked when obtaining a history from Ms. Campbell?

2. You are assigned to assist the physician performing a lumbar puncture on Mr. Pickens. What special precautions would you take when preparing samples of CSF for laboratory analysis? Why are these precautions necessary?

3. Mr. Thomas had a cerebral angiogram and has returned to his room. What observations or assessments are performed following this procedure?

43/ Caring for Clients with Central and Peripheral Nervous System Disorders

Some disorders of the central and peripheral nervous system are life-threatening; others, while not life-threatening, have a profound effect on the individual. When any part of the central or peripheral nervous system is damaged, removed, or destroyed, a permanent neurologic deficit can occur.

The following questions deal with the content of Chapter 43.

I. MULTIPLE CHOICE QUESTIONS

Circle the number of the most appropriate answer.

Mr. Ervin is admitted with a diagnosis of a possible brain tumor. On examination he is lethargic and responds poorly to questions. The physician states that Mr. Ervin may be developing increased intracranial pressure (ICP).

1. When assessing Mr. Ervin for signs of increased ICP, the nurse looks for one of the earliest signs of this disorder which is
   1. decortical posturing
   2. a change in the heart rate
   3. assuming a fetal position
   4. a change in the LOC

   Nursing Process: Collecting Data
   Client Need: Physiological Integrity

2. Mr. Ervin's respirations become shallow and rapid, building in intensity and depth, and followed by periods of apnea. The nurse charts this pattern of respirations as ____ respirations.
   1. apnea/dypsnea
   2. Cheyne-Stokes
   3. dypsnea/apnea
   4. Stokes-Adams

   Nursing Process: Implementation
   Client Need: Safe, Effective Care Environment

3. During a report to the next shift, a nurse asks if drugs can be given to reduce cerebral edema and decrease ICP. The most correct response is that cerebral edema may be reduced following the administration of
   1. osmotic diuretics, corticosteroids
   2. vasopressors, anticonvulsants
   3. anticholinergics, tranquilizers
   4. thiazide diuretics, adrenergic agents

   Nursing Process: Implementation
   Client Need: Safe, Effective Care Environment

4. When developing a plan of care for Mr. Ervin, the nurse may help decrease his ICP by
   1. placing him in a full Fowler's position
   2. reducing or eliminating environmental stressors
   3. administering oxygen
   4. encouraging coughing and deep breathing

   Nursing Process: Implementation
   Client Need: Physiological Integrity

5. The impact of the diagnosis has produced a pronounced emotional response. To help Mr. Ervin during this difficult period, the nurse can
   1. allow him time to verbalize his concerns and talk about the situation
   2. give him literature about chemotherapy and radiation therapy
   3. encourage him to socialize with other clients
   4. arrange a visit to the radiation therapy department

   Nursing Process: Implementation
   Client Need: Psychosocial Integrity

Mr. Grant, age 69, has Parkinsonism, an extrapyramidal disorder. He is admitted to the hospital for evaluation of his various problems including fever, multiple pressure ulcers, possible bladder infection, and weight loss. The physician states that he is in the advanced stage of the disease.

6. At a team conference Parkinson's disease is discussed. The nurse is correct in saying that this disorder affects primarily the
   1. midbrain and cerebellum
   2. basal ganglia and their connections
   3. corpus callosum
   4. thalamus and hypothalamus

   Nursing Process: Implementation
   Client Need: Safe, Effective Care Environment

7. When developing a plan of care, the nurse must be aware of the fact that clients with Parkinsonism are subject to
   1. respiratory problems
   2. bleeding disorders
   3. weight gain
   4. leukemia

   Nursing Process: Planning
   Client Need: Safe, Effective Care Environment

8. The initial assessment of Mr. Grant includes a complete neurologic examination to determine
   1. the effects of the disorder on his ability to function
   2. how well he accepts his disease
   3. if his weight loss is due to some other disease or disorder
   4. how he relates to his family

   Nursing Process: Collecting Data
   Client Need: Physiological Integrity

9. One of the major goals Mr. Grant may have is to
   1. understand the purpose of all available treatment modalities
   2. increase his muscle tone and mass and lose excess weight
   3. improve his physical mobility
   4. eliminate the symptoms of the disorder by means of a specialized exercise program

   Nursing Process: Implementation
   Client Need: Health Promotion/Maintenance

10. To prevent problems associated with Parkinsonism, nursing management of Mr. Grant focuses on
    1. eliminating the cause of the tremors
    2. encouraging independence and prolonging dependence
    3. encouraging him to accept his disabilities
    4. encouraging him to improve his ability to walk

    Nursing Process: Planning
    Client Need: Physiological Integrity

11. Which of the following may help prevent muscle contractures in this client?
    1. tepid tub baths twice daily
    2. application of hot soaks to the affected muscles
    3. muscle relaxants
    4. active or passive range-of-motion exercises

    Nursing Process: Implementation
    Client Need: Physiological Integrity

12. Since Mr. Grant has difficulty chewing and swallowing, the nurse
    1. places a suction machine in his room
    2. asks the family to feed Mr. Grant
    3. places him in a chair before meals
    4. restricts his diet to liquids

    Nursing Process: Implementation
    Client Need: Physiological Integrity

Ms. Burke is a 44-year-old secretary who has been admitted to the hospital for evaluation of her dizziness and the recent occurrence of a convulsive seizure. It is determined that Ms. Burke has grand mal epilepsy.

13. At a team conference the nurse is asked to define a seizure. The most correct description is that a seizure is a(n)
    1. abnormal electrical disturbance in one or more specific areas of the brain
    2. interruption of one or more cranial nerve pathways
    3. decrease in electrical activity of the brain
    4. electrical stimulation of higher sensory nerve centers

    Nursing Process: Implementation
    Client Need: Safe, Effective Care Environment

14. If in the room when Ms. Burke has a seizure, the nurse first
    1. applies wrist restraints to prevent injury
    2. places Ms. Burke on her back to prevent airway obstruction
    3. gives oxygen by mask to relieve cyanosis
    4. turns Mrs. Burke on her side to keep the airway patent

    Nursing Process: Implementation
    Client Need: Physiological Integrity

15. If Ms. Burke has a seizure, the nurse records
    1. Ms. Burke's blood pressure during the seizure
    2. the type of body movements during the seizure
    3. what Ms. Burke says she remembers about the seizure
    4. if Ms. Burke says she had pain during the seizure

    Nursing Process: Collecting Data
    Client Need: Physiological Integrity

16. The discharge teaching plan for Ms. Burke includes the danger of omitting or stopping the prescribed drug or drugs. The nurse emphasizes and describes that if she were to omit or suddenly stop her medication, ____ may occur.
    1. status epilepticus
    2. focal seizures
    3. gingival hyperplasia
    4. a change in her EEG pattern

    Nursing Process: Implementation
    Client Need: Health Promotion/Maintenance

Individual Questions

17. During a report to the next shift, a nurse asks what the term *nuchal rigidity* means. The most correct response is that this term is used to describe
    1. difficulty in focusing the eyes, inability to see close objects
    2. stiffness in the arms and legs with loss of muscle tone
    3. pain and stiffness of the neck, inability to place the chin on the chest
    4. inability to turn the head to the side, loss of speech

    Nursing Process: Implementation
    Client Need: Safe, Effective Care Environment

18. When the client has meningitis, the nurse
    1. keeps the client in a side-lying position
    2. forces fluids up to 3000 mL/day
    3. encourages a diet high in proteins
    4. monitors the LOC at frequent intervals

    Nursing Process:
    Client Need: Physiological Integrity

19. A client admitted today with the diagnosis of Guillain-Barré syndrome is closely observed for
    1. any signs of respiratory distress
    2. a marked increase in the blood pressure
    3. signs of skin breakdown
    4. changes in bowel function

    Nursing Process: Collecting Data
    Client Need: Physiological Integrity

20. At a team conference a nurse asks, "What part of the nervous system is affected when a client has Guillain-Barré syndrome?" The most correct response is that this disorder affects the
    1. midbrain and cerebellum
    2. central nervous system and basal ganglia
    3. thalamus and hypothalamus
    4. peripheral nerves and spinal nerve roots

    Nursing Process: Implementation
    Client Need: Safe, Effective Care Environment

21. Which one of the following may be instituted if the client has the potential to develop seizures following an infectious disorder of the central nervous system?
    1. perform ADL early in the morning
    2. encourage an adequate fluid intake
    3. keep activities and noise to a minimum
    4. keep the head of the bed raised 45°

    Nursing Process: Implementation
    Client Need: Safe, Effective Care Environment

22. Which one of the following is contraindicated if a client has increased ICP due to cerebral edema?
    1. doing position changes every 2 hours
    2. monitoring vital signs
    3. elevating the head of the bed
    4. suctioning

    Nursing Process: Implementation
    Client Need: Safe, Effective Care Environment

23. When there is a potential for increased ICP, the nurse advises the client to
    1. avoid straining to have a bowel movement
    2. drink extra fluids
    3. eat a diet high in carbohydrates
    4. sit on the edge of the bed several times a day

    Nursing Process: Implementation
    Client Need: Safe, Effective Care Environment

24. The first step in planning the management of the client with multiple sclerosis is
    1. determining the stage of the disease
    2. identification of the client's needs
    3. evaluating the client's sleep pattern
    4. reviewing all diagnostic tests

    Nursing Process: Planning
    Client Need: Physiological Integrity

25. At a team conference a nurse asks what drug is used in the treatment of myasthenia gravis. The correct reply is
    1. dopamine
    2. an anticholinesterase drug
    3. an adrenergic drug
    4. norepinephrine

    Nursing Process: Implementation
    Client Need: Safe, Effective Care Environment

26. Which of the following may be seen if the dose of the drug used in the treatment of myasthenia gravis is too high?
    1. excessive salivation, flaccid muscles
    2. abdominal distention, hypertension
    3. tachycardia, dyspnea
    4. clenched jaw, muscle rigidity

    Nursing Process: Collecting Data
    Client Need: Physiological Integrity

27. At a team conference a nurse asks, "What are the problems associated with the late stages of amyotrophic lateral sclerosis?" The most correct answer is
    1. hypertension and cardiac failure
    2. respiratory failure and total paralysis
    3. hypovolemia and paralytic ileus
    4. renal failure and seizures

    Nursing Process: Implementation
    Client Need: Safe, Effective Care Environment

28. Clients with a neuromuscular disorder are closely observed for
    1. nuchal rigidity
    2. urinary incontinence
    3. choking when swallowing liquids
    4. an increase in the urinary output

    Nursing Process: Collecting Data
    Client Need: Physiological Integrity

29. Clients with a neuromuscular disorder are observed for signs and symptoms of a respiratory infection because of
    1. their inability to clear respiratory secretions
    2. a rise in their PaO_2
    3. renal failure
    4. an impairment in their immune system

    Nursing Process: Collecting Data
    Client Need: Physiological Integrity

30. When teaching the client with trigeminal neuralgia, the nurse can suggest
    1. avoiding breezes, drafts, excessive talking
    2. eating a diet high in proteins and antioxidants
    3. exercising two to three times a day
    4. avoiding exposure to the sun and warm weather

    Nursing Process: Implementation
    Client Need: Health Promotion/Maintenance

31. Following surgery on the mandibular branch of the trigeminal nerve performed to relieve the pain associated with trigeminal neuralgia, the client is encouraged to
    1. ambulate shortly after surgery
    2. concentrate on chewing, eating, and swallowing
    3. chew on the operative side
    4. warm all food to 110°–120°

    Nursing Process: Implementation
    Client Need: Health Promotion/Maintenance

32. Which one of the following may be used when ptosis and a diminished blink reflex occur in the client with Bell's palsy?
    1. application of glycerin to the eyelids
    2. tape placed over the eyelid to keep it open
    3. an eye patch during the day and protective eye shield at night
    4. warm saline eye soaks

    Nursing Process: Implementation
    Client Need: Safe, Effective Care Environment

33. When a client has a cranial nerve disorder, the food remaining in the mouth after eating may be removed by
    1. using a small forceps
    2. suctioning the oral cavity
    3. offering a mouthwash containing alcohol
    4. using cotton-tipped applicators

    Nursing Process: Implementation
    Client Need: Safe, Effective Care Environment

34. A client in the outpatient clinic is being treated for TMJ (temporomandibular joint syndrome). To prepare a teaching plan, the nurse checks a reference book regarding
    1. postoperative care following removal of the affected joint
    2. hot water mouth irrigations
    3. the method of injecting an antibiotic into the joint
    4. transcutaneous electrical nerve stimulation (TENS)

    Nursing Process: Implementation
    Client Need: Safe, Effective Care Environment

35. A client is diagnosed as having Huntington's disease. At a team conference a nurse asks what part of and how the nervous system is affected by this disorder. The most correct response is

   1. degeneration of the basal ganglia and portions of the cerebral cortex
   2. degeneration of the thalamus and hypothalamus
   3. loss of myelin and the neurilemma from nerve sheaths
   4. absence of acetylcholine from parasympathetic nerve endings

   Nursing Process: Implementation
   Client Need: Safe, Effective Care Environment

II. CRITICAL THINKING EXERCISES

1. Your neighbor Liz is a college student. She was home on spring break and when she returned to school, she became ill and was diagnosed as having meningococcal meningitis. What medical advice would you give her family?

2. Ms. Coleman, age 21, developed grand mal epilepsy following a severe head injury. Although her seizures have been controlled with medication, she periodically stops taking her medication and the seizures return. When talking to Ms. Coleman, she tells you that she doesn't believe she has epilepsy and doesn't need medication. How would you approach this problem of client noncompliance?

3. Your friend Joy Peterson has multiple sclerosis. She is totally dependent on others for her care. A personal care aide is helping Ms. Peterson care for her daughter. When visiting one day, you help turn Joy on her side and note a reddened area on her sacrum. What suggestions could you give Ms. Peterson and the personal care aide to prevent further problems in this area?

44/   Caring for Clients with Cerebrovascular Disorders

Cerebrovascular disease is one of the major medical problems affecting adults. The frequency of cerebrovascular disease increases with age, but these disorders can be found in the young as well as the elderly.

The following questions deal with the content of Chapter 44.

I. MULTIPLE CHOICE QUESTIONS

Circle the number of the most appropriate answer.

Ms. Reese, age 72, is admitted to the hospital by ambulance. Her husband called 911 because she seemed to be suddenly incoherent and was having trouble speaking and moving her left side. Shortly after admission, the diagnosis of a stroke was made by the physician.

1. When talking to the nurse assistant, the nurse explains that a common cause of stroke in the elderly is
    1. untreated varicose veins
    2. hypotension related to medications
    3. atrial fibrillation accompanied by embolus formation
    4. ventricular bradycardia due to heart block

    Nursing Process: Implementation
    Client Need: Safe, Effective Care Environment

2. When performing an initial neurologic assessment on Ms. Reese, the nurse is aware that symptoms of this disorder are
    1. specific and most always the same
    2. not life-threatening
    3. depend on the site of the CVA
    4. depend on the age of the client

    Nursing Process: Collecting Data
    Client Need: Physiological Integrity

3. The nurse helps with planning short-term goals which include
    1. prevention of paralysis
    2. initiation of active exercises on the paralyzed side
    3. relief of pain on the paralyzed side
    4. prevention of contractures and joint deformities

    Nursing Process: Planning
    Client Need: Physiological Integrity

4. Which of the following may be used to help maintain a patent airway until Ms. Reese is more alert?
   1. keeping her in a supine position
   2. suctioning her oral cavity
   3. raising the foot of the bed
   4. keeping her only on the unaffected side

Nursing Process: Implementation
Client Need: Physiological Integrity

5. Ms. Reese had an indwelling catheter inserted at the time of admission. Two weeks later the physician orders the catheter to be removed. At this time the nurse can
   1. get her out of bed at frequent intervals and encourage ambulation
   2. offer the bedpan at 1- to 2-hour intervals and encourage her to void
   3. add more fluids to her meal tray
   4. restrict fluids during the morning hours

Nursing Process: Implementation
Client Need: Health Promotion/Maintenance

6. Ms. Reese is scheduled to be discharged in 1 week. Discharge planning includes
   1. encouraging the family to openly discuss problems created by Ms. Reese's illness
   2. plans to have her transferred to a nursing home
   3. encouraging Mrs. Reese to assume all responsibility for her own care
   4. discussion of the cost of hospitalization

Nursing Process: Implementation
Client Need: Psychosocial Integrity

Ms. Eaton, age 19, is admitted to the emergency department after experiencing a severe headache, visual disturbances, and nausea. Following examination she is diagnosed as having a leaking cerebral aneurysm and is admitted to ICU.

7. Immediately after Ms. Eaton is admitted to ICU, the nurse
   1. suctions her oral cavity to remove all secretions
   2. encourages her to change her position frequently
   3. institutes seizure precautions
   4. encourages her to drink extra fluids

Nursing Process: Implementation
Client Need: Physiological Integrity

8. Ms. Eaton is
   1. closely observed for signs of increased ICP
   2. encouraged to cough and deep breathe every 2 hours
   3. suctioned at frequent intervals
   4. encouraged to exercise her extremities frequently

Nursing Process: Implementation
Client Need: Physiological Integrity

9. Ms. Eaton experiences sensory deprivation. The nurse can relieve this problem by
   1. giving her a newspaper to read
   2. briefly discussing major news events
   3. asking the family to visit more often
   4. encouraging her to participate in her ADL

Nursing Process: Implementation
Client Need: Psychosocial Integrity

10. If Ms. Eaton is not to be turned every 2 hours, pressure ulcers can be prevented by
    1. passive range-of-motion exercises
    2. placing an incontinence pad under her hips
    3. massaging bony prominences
    4. use of a flotation mattress

Nursing Process: Implementation
Client Need: Physiological Integrity

Mr. Forman, age 61, has been showing signs of mental changes such as confusion and memory loss for 3 years. Recently, he has begun to wander away from home and requires supervision of a family member 24 hours a day. Following confirmation of a diagnosis of Alzheimer's disease and discussion with family members, the physician suggests transfer to a nursing home.

11. When explaining Alzheimer's disease to Mr. Forman's family, the nurse is correct in stating that this disorder is characterized by a(n)
    1. regeneration of nerve cells in association and memory areas
    2. decrease in the size of the cerebral cortex and degeneration of nerve cells
    3. sudden change in motor skills and sensory activity
    4. increase in cognitive abilities

    Nursing Process: Implementation
    Client Need: Health Promotion/Maintenance

12. When discussing Alzheimer's disease during a team conference, the nurse is correct in stating that treatment
    1. includes administration of dopamine
    2. is moderately successful if the disease is recognized in its early stages
    3. may require surgical intervention if medical treatment is not successful
    4. is mainly supportive

    Nursing Process: Implementation
    Client Need: Safe, Effective Care Environment

13. Assessment of Mr. Forman includes evaluation of his
    1. electrolyte status
    2. cognitive and motor skills
    3. desire to get better
    4. acceptance of nursing home care

    Nursing Process: Evaluation
    Client Need: Physiological Integrity

14. The nursing diagnoses for Mr. Forman will depend on the
    1. findings of laboratory and diagnostic tests
    2. physician's neurologic examination
    3. results of an MRI or CT scan
    4. assessments made during an initial assessment

    Nursing Process: Planning
    Client Need: Safe, Effective Care Environment

15. Mr. Forman exhibits a great deal of anxiety at certain times during the day. The nurse may be able to reduce Mr. Forman's anxiety by
    1. maintaining a structured daily routine
    2. explaining all treatments and drug therapies
    3. keeping him away from other clients until his anxiety begins to decrease
    4. suggesting that he become more involved in his daily activities

    Nursing Process: Implementation
    Client Need: Psychosocial Integrity

16. Mr. Forman becomes angry and uncooperative when he has to dress or take a shower. At this time the nurse may find it necessary to
    1. force him to at least bathe every other day
    2. suggest that he put on some of his regular clothing
    3. delay or change the situation until he begins to accept this part of his daily routine
    4. show him that other clients with the same problem are capable of getting dressed and bathing

    Nursing Process: Implementation
    Client Need: Psychosocial Integrity

17. At times, Mr. Forman appears to be unable to make his needs known. When this occurs, the nurse can
    1. provide him with a pad and pen so he can communicate with others
    2. take the time to understand what Mr. Forman is trying to say
    3. encourage him to speak slowly and clearly
    4. encourage him to ask questions only when he feels that he can remember what he wants to say

    Nursing Process: Implementation
    Client Need: Safe, Effective Care Environment

18. Daily planning includes physical activity. When physical activity is limited and Mr. Forman responds poorly to stimulation in the environment, he may have a tendency to
    1. sleep during the day and remain awake at night
    2. become more confused during the evening hours
    3. become depressed
    4. show evidence of memory loss and disorientation

    Nursing Process: Planning
    Client Need: Safe, Effective Care Environment

Individual Questions

19. When a client has a history of migraine headaches, the nurse can suggest
    1. lying on the side with the knees flexed
    2. staying in a dark room and keeping noise to a minimum
    3. eliminating beverages or foods containing caffeine
    4. using distraction methods such as watching television

    Nursing Process: Implementation
    Client Need: Health Promotion/Maintenance

20. Transient ischemic attacks (TIAs) are discussed at a team conference. The nurse describes this disorder as
    1. brief, fleeting attacks of neurologic impairment
    2. characterized by an increase in blood pressure
    3. a variant type of epilepsy
    4. sensory impairment in higher cerebral centers

    Nursing Process: Implementation
    Client Need: Safe, Effective Care Environment

21. The nurse, describing treatment of TIAs during the team conference, includes
    1. anticoagulant therapy, carotid endarterectomy
    2. low-cholesterol diet, drugs to dissolve the carotid plaques
    3. antibiotic therapy, physical therapy
    4. anticonvulsant therapy, carotid artery ligation

    Nursing Process: Implementation
    Client Need: Safe, Effective Care Environment

22. When surgery on the carotid artery is performed as treatment for TIAs, the most important postoperative observation is checking the client for
    1. abdominal distention
    2. electrolyte imbalances
    3. signs of neurologic impairment
    4. respiratory alkalosis

    Nursing Process: Collecting Data
    Client Need: Physiological Integrity

II. CRITICAL THINKING EXERCISES

1. Ms. Killian is terminally ill with a frontal lobe brain tumor. She has difficulty performing simple tasks and has periods of confusion. At present, her pain is controlled with PCA. Based on these problems, what specific nursing management would you include in a plan of care for this client?

2. Mr. Wallace suddenly developed a severe headache followed by unconsciousness. He is admitted with a diagnosis of a ruptured cerebral aneurysm. What specific nursing tasks would you include in his care plan to ensure that he is kept as quiet as possible?

3. Mr. Gaines has Alzheimer's disease and is admitted for treatment of severe congestive heart failure. He is confused and not always cooperative when receiving various treatments such as complete bedrest and oral medications. He frequently attempts to get out of bed to go to the bathroom. What can you include in his nursing care plan to reduce his tendency to try and get out of bed to void?

4. Mr. Carnes, age 78, is a client in a nursing home. He had a CVA 1 year ago. This past week he has become withdrawn and does not want to get out of bed and participate in any activities. What nursing measures would you now add to his plan of care?

45/   Caring for Clients with Head and Spinal Cord Trauma

The skull protects the brain. Because of this protection, slight injuries do not affect the brain. A severe blow to the head can cause serious problems such as lacerations, bruises, hemorrhage, and edema of the brain and the tissues that surround the brain. Spinal cord trauma is serious and sometimes fatal. Causes of wounds include automobile accidents, falls, and gunshot wounds. The cervical and lumbar spines are the most common sites of injury.

The following questions deal with the content of Chapter 45.

I. MULTIPLE CHOICE QUESTIONS

Circle the number of the most appropriate answer.

A team conference is held for all members of a head and spinal cord trauma unit. Each member is encouraged to ask as well as answer questions. To prepare for the conference the team leader recommends several references.

1. The nurse is asked to give the cause of an epidural hematoma. The most correct reply is an epidural hematoma results from
    1. arterial bleeding on top of the dura
    2. bleeding from the cerebral veins
    3. bleeding in the circle of Willis
    4. arterial bleeding between the dura mater and pia mater

    Nursing Process: Implementation
    Client Need: Safe, Effective Care Environment

2. The nurse is asked to describe the *most important* nursing task in the management of a client with an epidural hematoma. The most correct response is
    1. checking the extremities for movement
    2. observing for signs of increased ICP
    3. observing for changes in the CVP
    4. checking the Babinski reflex

    Nursing Process: Collecting Data
    Client Need: Physiological Integrity

3. When asked to explain a contusion, the nurse states that a contusion
    1. results in the bruising of cerebral tissue
    2. causes major neurologic symptoms
    3. rarely causes symptoms
    4. results in severe bleeding under the dura

    Nursing Process: Implementation
    Client Need: Safe, Effective Care Environment

4. The nurse is asked to differentiate between epidural and subdural bleeding. The most correct response is that
    1. subdural bleeding is more serious than epidural bleeding
    2. epidural bleeding causes less pressure on the brain than subdural bleeding
    3. subdural bleeding is usually slower than epidural bleeding
    4. epidural bleeding has a lower fatality rate than subdural bleeding

    Nursing Process: Implementation
    Client Need: Safe, Effective Care Environment

5. The nurse is asked what may be used to determine and evaluate the LOC. The correct reply is the
    1. Wyandotte Emotional Scale
    2. Glasgow Coma Scale
    3. Fernandez Determination Levels
    4. Williams Evaluation Record

    Nursing Process: Evaluation
    Client Need: Physiological Integrity

6. The nurse is asked why a corticosteroid preparation is given shortly after trauma to the spinal cord. The most correct response is that this type of drug is given to
   1. relieve pain
   2. reduce spasms in the lower extremities
   3. reduce spinal cord edema
   4. aid in the location of the injury

   Nursing Process: Implementation
   Client Need: Safe, Effective Care Environment

7. The nurse is asked to describe the purpose of intervertebral discs. The best answer is that discs are composed of cartilage that
   1. acts as cushions between vertebrae
   2. protects spinal nerve roots
   3. decreases lower body movement
   4. nourishes the spinal cord

   Nursing Process: Implementation
   Client Need: Safe, Effective Care Environment

8. When asked to give the most common site of a herniated intervertebral disc, the nurse correctly replies the
   1. four lower thoracic discs
   2. three lower lumbar discs
   3. upper thoracic discs
   4. sacral discs

   Nursing Process: Implementation
   Client Need: Safe, Effective Care Environment

9. A nurse asks why diazepam (Valium) is being given to the client with a ruptured intervertebral disc. The most correct answer is that this drug
   1. relaxes smooth muscle
   2. reduces inflammation
   3. has skeletal-muscle-relaxing properties
   4. sedates clients in traction

   Nursing Process: Implementation
   Client Need: Safe, Effective Care Environment

Mr. Rodney is scheduled for a craniotomy for removal of a benign brain tumor. While Mr. Rodney is in surgery, a team conference is held to discuss Mr. Rodney's postoperative care.

10. When asked during a team conference to explain the reason Mr. Rodney received an osmotic diuretic and a corticosteroid before surgery, the nurse answers to
    1. reduce peripheral edema
    2. correct a fluid volume excess
    3. reduce cerebral edema and the ICP
    4. control the blood pressure

    Nursing Process: Implementation
    Client Need: Safe, Effective Care Environment

11. During the team conference a nurse asks why phenytoin (Dilantin) was ordered before and after Mr. Rodney's surgery. The most correct answer is that phenytoin
    1. reduces the risk of convulsive seizures
    2. prevents infection
    3. reduces intracranial pressure
    4. stops intracranial bleeding

    Nursing Process: Implementation
    Client Need: Safe, Effective Care Environment

12. Postoperative rehabilitation of Mr. Rodney is planned to begin
    1. 7 to 10 days after surgery
    2. as soon as he is able to get out of bed
    3. when he expresses a desire to perform more tasks
    4. as soon as he returns from surgery

    Nursing Process: Planning
    Client Need: Physiological Integrity

13. Twenty-four hours after surgery Mr. Rodney is conscious. At this time the nurse
    1. begins to force fluids
    2. encourages deep breathing every hour
    3. has Mr. Rodney turn on his operative side
    4. encourages coughing every hour to keep the airway patent

    Nursing Process: Implementation
    Client Need: Physiological Integrity

14. Mr. Rodney has limited movement of his left upper and lower extremities. Which of the following can be used to prevent complications associated with this problem?
    1. elevation of the head of the bed, sheepskin boots
    2. a flotation mattress, wrist restraints
    3. footboard, trochanter rolls
    4. raising the foot gatch, sheepskin pads

    Nursing Process: Implementation
    Client Need: Physiological Integrity

15. Mr. Rodney may potentially develop the syndrome of inappropriate secretion of antidiuretic hormone (SIADH) which is a secretion of excess antidiuretic hormone. He is observed for signs and symptoms of this disorder which include
    1. water retention
    2. dependent edema
    3. excessive diuresis
    4. low urine specific gravity

    Nursing Process: Collecting Data
    Client Need: Physiological Integrity

David and his father were in an automobile accident. David is believed to have suffered a severe spinal injury. Radiographs and a neurologic examination show that David has an injury to his spinal cord at the lower thoracic level, namely T9 and T10.

16. The most important nursing task immediately following David's admission to the emergency department is
    1. keeping his body and head in alignment and limiting all movement
    2. monitoring vital signs and response of his pupils to light
    3. reassuring him that the physician will examine him shortly
    4. using pulse oximetry to monitor his respirations

    Nursing Process: Implementation
    Client Need: Physiological Integrity

17. In the first weeks following the accident David is observed for signs of spinal shock which include
    1. diarrhea, tachycardia, change in the LOC
    2. hypotension, bradycardia, flaccid paralysis
    3. cool skin, diaphoresis, cardiac arrhythmias
    4. diuresis, cyanosis, spastic paralysis

    Nursing Process: Collecting Data
    Client Need: Physiological Integrity

18. David's spinal cord has been severed and he has permanent paraplegia. Which of the following may be used to increase strength and movement in his upper extremities?
    1. passive repetitive movements of his fingers and hands
    2. overhead bars or a trapeze
    3. massage to his arms and hands
    4. application of arm splints

    Nursing Process: Implementation
    Client Need: Physiological Integrity

Individual Questions

19. Which of the following instructions are given when a client seen in the emergency department for a concussion is to be discharged to the care of the family?
    1. let the client rest undisturbed for the next 24 hours
    2. observe for changes in behavior, speech, or other abnormality for 2-3 days
    3. wake the client every 15 minutes during the night
    4. keep the client awake and sitting in a chair the first night home

    Nursing Process: Implementation
    Client Need: Health Promotion/Maintenance

20. Following a significant head injury, clients are detained in the hospital and observed for signs of
    1. hypernatremia
    2. decreased ICP
    3. a fluid volume excess
    4. increased ICP

    Nursing Process: Collecting Data
    Client Need: Physiological Integrity

21. When assessing a client with a head injury, the nurse notes that clear cerebrospinal fluid is seen draining from the ear. The physician is notified at once because this may be an indication of a
    1. simple skull fracture
    2. epidural hematoma
    3. ruptured cerebral veins
    4. basilar fracture

    Nursing Process: Collecting Data
    Client Need: Physiological Integrity

22. Which one of the following is the *most important* when obtaining the initial history when the client has had a head injury?
    1. the time and cause of the injury
    2. who caused the injury
    3. why the injury occurred
    4. who was present at the time of the injury

    Nursing Process: Collecting Data
    Client Need: Physiological Integrity

23. When a client has had a head injury, a patent airway is essential because
    1. bronchial constriction may develop
    2. airway obstruction results in a decrease in carbon dioxide
    3. the brain is sensitive to a lack of oxygen
    4. the ICP will decrease

    Nursing Process: Implementation
    Client Need: Physiological Integrity

24. Which of the following is not performed if the client has increased ICP due to intracranial bleeding following a head injury?
    1. deep breathing every 1 to 2 hours
    2. turning the client on the uninjured side
    3. suctioning to clear the mouth of mucus
    4. monitoring intake and output

    Nursing Process: Implementation
    Client Need: Physiological Integrity

25. When assessing the head-injured client, mental changes may indicate
    1. increased ICP, pain
    2. increased cerebral perfusion, nausea
    3. nuchal rigidity, a full bladder
    4. decreased ICP, cerebral edema

    Nursing Process: Collecting Data
    Client Need: Physiological Integrity

26. Which one of the following areas of a spinal cord injury requires observing the client for the signs and symptoms of autonomic dysreflexia? Injury to the
    1. lumbar spine
    2. lumbar-sacral spine
    3. thoracic-lumbar spine
    4. cervical or high thoracic spine

    Nursing Process: Collecting Data
    Client Need: Physiological Integrity

27. If a client has the potential for developing autonomic dysreflexia, the nurse looks for
    1. hypotension, tachycardia, cyanosis
    2. severe hypertension, bradycardia, pale skin
    3. projectile vomiting, irregular pulse, urticaria
    4. skin rash, abdominal distention, diarrhea

    Nursing Process: Collecting Data
    Client Need: Physiological Integrity

28. When administering intramuscular or subcutaneous injections to the client with a spinal cord injury, the nurse should give the injection
    1. below the level of paralysis
    2. in the gluteus muscle
    3. above the level of paralysis
    4. in the vastus lateralis muscle

    Nursing Process: Implementation
    Client Need: Physiological Integrity

29. The most common type of pain described by the client with a ruptured intervertebral disc in the lumbar region is pain
    1. radiating along the inner thigh
    2. across the lower lumbar region
    3. radiating from the back to the anterior abdomen
    4. along the distribution of the sciatic nerve

    Nursing Process: Collecting Data
    Client Need: Physiological Integrity

30. Hypercalcemia in those with extended immobility may be prevented by
    1. encouraging foods low in fiber
    2. increasing the fluid intake to 3 L/day
    3. giving foods high in calcium
    4. adding foods low in vitamin D to the diet

    Nursing Process: Implementation
    Client Need: Physiological Integrity

31. During the immediate postoperative period the client having chemonucleolysis for a ruptured intervertebral disc is observed for
    1. an anaphylactic reaction
    2. wound infection
    3. excessive diuresis
    4. abdominal pain

    Nursing Process: Collecting Data
    Client Need: Physiological Integrity

II. CRITICAL THINKING EXERCISES

1. Mr. Neil, a 41-year-old construction worker, is admitted to the hospital because of a severe headache, diplopia, and bizarre behavior. His symptoms have been occurring for the past 6 months. What neurologic assessments would you perform? In order to obtain a more thorough history, what questions would you ask regarding his occupation?

2. Ms. Babcock was hit by a car and brought to the emergency department. The physician suspects an epidural hematoma, puts in a call for a neurosurgeon, and tells you to get Ms. Babcock ready for emergency burr holes. What preoperative preparations would you perform?

3. Robert, who is 19, is a paraplegic following a motorcycle accident 4 weeks ago. What devices or tasks could you use to prevent pressure ulcers from forming on his heels?

4. Two days ago Mr. Deaver incurred a moderately severe head injury and is admitted for observation. He is in a semi-private room. Both he and the other client, who had gallbladder surgery yesterday, ask for something for pain. Another nurse gave both clients the analgesics. After administering the drugs the nurse realizes that a medication error has been made. Mr. Deaver was given morphine 0.1 mg IM and the other client codeine sulfate 30 mg PO. Besides this being a serious medication error, what problems are associated with giving morphine to Mr. Deaver?

46/   Caring for Clients with Neurologic Deficits

The client with a neurologic deficit is faced with many problems. While the cause of the deficit may vary, the results are essentially the same: The client is unable to perform tasks in the same manner as before the deficit occurred.

Disorders that cause a neurologic deficit may begin slowly, have few or vague symptoms, and progress through stages of remission and exacerbation. The disorder may begin with a chronic phase, but then periodic episodes of an acute phase may be seen. Other neurologic disorders begin with an injury or a client appearing acutely ill and then may progress from an acute phase to a recovery phase to a chronic phase.

The following questions deal with the content of Chapter 46.

I. MULTIPLE CHOICE QUESTIONS

Circle the number of the most appropriate answer.

1. During the acute phase, basic rehabilitation is planned
   1. once vital signs are stable
   2. as soon as the client is admitted to the hospital
   3. when the cause of the neurologic deficit is known
   4. once permission is given by the physician

   Nursing Process: Planning
   Client Need: Physiological Integrity

2. The nurse recognizes the importance of reporting any changes in the client's blood pressure during the acute phase because maintaining the blood pressure is necessary to
   1. allow fluids to be administered intravenously
   2. prevent skin breakdown
   3. ensure adequate cerebral oxygenation
   4. fully aerate the lungs

   Nursing Process: Evaluation
   Client Need: Physiological Integrity

3. During the recovery phase rehabilitation of the client is planned to
   1. return the client to normal function
   2. meet the client's immediate and long-term needs
   3. prevent further neurologic deficits
   4. help the family accept the disability

   Nursing Process: Planning
   Client Need: Health Promotion/Maintenance

4. When explaining the chronic phase of a neurologic deficit to a nurse assistant during a team conference, the nurse describes this phase as one in which the client
   1. shows little or no evidence of improvement
   2. cannot profit from rehabilitation
   3. no longer requires a structured rehabilitation program
   4. receives most care from family members

   Nursing Process: Implementation
   Client Need: Safe, Effective Care Environment

5. Physical and psychological rehabilitation during the chronic phase is planned primarily to
   1. enhance full recovery
   2. prevent further paralysis
   3. prevent complications
   4. correct other medical problems

   Nursing Process: Planning
   Client Need: Physiological Integrity

6. Nursing management during the chronic phase is planned to
   1. return the client to normal or near-normal physical activity
   2. prevent further neurologic deficits
   3. identify the causes of the neurologic deficits
   4. prevent complications associated with permanent neurologic deficits

   Nursing Process: Planning
   Client Need: Physiological Integrity

7. Respiratory complications may be avoided by
   1. frequent position changes
   2. suctioning the oral cavity every hour
   3. increasing the fluid intake
   4. encouraging exercises of the extremities

   Nursing Process: Implementation
   Client Need: Physiological Integrity

8. Pain is evaluated carefully since it may be a warning
   1. that the analgesic is ineffective
   2. of an allergy to the analgesic
   3. of events such as an infection or distended bladder
   4. that the client should not be receiving a narcotic

   Nursing Process: Evaluation
   Client Need: Physiological Integrity

9. Contractures can be prevented by
   1. use of a flotation pad
   2. keeping the extremities in alignment
   3. encouraging active exercise of the paralyzed side
   4. use of sheepskin boots

   Nursing Process: Implementation
   Client Need: Physiological Integrity

10. During the chronic phase elastic stockings may be applied to
    1. prevent arterial aneurysms in the extremities
    2. maintain the blood pressure
    3. prevent edema
    4. enhance venous blood return to the major veins

    Nursing Process: Implementation
    Client Need: Physiological Integrity

11. Because severe, prolonged illness can result in the development of stress ulcers, the nurse includes in the plan of care

    1. inspection of the skin for evidence of breakdown
    2. periodic evaluation of the client's behavior
    3. inspection of each stool for evidence of bleeding
    4. measurement of the urinary output

    Nursing Process: Planning
    Client Need: Physiological Integrity

12. To prevent constipation the nurse adds to the care plan

    1. passive ROM exercises every 4 hours
    2. increasing the fluid intake by encouraging fluids
    3. encouraging recreational and diversional activities
    4. elimination of fiber from the diet

    Nursing Process: Planning
    Client Need: Physiological Integrity

13. When intermittent catheterization is used for urinary retention and incontinence, the nurse plans to perform the procedure every ____ hours throughout the waking hours.

    1. 2
    2. 4
    3. 6
    4. 8

    Nursing Process: Planning
    Client Need: Physiological Integrity

14. When a client is to be catheterized for residual urine, the nurse plans to catheterize the client

    1. every 4 to 8 hours
    2. immediately after the client voids
    3. 1 hour after the client voids
    4. every 2 hours

    Nursing Process: Planning
    Client Need: Physiological Integrity

15. The temperature of the enema solution administered to a paraplegic or quadriplegic client is checked immediately prior to administration because the

    1. solution must be cold in order to be effective
    2. solution must be above 110° in order to be effective
    3. bowel mucosa may be affected if the solution is body temperature
    4. client cannot feel if the solution is too warm

    Nursing Process: Implementation
    Client Need: Physiological Integrity

16. If the client quickly expels a suppository used to establish a regular voiding pattern the nurse can

    1. tape the buttocks together to help retain the suppository
    2. place the client in a supine position and place a pad under the buttocks
    3. insert a small cotton ball into the rectum just beyond the rectal sphincter
    4. insert a rectal tube 3 inches beyond the rectal sphincter

    Nursing Process: Implementation
    Client Need: Physiological Integrity

17. The nurse can reduce anxiety associated with problems such as difficulty breathing or swallowing by

    1. frequent nurse-client contact
    2. offering to stay with the client until anxiety is relieved
    3. asking the family to spend more time with the client
    4. having another client sit by the bedside

    Nursing Process: Implementation
    Client Need: Psychosocial Integrity

18. When doing discharge teaching, which type of food can the nurse recommend to the family to keep tissues healthy, prevent or heal pressure ulcers, and increase the ability of tissues to heal?

    1. carbohydrates
    2. fats
    3. proteins
    4. vitamin B

    Nursing Process: Implementation
    Client Need: Health Promotion/Maintenance

II. CRITICAL THINKING EXERCISES

1. A bowel training program is to be started for Mr. Graves who is paralyzed from the waist down following a swimming pool accident. What data would you first attempt to obtain before beginning a bowel training program? Why is this information necessary?

2. A bladder training program is to be started for Ms. Roberts who has had a CVA. Ms. Roberts has not been totally incontinent and does have some control over her voiding. She requires assistance in getting out of bed and has been using a bedside commode during the day and a bedpan at night. What initial steps of a training program would you include in her plan of care? If the Credé maneuver is to be used, how would you demonstrate this to her?

3. Mr. Morrow had a CVA 6 months ago and has regained partial use of his right arm and leg. He is right-handed and has difficulty with tasks such as eating and combing his hair. How could you modify the things used for ADL so that Mr. Morrow will regain some ability to perform one or more of these basic activities?

X   Caring for Clients with Sensory Problems

47/   Introduction to the Special Senses

The eye is the sense organ for sight. The ear is the sense organ for hearing and equilibrium. In order for images to be seen, sound to be heard, and balance maintained, sensory information is transmitted over neural pathways to the brain.

The following questions deal with the content of Chapter 47.

I. MULTIPLE CHOICE QUESTIONS

Circle the number of the most appropriate answer.

Margaret Sawyer, 75 years of age, is being interviewed by the nurse prior to being examined by an ophthalmologist. The nurse makes an attempt to provide her with as much health teaching as possible so that she can understand the plan for her care.

1. The nurse would be most correct in explaining that the structures in the eye are anatomically divided into the
   1. right and left orbits
   2. upper and lower segments
   3. visual and sensory pathways
   4. anterior and posterior chambers

   Nursing Process: Implementation
   Client Need: Health Promotion/Maintenance

2. The best evidence that the client has understood the nurse's explanation of vision is if the client indicates that the structure of the eye that converts light to electrical energy is called the
   1. sclera
   2. choroid
   3. retina
   4. lens

   Nursing Process: Evaluation
   Client Need: Health Promotion/Maintenance

3. During Ms. Sawyer's physical assessment, if the nurse felt a need to assess for jaundice, the structure that would be most appropriate to inspect is the
   1. iris
   2. sclera
   3. cornea
   4. conjunctiva

   Nursing Process: Implementation
   Client Need: Physiological Integrity

4. The nurse would be most accurate in telling Ms. Sawyer that colors are perceived due to the function of retinal nerve cells called
   1. macula
   2. trabeculae
   3. rods
   4. cones

   Nursing Process: Implementation
   Client Need: Health Promotion/Maintenance

5. Ms. Sawyer understands the nurse's explanation of accommodation if she refers to it as a process in which the
   1. choroid turns darker
   2. iris gets thinner
   3. lens changes shape
   4. pupil becomes smaller

   Nursing Process: Evaluation
   Client Need: Health Promotion/Maintenance

Nurses who are employed in an ear, nose, and throat clinic attend a team conference to review the anatomy of the ear and the types of tests that clients commonly undergo.

6. During the conference, the best evidence that a nurse understands the structure ultimately responsible for transmitting sound into electrical energy and sending it to the brain is the correlation of this function with the
   1. cochlear branch of the vestibulocochlear nerve
   2. afferent branch of the glossopharyngeal nerve
   3. efferent branch of the hypoglossal nerve
   4. postsynaptic branch of the trigeminal nerve

   Nursing Process: Implementation
   Client Need: Safe, Effective Care Environment

7. When asked during the conference to identify the waxy substance that lubricates the ear canal, the correct answer is
   1. aqueous fluid
   2. vitreous fluid
   3. cerumen
   4. sebum

   Nursing Process: Implementation
   Client Need: Safe, Effective Care Environment

8. The leader asks one of the nurses attending the conference to identify the structure that connects the pharynx with the middle ear. The correct answer is the
   1. eustachian tube
   2. semicircular canals
   3. acoustic meatus
   4. fovea centralis

   Nursing Process: Implementation
   Client Need: Safe, Effective Care Environment

Individual Questions

9. When the nurse examines a client's eyes with an ophthalmoscope, the macula is best identified as an area in the retina in which
   1. there are no blood vessels
   2. the iris meets the cornea
   3. there is a ring of drainage channels
   4. many blood vessels enter the eye

   Nursing Process: Assessment
   Client Need: Physiological Integrity

10. The family history is especially important for the nurse to assess to determine a client's predisposition to developing
    1. cataracts
    2. glaucoma
    3. conjunctivitis
    4. astigmatism

    Nursing Process: Assessment
    Client Need: Safe, Effective Care Environment

11. When inspecting the eyes, the nurse shines a light into each eye and expects that
    1. tears will be produced
    2. the eyelid will open widely
    3. the pupils will get smaller
    4. the lens will look opaque

    Nursing Process: Assessment
    Client Need: Physiological Integrity

12. If a client with an eye abrasion is examined after fluorescein dye eyedrops have been instilled, the area of trauma will most likely appear
    1. bright yellow-green
    2. dull purplish-red
    3. light grayish-white
    4. dark bluish-black

    Nursing Process: Assessment
    Client Need: Physiological Integrity

13. A client asks the nurse to explain what the physician meant when she was told she had 20/70 vision in her right eye. The best answer is that the client can see
    1. at 70 feet what others with normal vision see at a distance of 20 feet
    2. at 20 feet what others with normal vision see at a distance of 70 feet
    3. letters that are between 20 to 70 millimeters in size
    4. clearly within a range of 20 to 70 feet from the eyes

    Nursing Process: Implementation
    Client Need: Health Promotion/Maintenance

14. To examine a client's ability to see in the distance, the nurse would plan to use a(n)
    1. Ishihara plate
    2. Jaeger chart
    3. Snellen chart
    4. Goldmann perimeter

    Nursing Process: Planning
    Client Need: Safe, Effective Care Environment

15. If a nurse utilized Ishihara plates during the assessment of a client's vision, the most appropriate instruction would be to ask the client to
    1. read the largest line of print possible
    2. read the smallest line of print possible
    3. identify the number within a colored circle
    4. indicate how many fingers are being held up

    Nursing Process: Implementation
    Client Need: Safe, Effective Care Environment

16. During a routine ophthalmic evaluation, the instrument the nurse would plan on having in readiness so the physician can measure the client's intraocular pressure is a(n)
    1. slit lamp
    2. retinoscope
    3. ophthalmoscope
    4. tonometer

    Nursing Process: Planning
    Client Need: Safe, Effective Care Environment

17. A client tells the nurse that he hears noises like buzzing or whistling which no one else hears. The best term to use when documenting this finding is
    1. fremitus
    2. tinnitus
    3. tenesmus
    4. crepitus

    Nursing Process: Implementation
    Client Need: Safe, Effective Care Environment

18. Which one of the following findings is most indicative that a client has had a hearing impairment since early childhood? The client
    1. has seasonal allergies
    2. uses a hearing aid
    3. mispronounces words
    4. has impacted cerumen

    Nursing Process: Assessment
    Client Need: Physiological Integrity

19. To grossly test a client's hearing, it would be appropriate to have the client
    1. repeat words whispered from a distance of 1 or 2 feet
    2. listen and identify some common sounds, like a fire engine
    3. adjust the sound on the television to a comfortable level
    4. identify a familiar tune whistled or hummed by the nurse

    Nursing Process: Assessment
    Client Need: Physiological Integrity

20. When a nurse reviews the results of a client's audiometric examination, which one of the following indicates that the client has profoundly impaired hearing? The client hears sounds at the level of
    1. 0–25 dB
    2. 31–55 dB
    3. 56–70 dB
    4. 91–110 dB

    Nursing Process: Assessment
    Client Need: Physiological Integrity

21. When reporting to the nurses on the next shift, a nurse uses which term as most appropriate for describing the quivering movement of the eyes which occurred when a client underwent a caloric stimulation test?
    1. nystagmus
    2. tremulous
    3. oculogyrus
    4. monomphalus

    Nursing Process: Implementation
    Client Need: Safe, Effective Care Environment

22. Which location would be appropriate to palpate when examining a client with symptoms of ear discomfort?
    1. behind the ear
    2. tympanic membrane
    3. oval window
    4. within the ear

    Nursing Process: Assessment
    Client Need: Physiological Integrity

23. When using an otoscope, the normal appearance of the tympanic membrane is
    1. pearly gray
    2. beefy red
    3. metallic blue
    4. creamy yellow

    Nursing Process: Assessment
    Client Need: Physiological Integrity

24. A client's pupils have been dilated to facilitate an ophthalmic examination. Which one of the following would be most appropriate for preventing discomfort following the test?
    1. open the shades to provide more light
    2. patch both eyes for at least 24 hours
    3. furnish the client with dark glasses
    4. place the client in a supine position

    Nursing Process: Implementation
    Client Need: Physiological Integrity

25. A nursing assistant is to ambulate a client whose eyes are bilaterally patched. Which instruction by the nurse is most appropriate?
    1. "Have the client take your elbow and follow you."
    2. "Take the client's elbow and walk beside him."
    3. "Describe the environment and let the client walk independently."
    4. "Watch the client from afar and warn him if there are any hazards in the way."

    Nursing Process: Implementation
    Client Need: Safe, Effective Care Environment

26. When caring for a client who has both eyes patched, which one of the following actions should take place first? The nurse should
    1. touch the client before speaking
    2. check the client's wristband
    3. speak upon entering the room
    4. raise the head of the bed

    Nursing Process: Implementation
    Client Need: Psychosocial Integrity

27. To facilitate communication with a client whose hearing is mildly impaired, it would be best to
    1. shout into the affected ear
    2. reduce unnecessary noise
    3. use pantomime as much as possible
    4. ask if the client understands sign language

    Nursing Process: Implementation
    Client Need: Safe, Effective Care Environment

II. CRITICAL THINKING EXERCISES

1. When examining Mr. Mark Stevens, 27 years old, the nurse observes that his eyes do not appear symmetrical. How would the nurse proceed to determine whether Mr. Stevens' extraocular muscles are functioning properly?

2. How would a Rinne and Weber test be performed?

3. What information would be appropriate to tell a client who is given fluorescein dye intravenously during a diagnostic eye examination?

4. When preparing a client with a hearing impairment for a diagnostic test, what actions would help facilitate the client's comprehension of the instructions?

48/   Caring for Clients with Disorders of the Eye and Ear

Vision and hearing disorders are common among adults. Refraction errors and some forms of hearing loss may be corrected with optical lenses or hearing aids. More serious diseases of the eye and ear require medical and surgical treatment. The nurse's role includes assessing vision and hearing, referring clients with problems to specialized professionals for further diagnostic tests, implementing first aid measures for clients who sustain trauma, administering medically prescribed therapy, caring for surgically treated clients, and providing health teaching.

The following questions deal with the content of Chapter 48.

I. MULTIPLE CHOICE QUESTIONS

Circle the number of the most appropriate answer.

1. A client is interested in making an appointment with a physician who specializes in diagnosing and treating eye disorders. It would be most appropriate for the nurse to refer the client to a(n)
    1. optometrist
    2. optician
    3. ophthalmologist
    4. ocularist

    Nursing Process: Implementation
    Client Need: Safe, Effective Care Environment

2. The nurse would be most correct in explaining to a client who requires reading glasses at age 40, that the visual impairment that results in a gradual loss of elasticity of the lens as individuals age is called
    1. astigmatism
    2. myopia
    3. presbyopia
    4. hyperopia

    Nursing Process: Implementation
    Client Need: Safe, Effective Care Environment

3. When assessing a client with hyperopia, which one of the following is the nurse likely to observe? The client
    1. brings objects close to the eyes to see them
    2. wears thick, concave-shaped corrective lenses
    3. sees halos around lights, especially at night
    4. sees objects at a distance with greater clarity

    Nursing Process: Assessment
    Client Need: Physiological Integrity

4. The nurse would be most correct in explaining to a client that refractive errors, like hyperopia, are usually managed with
   1. laser therapy
   2. corrective lenses
   3. ophthalmic drugs
   4. corneal transplants

   Nursing Process: Implementation
   Client Need: Safe, Effective Care Environment

5. A visually impaired client needs more teaching if he says that at a rehabilitation center for the blind, he may be able to learn
   1. skills for independent living
   2. how to drive an automobile
   3. use a cane for mobility
   4. read and write Braille

   Nursing Process: Evaluation
   Client Need: Health Promotion/Maintenance

6. A client understands the physician's explanation of an incisional radial keratotomy if he says that
   1. the cornea will be reshaped to eliminate the need for glasses
   2. the lens will be shattered and removed by suction
   3. an additional drainage channel will be made in the iris
   4. fluid will be drained from between the retina and choroid

   Nursing Process: Evaluation
   Client Need: Safe, Effective Care Environment

7. If a client with a visual impairment cannot read the letters on a Snellen chart or perceive motion, what else would be most important for the nurse to assess at this time?
   1. depth perception
   2. color perception
   3. ability to see light
   4. ability to see numbers

   Nursing Process: Assessment
   Client Need: Physiological Integrity

8. Which one of the following would be most important to preserve when caring for a client with a visual impairment?
   1. independence
   2. creativity
   3. skin integrity
   4. motor skills

   Nursing Process: Planning
   Client Need: Safe, Effective Care Environment

9. When providing a dietary tray for a client who is visually impaired, the best nursing approach would be to
   1. feed the client
   2. observe how the client eats
   3. open containers and describe where food is located
   4. combine all the food together and serve it in a bowl

   Nursing Process: Implementation
   Client Need: Physiological Integrity

10. A client has just been told that his vision is not likely to be restored. The best nursing approach at this time is to
    1. try to cheer the client with something pleasant
    2. acknowledge the grief that the client is feeling
    3. explain all of the benefits available to the disabled
    4. inform the client of his anti-discrimination rights

    Nursing Process: Implementation
    Client Need: Psychosocial Integrity

11. To improve a permanently blind client's self-esteem, it would be best for the nurse to
    1. delay offering help until the client asks for assistance
    2. teach the client several rehabilitation skills each day
    3. refer the client for disability insurance
    4. call attention to the client's competencies

    Nursing Process: Implementation
    Client Need: Psychosocial Integrity

12. Which one of the following would be the best nursing intervention to add to the plan of care for a client who is visually impaired?
    1. encourage the client to be up and about
    2. keep overhead lights dimly lit at all times
    3. keep room furniture in the same location
    4. leave doors partially open on all rooms

    Nursing Process: Planning
    Client Need: Safe, Effective Care Environment

13. Which of the following could the nurse inform a visually impaired client are available at most public libraries?
    1. Braille typewriters and books in Braille
    2. books in large print and audiocassettes
    3. card catalogs with voice-assisted directories
    4. optical scanners with synthesized voice

    Nursing Process: Implementation
    Client Need: Health Promotion/Maintenance

14. A client has just received a pair of corrective eyeglasses with plastic lenses. Which of the following instructions is appropriate for their care?
    1. store glasses in a case when not worn
    2. clean the lenses once each week
    3. use hot water and bleach for cleaning
    4. dry the lenses with paper tissues

    Nursing Process: Implementation
    Client Need: Health Promotion/Maintenance

15. Which one of the following is most indicative that a client has sustained a fracture of the bony orbit around the eye?
    1. The client cannot read the Snellen chart.
    2. The client describes seeing double images.
    3. There is blood beneath the conjunctiva.
    4. The pupil does not respond to light.

    Nursing Process: Assessment
    Client Need: Physiological Integrity

16. If a client is brought to the hospital following an eye injury, which of the following would the nurse have in readiness so that the physician could locate a possible foreign body?
    1. tonometer
    2. retinoscope
    3. a strong magnet
    4. fluorescein dye

    Nursing Process: Planning
    Client Need: Safe, Effective Care Environment

17. If a client sustains an eye injury at work, but resists letting the industrial nurse assess it, the best action the nurse can take is to
    1. loosely patch the eye and contact the physician
    2. hold the eyelid apart and inspect the eye
    3. press on the eyelid to assess discomfort
    4. tape the eyelid tightly shut and send to the ER

    Nursing Process: Implementation
    Client Need: Physiological Integrity

18. If a chemical is splashed into the eye, the most appropriate first aid measure the nurse could perform is to
    1. inspect the cornea for redness
    2. flush the eye with tap water
    3. cover the eye with a sterile patch
    4. instill topical anesthetic eye drops

    Nursing Process: Implementation
    Client Need: Physiological Integrity

19. Which one of the following is the most important nursing action for reducing the potential for an eye infection?
    1. take the client's temperature daily
    2. monitor the client's white cell count
    3. keep the eye patched while injured
    4. perform thorough handwashing

    Nursing Process: Implementation
    Client Need: Safe, Effective Care Environment

20. Where is the best location for instilling eye medications?
    1. directly onto the exposed cornea
    2. in the nasal corner of the eyelid
    3. within the lower conjunctival sac
    4. in the outer corner of the eyelid

    Nursing Process: Implementation
    Client Need: Physiological Integrity

21. When irrigating the eye, the flow of the solution is instilled
    1. in a temporal to nasal direction
    2. in a nasal to temporal direction
    3. under the upper conjunctival sac
    4. within the lower conjunctival sac

    Nursing Process: Implementation
    Client Need: Safe, Effective Care Environment

22. If a client has an infectious type of conjunctivitis, which of the following would be the best recommendation?
    1. consume fruits and vegetables that are high in vitamin A
    2. wash your face morning and night with antibacterial soap
    3. do not share face cloths and towels in common with others
    4. get a minimum of at least 8 hours of sleep each night

    Nursing Process: Implementation
    Client Need: Health Promotion/Maintenance

23. If a client describes symptoms of photophobia, which one of the following would be most appropriate to recommend?
    1. patching the eyes bilaterally
    2. wearing darkened sunglasses
    3. staying indoors on sunny days
    4. instilling saline eyedrops

    Nursing Process: Implementation
    Client Need: Health Promotion/Maintenance

24. If a client had blepharitis, which assessment finding is the nurse most likely to obtain? The client
    1. describes having double vision
    2. has severe eye pain in both eyes
    3. has patchy flakes on the eyelashes
    4. has difficulty reading small print

    Nursing Process: Assessment
    Client Need: Physiological Integrity

25. In regard to the laboratory test result on the culture taken from a client's sty (hordeolum), the microorganism that is most likely causing the disorder is
    1. *Neisseria gonorrhoeae*
    2. *Chlamydia trachomatis*
    3. *Mycobacterium tuberculosis*
    4. *Staphylococcus aureus*

    Nursing Process: Assessment
    Client Need: Physiological Integrity

26. The best evidence that a client understands the primary treatment for a chalazion is if he states he should
    1. keep his eye patched
    2. massage the eyelid
    3. instill mydriatic drops
    4. apply antibiotic ointment

    Nursing Process: Evaluation
    Client Need: Health Promotion/Maintenance

27. What health teaching is most appropriate for a client who has frequent conjunctivitis?
    1. stop using mascara
    2. wear a sleep mask
    3. avoid direct sunlight
    4. give up your pet cat

    Nursing Process: Implementation
    Client Need: Health Promotion/Maintenance

28. The most common chief complaint of a client with macular degeneration is that
    1. there are frequent headaches
    2. the eyes tear continuously
    3. central vision is lost
    4. peripheral vision is lost

    Nursing Process: Assessment
    Client Need: Physiological Integrity

29. A client with open-angle glaucoma makes all of the following statements. Which one indicates that the client needs more teaching? The client says
    1. glaucoma results from high intraocular pressure
    2. there is an excess of aqueous fluid in the eye
    3. if untreated, the disease can lead to blindness
    4. his vision will improve with corrective lenses

    Nursing Process: Evaluation
    Client Need: Health Promotion/Maintenance

30. The client with glaucoma understands the effect of pilocarpine eye drops when he says this drug will
    1. dilate his pupils
    2. constrict his pupils
    3. elongate the eyeball
    4. shorten the eyeball

    Nursing Process: Evaluation
    Client Need: Health Promotion/Maintenance

31. A client with angle-closure glaucoma understands when to contact the physician if he says he should immediately report
    1. sudden loss of vision
    2. inability to see colors
    3. gaps in the visual field
    4. spots floating before his eyes

    Nursing Process: Evaluation
    Client Need: Health Promotion/Maintenance

32. If all of the following drugs are prescribed for a client with glaucoma, which one should the nurse withhold until checking with the physician?
    1. nafcillin (Unipen)
    2. cimetidine (Tagamet)
    3. codeine sulfate
    4. atropine sulfate

    Nursing Process: Implementation
    Client Need: Physiological Integrity

33. If a client with glaucoma makes all of the following statements, which one indicates that the client needs more teaching? The client says he should
    1. not lift heavy objects
    2. wear a Medic-Alert bracelet
    3. administer extra eyedrops if eye pain develops
    4. avoid straining when having a bowel movement

    Nursing Process: Evaluation
    Client Need: Health Promotion/Maintenance

34. During the postoperative care of a client who has had a cataract extracted, which one of the following is most important to report immediately?
    1. The client sees light with the operative eye.
    2. There is excessive tearing from the operative eye.
    3. There is pain within the operative eye.
    4. The operative eye looks red and irritated.

    Nursing Process: Implementation
    Client Need: Physiological Integrity

35. Following cataract surgery, which one of the following positions would be most appropriate for the client?
    1. keeping the head elevated
    2. maintaining a Sims' position
    3. laying on the operative side
    4. having the client lie prone

    Nursing Process: Implementation
    Client Need: Physiological Integrity

36. If the nurse observes a postoperative client with a cataract extraction doing all of the following, for which one would it be appropriate to intervene? The client
    1. watches television
    2. uses the telephone
    3. bends forward
    4. feeds himself

    Nursing Process: Implementation
    Client Need: Safe, Effective Care Environment

37. Which one of the following assessment findings is most indicative of a retinal detachment?
    1. The client sees flashes of light.
    2. The client cannot see light at all.
    3. The client has a rock-hard eyeball.
    4. The client's eye looks bloody.

    Nursing Process: Assessment
    Client Need: Physiological Integrity

38. Prior to a scleral buckling procedure, it would be most appropriate for the nurse to
    1. enforce strict bedrest before surgery
    2. provide assistance during ambulation
    3. let the client move about at will
    4. provide activity in a wheelchair

    Nursing Process: Implementation
    Client Need: Safe, Effective Care Environment

39. A client who is about to undergo an enucleation correctly understands the prosthetic replacement if he describes it as looking like a
    1. golf ball
    2. large marble
    3. painted shell
    4. stuffed olive

    Nursing Process: Evaluation
    Client Need: Safe, Effective Care Environment

40. It has been determined that a client has sensorineural hearing loss. If the client's history includes all of the following, which one is most likely the underlying cause for this client's hearing impairment?
    1. exposure to loud noise
    2. excessive cerumen
    3. rigid stapes
    4. seasonal allergies

    Nursing Process: Assessment
    Client Need: Safe, Effective Care Environment

41. One of the best techniques for communicating with a person who is hearing impaired is to
    1. face the client when speaking
    2. speak into the affected ear
    3. raise the volume of speech
    4. speak at a higher pitch

    Nursing Process: Implementation
    Client Need: Safe, Effective Care Environment

42. A client who has noticed some changes in hearing asks who he should see for an evaluation. It would be most appropriate to refer the client first to a(n)
    1. hearing aid representative
    2. speech pathologist
    3. otolaryngologist
    4. audiologist

    Nursing Process: Implementation
    Client Need: Safe, Effective Care Environment

43. When irrigating the ear to remove cerumen, it is best if the fluid is directed
    1. directly toward the ear drum
    2. toward the roof of the ear canal
    3. behind the auricle
    4. beneath the pinna

    Nursing Process: Implementation
    Client Need: Physiological Integrity

44. A client presents with a fever and pain within the ear. If the client's past history reveals all of the following, which one is the most likely cause for the diagnosis of otitis media at this time? The client has had
    1. a recent sore throat
    2. a recent fractured nose
    3. nasal polyps removed 2 years ago
    4. tonsils removed 20 years ago

    Nursing Process: Assessment
    Client Need: Safe, Effective Care Environment

45. Following an incision of the ear drum (tympanic membrane), which one of the following instructions is most appropriate?
    1. Expect that the drainage will be creamy white and then bloody.
    2. Pack a cotton plug tightly and deeply within the ear canal.
    3. Take the prescribed antibiotics until they are all gone.
    4. Do not remove the cotton plug under any circumstances.

    Nursing Process: Implementation
    Client Need: Health Promotion/Maintenance

46. When clarifying the physician's explanation of otosclerosis, the nurse would be accurate in telling a client that this condition involves bony overgrowth and fixation of the
    1. incus
    2. malleolus
    3. stapes
    4. cochlea

    Nursing Process: Implementation
    Client Need: Health Promotion/Maintenance

47. Before having surgery for otosclerosis, a client should be told that immediately after surgery hearing may temporarily be the same or worse than before due to
    1. swelling, packing, or accumulated drainage
    2. chipped pieces of bone that must be absorbed
    3. swelling of the vestibulocochlear nerve
    4. surgical trauma to the oval window

    Nursing Process: Implementation
    Client Need: Safe, Effective Care Environment

48. The nurse would be most correct in assessing a client for facial nerve damage following surgery for otosclerosis by observing the client's ability to
    1. talk
    2. smile
    3. sneeze
    4. smell

    Nursing Process: Assessment
    Client Need: Physiological Integrity

49. The best postoperative position for a client following surgery for otosclerosis is
    1. with the operative ear upward
    2. lying on the operative ear
    3. sitting with the head elevated
    4. lying flat with the legs raised

    Nursing Process: Planning
    Client Need: Physiological Integrity

50. If a client with Meniere's disease made all of the following statements, which one indicates that the client needs more teaching? The client says,
    1. "My symptoms occur when fluid builds within my inner ear"
    2. "This disease causes nausea, vomiting, and dizziness"
    3. "Between the periodic attacks, my hearing will remain normal"
    4. "I may need surgery, but it will result in permanent deafness"

    Nursing Process: Evaluation
    Client Need: Health Promotion/Maintenance

II. CRITICAL THINKING EXERCISES

1. A client becomes suddenly blind. What rehabilitation services might be available to this person?

2. What nursing actions would promote communication with a client who has a hearing impairment?

3. What kind of health teaching would be appropriate for a client who has a perforated tympanic membrane?

4. What should the plan of care include for a client following ear surgery?

XI Caring for Clients with Gastrointestinal Problems

49/ Introduction to the Gastrointestinal System and Accessory Structures

Clients with GI disorders have a wide variety of health problems that involve disturbances in ingesting and digesting food, absorbing nutrients, and eliminating waste products from the GI tract. Gastrointestinal problems may be caused by physical or emotional factors. Many GI disturbances cannot be neatly classified as emotional or physical in origin; these illnesses seem to stem from both psychological and physiologic malfunctions, which tend to interact.

The following questions deal with the content of Chapter 49.

I. MULTIPLE CHOICE QUESTIONS

Circle the number of the most appropriate answer.

A nurse has organized a weekly group meeting for hospitalized clients who wish to know more about nutrition, the gastrointestinal system, and a variety of disorders that affect this system.

1. The nurse would be most correct in telling the group that the substance that undergoes partial digestion when it is mixed with secretions from the salivary glands is
   1. protein
   2. starch
   3. simple sugars
   4. saturated fats

   Nursing Process: Implementation
   Client Need: Health Promotion/Maintenance

2. A client demonstrates correct understanding of how food and gastrointestinal contents move through the GI tract by using the term
   1. homeostasis
   2. anastomosis
   3. peristalsis
   4. synarthrosis

   Nursing Process: Evaluation
   Client Need: Health Promotion/Maintenance

3. The nurse asks if anyone in the group can identify the name of the narrow blind tube that is attached near the junction where the small intestine joins the large intestine. The correct answer the nurse is looking for is the
   1. spleen
   2. gallbladder
   3. ampulla
   4. appendix

   Nursing Process: Assessment
   Client Need: Health Promotion/Maintenance

4. The nurse asks the group to speculate on which accessory structure to the gastrointestinal system is the largest glandular organ in the body. The nurse would be correct in agreeing with the client who says it is the
   1. liver
   2. spleen
   3. pancreas
   4. gallbladder

   Nursing Process: Implementation
   Client Need: Health Promotion/Maintenance

Individual Questions

5. A client needs additional teaching if he identifies that the liver produces
   1. fibrinogen
   2. prothrombin
   3. insulin
   4. bile

   Nursing Process: Evaluation
   Client Need: Health Promotion/Maintenance

6. When the nurse is asked what stimulates the gallbladder to release bile, she gives the correct answer as
   1. hydrochloric acid
   2. fatty food
   3. insulin
   4. peristalsis

   Nursing Process: Assessment
   Client Need: Health Promotion/Maintenance

7. Which one of the following assessments is the best indicator of whether the client's nutrition is adequate?
   1. obtaining a diet history
   2. listening to bowel sounds
   3. asking about appetite
   4. weighing the client

   Nursing Process: Assessment
   Client Need: Safe, Effective Care Environment

8. When assessing a dark-skinned client for jaundice, which structure would be most appropriate to inspect?
   1. urine
   2. tongue
   3. hard palate
   4. palatine tonsils

   Nursing Process: Assessment
   Client Need: Physiological Integrity

9. To whom would it be most appropriate to report that a hospitalized client has no teeth or dentures?
   1. the client's dentist
   2. a medical social worker
   3. the discharge planner
   4. a hospital dietitian

   Nursing Process: Implementation
   Client Need: Safe, Effective Care Environment

10. After inspecting the abdomen of a new client, which assessment technique is used next?
    1. light palpation
    2. deep palpation
    3. auscultation
    4. percussion

    Nursing Process: Assessment
    Client Need: Safe, Effective Care Environment

11. Which one of the following would be essential when examining a client's anorectal area?

   1. absorbent pads
   2. sterile lubricant
   3. clean gloves
   4. applicator sticks

   Nursing Process: Planning
   Client Need: Safe, Effective Care Environment

12. When auscultating the abdomen, the normal frequency of sounds emanating from the bowel is every

   1. 1 to 5 seconds
   2. 5 to 30 seconds
   3. 30 to 45 seconds
   4. 45 to 60 seconds

   Nursing Process: Assessment
   Client Need: Physiological Integrity

13. Which one of the following would be most important following the completion of an upper GI series?

   1. taking vital signs
   2. providing hygiene
   3. monitoring bowel elimination
   4. ambulating the client

   Nursing Process: Planning
   Client Need: Safe, Effective Care Environment

14. Before a client undergoes a lower GI series, the nurse could expect that the client's preparation will include

   1. administration of a sedative
   2. fasting from food and water
   3. a laxative and cleansing enemas
   4. starting an intravenous infusion

   Nursing Process: Planning
   Client Need: Safe, Effective Care Environment

15. Which one of the following sensitivities is most important to report before a client undergoes cholangiography?

   1. morphine
   2. penicillin
   3. iodine
   4. aspirin

   Nursing Process: Implementation
   Client Need: Safe, Effective Care Environment

16. If a client vomits the capsules used for an oral cholescystography, it would be most appropriate for the nurse to

   1. restrict the client's food intake
   2. limit the client's activity
   3. insert a nasogastric tube
   4. notify the radiology department

   Nursing Process: Implementation
   Client Need: Safe, Effective Care Environment

17. Which one of the following nursing measures would be appropriate to plan for the care of a client following a cholangiography?

   1. aspirating stomach secretions
   2. providing a high fluid intake
   3. withholding food for several hours
   4. keeping the head of the bed elevated

   Nursing Process: Planning
   Client Need: Safe, Effective Care Environment

18. It would be most appropriate for the nurse to tell clients who have undergone a barium enema to

   1. decrease their fluid intake for 24 hours
   2. expect light-colored stools for a few days
   3. watch for the appearance of bile in stools
   4. increase their intake of fiber for a week

   Nursing Process: Implementation
   Client Need: Safe, Effective Care Environment

19. If a client who is scheduled for an MRI of the abdomen made all of the following statements, which one indicates that the client needs more teaching? The client says he will
    1. be asked to drink barium just before the examination
    2. require cleansing enemas to remove stool and gas
    3. need to remove all metal objects from his person
    4. have to lie still while within the testing chamber

    Nursing Process: Evaluation
    Client Need: Safe, Effective Care Environment

20. Which one of the following instructions is most appropriate for a client undergoing an ultrasonography of the abdomen?
    1. "You may hear repetitive clicking noises during the test."
    2. "To avoid inaccurate findings, don't drink through a straw."
    3. "Be sure to remove your wrist watch before the examination."
    4. "Your body will be rotated within a circular chamber."

    Nursing Process: Implementation
    Client Need: Safe, Effective Care Environment

21. Clients having a liver biopsy are instructed to
    1. lie on their right side for 2 or 3 hours
    2. remain upright in bed for 2 or 3 hours
    3. cough and deep breath hourly for 24 hours
    4. ambulate frequently during the next 24 hours

    Nursing Process: Implementation
    Client Need: Safe, Effective Care Environment

22. It would be most appropriate for the nurse to assess for which one of the following complications following a liver biopsy?
    1. infection
    2. bleeding
    3. coma
    4. shock

    Nursing Process: Assessment
    Client Need: Physiological Integrity

23. After an endoscopic examination of the esophagus or stomach, before the client is allowed to eat or drink, the nurse must establish that
    1. bowel sounds are present
    2. peristalsis has resumed
    3. there is a gag reflex
    4. no nausea exists

    Nursing Process: Implementation
    Client Need: Safe, Effective Care Environment

24. A nurse collects a stool sample for a culture and examination for ova and parasites. What action is most appropriate next?
    1. spray the sample with a fixative solution
    2. cover the sample with formaldehyde
    3. take the sample to the lab while warm
    4. refrigerate the sample for 8 hours

    Nursing Process: Implementation
    Client Need: Safe, Effective Care Environment

25. A client receives midazolam (Versed) prior to and during an endoscopic examination. It would be most appropriate for the nurse to plan on monitoring the client for which one of the following complications?
    1. tachyarrhythmias
    2. anaphylaxis
    3. respiratory depression
    4. hypovolemic shock

    Nursing Process: Planning
    Client Need: Safe, Effective Care Environment

26. A client who is scheduled for an endoscopic retrograde cholangiopancreatography (ERCP) says to the nurse, "I'm afraid I may not wake up from this." The best response the nurse could make is,
    1. "Nonsense, you'll be awake the entire time."
    2. "This test isn't as dangerous as you think."
    3. "You'll see how foolish you are by tonight."
    4. "What kinds of concerns are you having?"

    Nursing Process: Implementation
    Client Need: Psychosocial Integrity

II. CRITICAL THINKING EXERCISES

1. If a client indicated that the reason he is seeking treatment is to find the cause of his indigestion, what additional questions would help the physician in diagnosing the client's problem?

2. Following an endoscopic examination of upper gastrointestinal structures, what nursing care would be appropriate?

3. What test preparations would be appropriate when a client is scheduled for a gastric analysis?

50/ Caring for Clients with Disorders of the Upper Gastrointestinal Tract

Disorders of the upper gastrointestinal tract are common. The nurse is often called on to manage the care of clients with disorders affecting eating and digestion. These problems and their treatment approaches are commonly addressed in the nursing care plans of clients who have upper GI disorders. The client with an upper gastrointestinal disorder may require intensive medical and sometimes surgical management.

The following questions deal with the content of Chapter 50.

I. MULTIPLE CHOICE QUESTIONS

Circle the number of the most appropriate answer.

Martin O'Brien, a 41-year-old accountant, has been diagnosed as having a peptic ulcer. At present he is being treated conservatively.

1. If Mr. Martin is typical of others with peptic ulcer disease, he experiences pain most often
    1. while eating a high-fat meal
    2. after eating fresh produce
    3. after finishing a meal
    4. when his stomach is empty

    Nursing Process: Assessment
    Client Need: Physiological Integrity

2. It would be accurate for the nurse to explain that among those who develop peptic ulcer disease, the protective layer of mucus may be eroded by the enzymatic action of a particular bacteria known as
    1. *Staphylococcus aureus*
    2. *Cryptococcus neoformans*
    3. *Pseudomonas aeurginosa*
    4. *Helicobactor pylori*

    Nursing Process: Implementation
    Client Need: Health Promotion/Maintenance

3. Which of the following complications would it be most appropriate for the nurse to monitor to detect when caring for Ms. O'Brien?
    1. hemorrhage, obstruction, and perforation
    2. pain, bleeding, and constipation
    3. anorexia, weight loss, and vomiting
    4. abdominal distention and flatulence

    Nursing Process: Assessment
    Client Need: Physiological Integrity

4. The physician prescribes cimetidine (Tagamet), a histamine H_2-receptor antagonist. The best evidence that Ms. O'Brien understands the action of this drug is the statement that it
    1. promotes digestion of food
    2. neutralizes stomach acid
    3. relieves gastric dilation
    4. decreases hydrocholoric acid

    Nursing Process: Evaluation
    Client Need: Health Promotion/Maintenance

5. Evidence that Ms. O'Brien's ulcer is bleeding include
    1. coffee-ground-appearing emesis and black stools
    2. greenish-yellow emesis and tarry stools
    3. clear mucoid emesis and bright bloody stools
    4. coffee-ground emesis and clay-colored stools

    Nursing Process: Assessment
    Client Need: Physiological Integrity

Mr. Morgan Wilson, age 46, is an executive at a small manufacturing company. He has self-treated his symptoms of chronic gastritis for several years. Since his symptoms have become worse, he has made an appointment with a physician.

6. The nurse interviews Mr. Wilson to collect a data-base of information. If Mr. Wilson has a peptic ulcer, he will most likely describe the location of his pain as
   1. being in the mid-epigastrium
   2. radiating to the left shoulder
   3. penetrating toward his back
   4. centering in the mid-abdomen

   Nursing Process: Assessment
   Client Need: Physiological Integrity

7. Which one of the following statements is the best evidence that Mr. Wilson understands the action of the drug sucralfate (Carafate) which the physician has prescribed? Mr. Wilson says this drug will
   1. decrease gastric motility
   2. form a seal over the ulcer
   3. buffer the stomach's acid
   4. sustain gastric mucus

   Nursing Process: Evaluation
   Client Need: Health Promotion/Maintenance

Mr. Wilson does not comply with medical treatment and is admitted for a gastrojejunostomy (Billroth II) procedure.

8. Prior to surgery the nurse inserts a nasogastric tube and administers liquid antacid depending upon the gastric pH. In withdrawing a sample of gastric secretions, which one of the following actions is most appropriate? The nurse
   1. flushes the tube with saline
   2. offers the client ice chips
   3. uses a clean syringe for aspiration
   4. places the client on his left side

   Nursing Process: Implementation
   Client Need: Safe, Effective Care Environment

9. Mr. Wilson is returned from surgery with the nasogastric tube connected to low, intermittent suction. If all of the following are observed, for which one should the nurse intervene? The client
   1. requests pain medication every 4 to 6 hours
   2. has a urine output of 1000 mL in 24 hours
   3. consumes the equivalent of 1000 mL of ice chips
   4. has greenish-brown drainage from the NG tube

   Nursing Process: Evaluation
   Client Need: Physiological Integrity

10. After Mr. Wilson resumes eating, which one of the following symptoms is an indication that he may be experiencing dumping syndrome? Mr. Wilson tells the nurse he feels
    1. warm and looks flushed before eating
    2. cold and shivers before eating
    3. weak and dizzy after eating
    4. nauseous and vomits after eating

    Nursing Process: Assessment
    Client Need: Physiological Integrity

11. Which one of the following is most appropriate to tell Mr. Wilson to reduce or eliminate the symptoms associated with the dumping syndrome?
    1. eat carbohydrates, especially simple sugars, in moderation
    2. drink a large volume of fluids, like water, with each meal
    3. remain seated or ambulate for 30 minutes after each meal
    4. consume three meals each day and avoid in-between snacks

    Nursing Process: Implementation
    Client Need: Health Promotion/Maintenance

Individual Questions

12. The most striking characteristic of simple anorexia is that the client
    1. experiences chronic nausea
    2. has no desire for food
    3. suffers bouts of vomiting
    4. fasts to lose weight

    Nursing Process: Assessment
    Client Need: Physiological Integrity

13. Which one of the following nursing approaches is more likely to promote the consumption of food when a client has simple anorexia?
    1. serve small portions of food
    2. avoid distractions during meals
    3. serve foods that do not require chewing
    4. calorie-load the last meal of the day

    Nursing Process: Implementation
    Client Need: Physiological Integrity

14. If a client has anorexia nervosa, which one of the following is a common associated finding? The client tends to be
    1. perfectionistic
    2. antagonistic
    3. argumentative
    4. irresponsible

    Nursing Process: Assessment
    Client Need: Psychosocial Integrity

15. When examining a severely emaciated client with anorexia nervosa, the nurse is most likely to note the presence of
    1. petechiae
    2. lanugo
    3. keloids
    4. striae

    Nursing Process: Assessment
    Client Need: Physiological Integrity

16. The best evidence that a client with anorexia nervosa has hypokalemia is that the EKG rhythm strip shows
    1. prolonged PR intervals
    2. tall peaked T waves
    3. wide QRS complexes
    4. absence of P waves

    Nursing Process: Assessment
    Client Need: Physiological Integrity

17. The nurse removes a tray of uneaten food left untouched by a client with anorexia nervosa. The most appropriate nursing action would be to
    1. remind the client of the contract agreement
    2. make one last attempt to coax the client to eat
    3. remove the tray without making any comments
    4. explain that the physician will be informed

    Nursing Process: Implementation
    Client Need: Psychosocial Integrity

18. A client with anorexia nervosa consumes most of the food served at the noon meal. At this time, it would be most important for the nurse to
    1. weigh the client now and again 2 hours later
    2. observe the client closely for several hours
    3. comment on how attractive the client looks
    4. let the client leave the unit for a walk

    Nursing Process: Implementation
    Client Need: Psychosocial Integrity

19. A client with bulimia is most likely to manifest secretive food binges followed by
    1. starvation
    2. purging
    3. normal eating
    4. dislike for food

    Nursing Process: Assessment
    Client Need: Physiological Integrity

20. Which one of the following assessment findings is associated more with bulimia than any other type of eating disorder?

    1. The client is concerned about being fat.
    2. The client hides food to avoid eating it.
    3. The client's tooth enamel is eroded.
    4. The client has lost 25% body weight.

    Nursing Process: Assessment
    Client Need: Physiological Integrity

21. Which is the best technique for assessing obesity?

    1. weighing a client
    2. obtaining a dietary history
    3. measuring skinfold thickness
    4. measuring abdominal girth

    Nursing Process: Assessment
    Client Need: Physiological Integrity

22. To achieve a weight loss of 1 pound per week, the nurse would be most correct in helping clients reduce their usual intake of calories per day by

    1. 500 calories
    2. 1000 calories
    3. 1500 calories
    4. 1800 calories

    Nursing Process: Implementation
    Client Need: Physiological Integrity

23. After a period of not eating, which one of the following groups of foods might a client with nausea and vomiting tolerate best?

    1. juice, poached eggs, coffee
    2. tea, dry toast, crackers
    3. egg nog, milk shakes, gelatin
    4. baked chicken, potatoes, corn

    Nursing Process: Implementation
    Client Need: Physiological Integrity

24. A client is referred to a physician by a dentist who has detected a suspicious lesion on the client's lip. If the lesion is cancerous, which of the following is a common finding in the client's history? The client is likely to

    1. bite his or her fingernails
    2. be someone who smokes a pipe
    3. prefer eating spicy foods
    4. neglect his or her oral hygiene

    Nursing Process: Assessment
    Client Need: Physiological Integrity

25. The nurse would be most correct in explaining to a client with oral cancer that the white patch on the inner cheek is referred to as

    1. leukorrhea
    2. leukopenia
    3. leukoplakia
    4. leukorrhagia

    Nursing Process: Implementation
    Client Need: Health Promotion/Maintenance

26. In planning the care of a client with oral cancer, which one of the following has the highest priority?

    1. helping the client cope
    2. supporting communication
    3. maintaining a patent airway
    4. improving body image

    Nursing Process: Planning
    Client Need: Safe, Effective Care Environment

27. Once a nasogastric tube is in the nasopharynx, to promote advancement into the stomach, the nurse should ask the client to

    1. hyperextend the neck
    2. stick out the tongue
    3. open the mouth and say, "Ahhh"
    4. lower the chin to the chest

    Nursing Process: Implementation
    Client Need: Physiological Integrity

28. Which one of the following is an indication that a nasogastric tube has entered the lungs rather than the stomach? The client
    1. belches
    2. vomits
    3. cannot speak
    4. asks for food

    Nursing Process: Assessment
    Client Need: Physiological Integrity

29. After completion of a bolus nasogastric tube feeding, it would be most appropriate for the nurse to
    1. keep the client in a Fowler's position
    2. leave the tube unclamped for 30 minutes
    3. instill air to clear the tube of formula
    4. connect the tube to low, intermittent suction

    Nursing Process: Implementation
    Client Need: Safe, Effective Care Environment

30. When measuring the gastric residual before administering a tube feeding, the nurse would be most correct in
    1. disposing of the aspirated residual
    2. adding the residual to the formula
    3. reinstilling the gastric residual
    4. sending the residual to the laboratory

    Nursing Process: Implementation
    Client Need: Safe, Effective Care Environment

31. To avoid conditions that promote bacterial growth in formula that infuses by continuous flow, the nurse should hang only the volume that will instill in the next
    1. 2 hours
    2. 4 hours
    3. 8 hours
    4. 12 hours

    Nursing Process: Implementation
    Client Need: Safe, Effective Care Environment

32. A client who receives medications through a nasogastric tube has all of the following drugs ordered. For which one should the nurse call the physician concerning a revision in the drug regimen?
    1. digoxin (Lanoxin) elixir
    2. enteric-coated aspirin
    3. ampicillin (Omnipen) suspension
    4. furosemide (Lasix) tablets

    Nursing Process: Implementation
    Client Need: Physiological Integrity

33. The best evidence that a client with a hiatal hernia understands the rationale for sleeping with the head of the bed elevated is the statement that this measure will
    1. prevent stomach acid from refluxing into the esophagus
    2. allow the esophagus to move up into the thoracic cavity
    3. decrease gastric secretions from accumulating
    4. reduce the reflux of chyme into the stomach

    Nursing Process: Evaluation
    Client Need: Health Promotion/Maintenance

34. Which one of the following symptoms occurs early in the development of esophageal cancer?
    1. nausea
    2. vomiting
    3. difficulty swallowing food
    4. pain in the epigastric region

    Nursing Process: Assessment
    Client Need: Physiological Integrity

35. Which one of the following beverages would the nurse be most correct in telling a client with gastritis to avoid?
    1. orange juice
    2. carbonated drinks
    3. alcohol
    4. lemonade

    Nursing Process: Implementation
    Client Need: Health Promotion/Maintenance

36. The best evidence that a client with cancer of the stomach has correctly understood the prognosis of this condition is the statement that
    1. diet and drug therapy can control metastasis
    2. malignant cells can be destroyed with a laser
    3. chemotherapy may be used to abolish the tumor
    4. surgery is the only curative treatment measure

    Nursing Process: Evaluation
    Client Need: Health Promotion/Maintenance

37. A client provides all the following information in a health history. It would be appropriate for the nurse to identify which one of them as a health risk predisposing to cancer of the stomach? The client says that he
    1. eats charcoaled meat at least once a week
    2. has an intolerance for milk and dairy products
    3. includes cooked greens in his diet weekly
    4. prefers canned fruit rather than fresh

    Nursing Process: Implementation
    Client Need: Health Promotion/Maintenance

38. If a client with a stomach disorder undergoes surgery that includes a gastrectomy, it would be appropriate for the nurse to advise the client that a vitamin that will need life-long replacement is
    1. vitamin A
    2. vitamin B_{12}
    3. vitamin D
    4. vitamin K

    Nursing Process: Implementation
    Client Need: Health Promotion/Maintenance

II. CRITICAL THINKING EXERCISES

1. Anne Jamieson, 18 years of age, has been hospitalized on a special eating disorders unit and is being treated for anorexia nervosa. In a contract between Anne and her primary nurse, Anne has agreed to gain 2 pounds this week. If she does so, she may have unlimited phone privileges; if not, she may not use the telephone until she meets the goal weight. When Anne is weighed, the scale indicates that she has gained 1.5 pounds. Anne begs the nurse to let her make one last phone call. What response would be most appropriate?

2. What purpose is served by using a double lumen sump tube for gastric decompression?

3. A client who has just started receiving continuous nasoenteral tube feedings develops diarrhea. What can be done to eliminate the client's frequent stools?

4. What techniques might help a client with a hiatal hernia avoid gastroesophageal reflux?

51/ Caring for Clients with Disorders of the Lower Gastrointestinal Tract

The material that moves down the large intestine is composed of food residues, microorganisms, digestive juices, and mucus that is secreted in the large intestine. Disorders of the lower gastrointestinal tract generally affect the movement of feces toward the anus, absorption of water and electrolytes, and the elimination of dietary wastes.

The following questions deal with the content of Chapter 51.

I. MULTIPLE CHOICE QUESTIONS

Circle the number of the most appropriate answer.

1. When discussing bowel elimination with a client, the nurse would be most correct in explaining that the major indicators for constipation or diarrhea are the
   1. consistency of stools and their ease of passage
   2. number of stools and the frequency of passage
   3. color of stools and the number of stools per day
   4. odor to the stools and the shape of the stools

   Nursing Process: Implementation
   Client Need: Health Promotion/Maintenance

2. For bulkier, yet more moist stool, the nurse would be most correct in advising a client to consume foods that are high in

   1. water-soluble vitamins
   2. beta carotene
   3. fiber
   4. starch

   Nursing Process: Implementation
   Client Need: Health Promotion/Maintenance

3. Which one of the dietary choices listed below would be *least* appropriate for promoting bulkier stools and resolving a client's constipation?

   1. brown rice
   2. split peas
   3. raisins
   4. cheese

   Nursing Process: Implementation
   Client Need: Health Promotion/Maintenance

4. A client who is constipated should be advised against straining to expel stool since this can lead to

   1. colitis
   2. hemorrhoids
   3. diverticula
   4. appendicitis

   Nursing Process: Implementation
   Client Need: Health Promotion/Maintenance

5. When assessing a client who has diarrhea, which one of the following is a common finding? The client has

   1. a feeling of rectal fullness
   2. abdominal distention
   3. hyperperistalsis
   4. rectal bleeding

   Nursing Process: Assessment
   Client Need: Physiological Integrity

6. A food source that may help a client restore proper balance of intestinal bacteria being purged through diarrhea is

   1. buttermilk
   2. mushrooms
   3. bananas
   4. broccoli

   Nursing Process: Implementation
   Client Need: Health Promotion/Maintenance

7. If enteric precautions are followed when emptying the bedpan of a client with diarrhea, the nurse would

   1. clean the bedpan with povidone iodine (Betadine)
   2. don a mask, goggles, and moisture-resistant apron
   3. wear a gown and gloves, and perform thorough handwashing
   4. avoid touching any areas that were in contact with the client

   Nursing Process: Implementation
   Client Need: Safe, Effective Care Environment

8. For the client who is recovering from diarrhea, which one of the following would be considered an appropriate low-residue food that the client could consume?

   1. canned tuna
   2. steamed okra
   3. raw sprouts
   4. dried dates

   Nursing Process: Implementation
   Client Need: Physiological Integrity

9. A client with irritable bowel disorder needs more teaching if he says

   1. the disorder is sometimes called spastic colon
   2. there is no pathology to explain the symptoms
   3. the symptoms are probably due to an infectious microorganism
   4. it is characterized by periods of constipation and diarrhea

   Nursing Process: Evaluation
   Client Need: Health Promotion/Maintenance

10. When clarifying the physician's explanation for why surgery is not necessarily a curative form of treatment for Crohn's disease, the nurse would be most accurate in telling the client that the lesions
    1. generally become cancerous as the disease spreads
    2. gradually disappear as clients grow older
    3. occur in random patches throughout the intestinal tract
    4. are confined to the superficial muscular layer of bowel

    Nursing Process: Implementation
    Client Need: Health Promotion/Maintenance

11. If a client with Crohn's disease asks what the usual drug therapy includes for reducing intestinal inflammation of his type, the nurse would be most correct in identifying which one of the following drug categories?
    1. antidiarrheals, like loperamide (Imodium)
    2. corticosteroids, like dexamethasone (Decadron)
    3. cephalosporins, like cephradine (Velosef)
    4. salicylates, like acetylsalicylic acid (aspirin)

    Nursing Process: Implementation
    Client Need: Health Promotion/Maintenance

12. When assigned to a client with Crohn's disease, which one of the following would be the priority of care?
    1. assisting with hygiene
    2. providing physical rest
    3. meeting nutritional needs
    4. improving body image

    Nursing Process: Planning
    Client Need: Physiological Integrity

13. If a client with ulcerative colitis is typical of most others with this disease, the nurse is most likely to find that the client has
    1. nausea and vomiting
    2. bloody diarrhea
    3. lactose intolerance
    4. insidious weight gain

    Nursing Process: Assessment
    Client Need: Physiological Integrity

14. A client with ulcerative colitis is to undergo a total colectomy as surgical treatment for the disorder. The best evidence that the client understands what this procedure involves is the statement,
    1. "I won't have diarrhea anymore."
    2. "I will eliminate stool through an ileostomy."
    3. "The surgery will slow the process from spreading to my ileum."
    4. "Once my incision heals, I'll have normal bowel elimination."

    Nursing Process: Evaluation
    Client Need: Safe, Effective Care Environment

15. If a client requires total parenteral nutrition during an acute episode of ulcerative colitis, which additional nursing action should the nurse plan to perform?
    1. measure the pH of gastric secretions
    2. check the specific gravity of urine
    3. monitor the blood glucose level
    4. test the urine for ketones

    Nursing Process: Planning
    Client Need: Physiological Integrity

16. As appendicitis intensifies, the client will identify the location of the pain as being in the
    1. right upper quadrant of the abdomen
    2. right lower quadrant of the abdomen
    3. left upper quadrant of the abdomen
    4. left lower quadrant of the abdomen

    Nursing Process: Assessment
    Client Need: Physiological Integrity

17. When the nurse reviews the laboratory results of tests performed on a client with suspected appendicitis, which one of the following tends to confirm the diagnosis? The
    1. number of immature neutrophils is increased
    2. number of reticulocytes is increased
    3. red cell count is decreased
    4. hematocrit is elevated

    Nursing Process: Assessment
    Client Need: Physiological Integrity

18. Which group of assessment findings is most consistent with those associated with peritonitis?
    1. hypoactive bowel sounds, slow and irregular pulse
    2. hyperactive bowel sounds, vomiting, diarrhea
    3. abdominal pain, fever, rigid board-like abdomen
    4. lethargy, hypothermia, and slow respirations

    Nursing Process: Assessment
    Client Need: Physiological Integrity

19. When planning the care of a client who has the potential for developing peritonitis, which one of the following would be most important to assess?
    1. skin color
    2. pupil size
    3. bowel sounds
    4. capillary refill

    Nursing Process: Planning
    Client Need: Physiological Integrity

20. If a client with peritonitis undergoes surgical treatment, which one of the following is likely to be part of the client's care?
    1. nasoenteric tube feedings
    2. gastric decompression
    3. mechanical ventilation
    4. daily cleansing enemas

    Nursing Process: Planning
    Client Need: Physiological Integrity

21. If a client develops an obstruction in the upper areas of the intestine, which one of the following assessment findings is the nurse most likely to detect?
    1. vomiting fecal material
    2. foul odor to the breath
    3. difficulty swallowing
    4. flat, board-like abdomen

    Nursing Process: Assessment
    Client Need: Physiological Integrity

22. The nurse would be most correct in explaining to a client for whom an intestinal tube (Miller-Abbott) will be inserted that the bag on its distal end will be filled with
    1. water
    2. saline
    3. silver
    4. mercury

    Nursing Process: Implementation
    Client Need: Safe, Effective Care Environment

23. When is it appropriate for the nurse to stabilize the proximal end of an intestinal tube, such as the Miller-Abbott tube, to the client's nose?
    1. after the physician inserts the tube
    2. when the tube exits the pylorus
    3. at the point of the obstruction
    4. when the tip is in the duodenum

    Nursing Process: Planning
    Client Need: Safe, Effective Care Environment

24. A client with asymptomatic diverticulosis understands how to best prevent the pouch-like areas of intestine from becoming inflamed if he states,
    1. "If I eat fruit, it should be canned or steamed"
    2. "I should eat more whole grains and fresh produce"
    3. "It would be best to use refined flour and grains"
    4. "I should refrain from eating if constipation develops

    Nursing Process: Evaluation
    Client Need: Health Promotion/Maintenance

25. If a client develops diverticulitis, which one of the following changes in stool is common? The stool is commonly described as
    1. appearing clay-colored
    2. looking like currant jelly
    3. being stonelike in texture
    4. being coated with mucus

    Nursing Process: Assessment
    Client Need: Physiological Integrity

26. A client with a hernia tells the nurse that he is able to temporarily relieve the protrusion by applying pressure over it with his hands. When giving report to the nurses on the next shift, the nurse would be most correct in referring to this type of hernia as one that is
    1. incarcerated
    2. strangulated
    3. reducible
    4. alterable

    Nursing Process: Implementation
    Client Need: Safe, Effective Care Environment

27. A client with a hernia understands the health teaching provided by the nurse if he says he should avoid
    1. sitting for long periods of time
    2. eating fresh fruits and vegetables
    3. lying on his abdomen when sleeping
    4. straining during a bowel movement

    Nursing Process: Evaluation
    Client Need: Health Promotion/Maintenance

28. Following a herniorrhaphy, the postoperative care should include plans to
    1. perform deep-breathing exercises
    2. splint the incision while coughing
    3. maintain bedrest for at least 3 days
    4. take a tub bath for daily hygiene

    Nursing Process: Planning
    Client Need: Safe, Effective Care Environment

29. Which one of the following should the nurse monitor to detect following the surgical repair of an inguinal hernia on a male client?
    1. temporary impotence
    2. premature ejaculation
    3. edema of the scrotum
    4. sustained erection

    Nursing Process: Assessment
    Client Need: Physiological Integrity

30. A nurse who is volunteering during a community-wide screening for colorectal cancer would be correct in telling participants that one of the earliest warning signs of colorectal cancer is
    1. a lump within the tissue
    2. a change in bowel habits
    3. usual bleeding or discharge
    4. persistent indigestion

    Nursing Process: Implementation
    Client Need: Health Promotion/Maintenance

31. It would be essential to inform clients participating in colorectal cancer screening that before collecting a stool specimen they should abstain from red meat for 2 days as well as avoid eating
    1. beets
    2. watermelon
    3. broccoli
    4. asparagus

    Nursing Process: Implementation
    Client Need: Safe, Effective Care Environment

32. Which one of the following nursing measures would be most appropriate for the care of a client following a hemorrhoidectomy?
    1. sitting in a folding chair
    2. using a knee-chest position
    3. providing frequent Sitz baths
    4. applying ice to the rectal area

    Nursing Process: Planning
    Client Need: Physiological Integrity

33. Which one of the following is a common route of transmission for anorectal infections?
    1. consuming contaminated food and water
    2. swimming in polluted lakes or streams
    3. using toilets in public restrooms
    4. having unprotected anal intercourse

    Nursing Process: Assessment
    Client Need: Safe, Effective Care Environment

34. When assessing a client with a pilonidal sinus, the client would most likely have pain and swelling
    1. in and about the anus
    2. in the groin area
    3. at the base of the spine
    4. in the right lower quadrant

    Nursing Process: Assessment
    Client Need: Physiological Integrity

35. Which one of the following is a major factor in the development of a pilonidal sinus?
    1. chronic constipation
    2. prolonged sitting
    3. straining during defecation
    4. abundance of perianal hair

    Nursing Process: Assessment
    Client Need: Physiological Integrity

II. CRITICAL THINKING EXERCISES

1. A client in a nursing home who has a history of constipation suddenly begins to pass liquid stool. What further assessments are appropriate at this time?

2. How would you explain that the chronic use of laxatives or enemas contributes to constipation?

3. How does the dwell time of food residue within the intestine affect the stool's moisture content?

4. When assessing a client, the nurse finds that there are no bowel sounds present throughout the abdomen. If the client has an intestinal obstruction, what are some possible etiologies?

5. After the physician inserts a tube used for intestinal decompression, such as the Miller-Abbott tube, what are the responsibilities of the nurse?

52/ Caring for Clients with an Ileostomy or Colostomy

An *ostomy,* as used here, is the creation of an opening of the bowel onto the skin. Fecal material drains through the opening, which is called a *stoma.* Helping each client learn to manage this change in body function is an important nursing role.

The following questions deal with the content of Chapter 52.

I. MULTIPLE CHOICE QUESTIONS

Circle the number of the most appropriate answer.

Ms. Florence Flynn, age 44, has been treated for ulcerative colitis for 20 years. Recently, her diarrhea has become more frequent, she has lost weight, and blood and mucus appear in her stools. Following discussion with her physician she has given consent for a total colectomy and a conventional ileostomy.

1. Which one of the following statements indicates that Ms. Flynn needs more teaching? Ms. Flynn says,
   1. "I will have to wear an appliance at all times"
   2. "My stoma will be on my abdomen below the beltline"
   3. "I will probably eliminate formed stool"
   4. "My type of ostomy will be permanent"

   Nursing Process: Evaluation
   Client Need: Safe, Effective Care Environment

2. If Ms. Flynn reports taking all of the following drugs, which should the nurse check to see is being gradually tapered before surgery?
   1. loperamide (Imodium), an antidiarrheal
   2. Os-Cal, a nonprescription calcium product
   3. terfenadine (Seldane), an antihistamine
   4. prednisone (Deltasone), a corticosteroid

   Nursing Process: Implementation
   Client Need: Physiological Integrity

3. Before Ms. Flynn goes to surgery, the nurse describes how the stoma will appear. The best description is that the stoma will look
   1. bright red and will be larger than it will be later on
   2. purplish-blue and will be larger than it will be later on
   3. bright red and will be smaller than it will be later on
   4. purplish-blue and will be smaller than it will be later on

   Nursing Process: Implementation
   Client Need: Safe, Effective Care Environment

4. The physician prescribes kanamycin (Kantrex) preoperatively. When administering the drug, the nurse would be most correct in explaining to Ms. Flynn that this medication is prescribed to
   1. prevent postoperative pneumonia
   2. destroy bacteria within the bowel
   3. treat urinary tract infections
   4. reduce transient skin bacteria

   Nursing Process: Implementation
   Client Need: Health Promotion/Maintenance

5. Besides checking the stoma and abdominal incision after Ms. Flynn returns from the postanesthesia recovery room, what additional area of the body is most important to assess?
   1. rectal area
   2. urinary meatus
   3. vagina
   4. umbilicus

   Nursing Process: Assessment
   Client Need: Physiological Integrity

6. If Ms. Flynn resists deep breathing postoperatively, which item in the following list will best help her evaluate the effectiveness of her respiratory efforts?
   1. stethoscope
   2. incentive spirometer
   3. mechanical ventilator
   4. Swan-Ganz catheter

   Nursing Process: Planning
   Client Need: Physiological Integrity

7. If Ms. Flynn's ileal output exceeds her intake of fluid, besides a fluid volume deficit, which other complication should the nurse monitor to detect?
   1. respiratory alkalosis
   2. respiratory acidosis
   3. electrolyte imbalance
   4. hemolytic anemia

   Nursing Process: Assessment
   Client Need: Physiological Integrity

8. It would be appropriate to instruct Ms. Flynn that an ostomy appliance must be changed when it becomes tight, uncomfortable, or
   1. leaks
   2. fills with gas
   3. bulges under clothes
   4. emits an odor

   Nursing Process: Implementation
   Client Need: Health Promotion/Maintenance

Individual Questions

9. Which one of the following is a priority when planning the care of a client with an ileostomy?
    1. reducing social isolation
    2. maintaining skin integrity
    3. promoting physical mobility
    4. relieving unrealistic fears

    Nursing Process: Planning
    Client Need: Safe, Effective Care Environment

10. A nursing assistant asks the nurse to explain what the physician meant when he said a client would be returned postoperatively with a matured stoma. The nurse would be most correct in explaining that a matured stoma is one in which the bowel is
    1. opened when peristalsis resumes
    2. allowed to heal before it is opened
    3. everted during surgery and sutured to the skin
    4. conditioned to avoid the need for an appliance

    Nursing Process: Implementation
    Client Need: Safe, Effective Care Environment

11. Which one of the following substances should the nurse plan to use to protect the skin around an ostomy appliance or fill in uneven skin surfaces where an ostomy appliance must be attached?
    1. mucilage
    2. white glue
    3. telfa pads
    4. karaya gum

    Nursing Process: Planning
    Client Need: Physiological Integrity

12. Which one of the following professionals would it be most appropriate to consult for problems concerning an ostomy?
    1. gastroenterologist
    2. enterostomal therapist
    3. psychiatrist
    4. dermatologist

    Nursing Process: Implementation
    Client Need: Safe, Effective Care Environment

13. If a client experiences a prolapse of the stoma, which of the following assessment findings will most likely be evident? The stoma will
    1. protrude several inches, look swollen and dusky blue
    2. protrude several inches, look swollen and bright red
    3. recede several inches, look swollen and dusky blue
    4. recede several inches, look swollen and bright red

    Nursing Process: Assessment
    Client Need: Physiological Integrity

14. The best substance to use for cleaning the skin around a stoma is
    1. soap and water
    2. tincture of benzoin
    3. povidone iodine
    4. hydrogen peroxide

    Nursing Process: Implementation
    Client Need: Physiological Integrity

15. To determine the size for the appliance opening or O-ring, it would be best for the nurse to measure the stoma with
    1. calipers
    2. a compass
    3. a stomal guide
    4. a tape measure

    Nursing Process: Implementation
    Client Need: Physiological Integrity

16. When changing an ostomy appliance, the opening in the faceplate or circumference of the O-ring should be the size of the stoma plus
    1. 1/8 inch
    2. 1/4 inch
    3. 1/2 inch
    4. 3/4 inch

    Nursing Process: Implementation
    Client Need: Physiological Integrity

17. A client with a conventional ileostomy demonstrates an understanding of the relationship of skin integrity to pouch volume with the statement that the appliance should be emptied when it becomes
    1. 1/4 full
    2. 1/3 full
    3. 1/2 full
    4. 3/4 full

    Nursing Process: Evaluation
    Client Need: Health Promotion/Maintenance

18. The nurse observes that a client with an ileostomy avoids looking at the ostomy while the nurse performs its initial care. What communication technique would be most therapeutic?
    1. "Why don't you watch me while I change the appliance?"
    2. "Dr. Alexander did one of the best surgical incisions I've seen."
    3. "Lots of clients learn to adjust to the presence of an ostomy."
    4. "Your stoma looks pinkish-red and moist, which is normal."

    Nursing Process: Implementation
    Client Need: Psychosocial Integrity

19. If a client with an ileostomy describes all of the following measures as techniques for reducing the formation of gas, which one indicates the client needs more teaching? The client says it would be best if he
    1. chewed food well
    2. ate at a slow pace
    3. did not chew gum
    4. drank with a straw

    Nursing Process: Evaluation
    Client Need: Health Promotion/Maintenance

20. If a client with an ileostomy mentions all of the following as measures to reduce odors, which one indicates that the client needs more teaching? The client says it would be appropriate to
    1. ingest a charcoal tablet daily
    2. use a plastic cover over the pouch
    3. take a nonprescription chlorophyll product
    4. change and clean the pouch periodically

    Nursing Process: Evaluation
    Client Need: Health Promotion/Maintenance

21. Immediately after surgery in which a continent ileostomy has been created, which one of the following is a sign that there may be an obstruction present?
    1. The stoma protrudes several inches.
    2. The stoma appears dusky blue.
    3. Stool leaks around the catheter.
    4. It is difficult to insert the catheter.

    Nursing Process: Assessment
    Client Need: Physiological Integrity

22. The client with a continent ileostomy has understood the treatment plan correctly if he says that the ileal catheter will be removed ____ after surgery.
    1. 2 to 3 days
    2. 4 to 6 days
    3. 8 to 10 days
    4. 10 to 14 days

    Nursing Process: Evaluation
    Client Need: Safe, Effective Care Environment

23. After the ileal catheter is removed from the reservoir of a continent ileostomy, the nurse should plan to intubate the stoma every
    1. morning
    2. evening
    3. 2 to 4 hours
    4. 8 to 10 hours

    Nursing Process: Implementation
    Client Need: Physiological Integrity

24. A client with a continent ileostomy has understood the instructions of the nurse if he says that when the reservoir is siphoned, the catheter is inserted to a depth of
    1. 1 to 2 inches
    2. 2 to 3 inches
    3. 3 to 4 inches
    4. 4 to 5 inches

    Nursing Process: Evaluation
    Client Need: Health Promotion/Maintenance

25. A client scheduled for an ileoanal reservoir understands an advantage of the procedure when compared to a conventional ileostomy when he says that this surgery will not affect his
    1. fertility
    2. body image
    3. fecal consistency
    4. fecal volume

    Nursing Process: Evaluation
    Client Need: Safe, Effective Care Environment

26. The best instruction for promoting sphincter control after an ileoanal reservoir has been created is to tell the client to
    1. sit on the toilet and relax the perineum for 10 seconds
    2. tighten the anus and hold the contraction for 10 seconds
    3. contract the abdominal muscles for a count of 10 seconds
    4. take a deep breath and exhale slowly for a count of 10

    Nursing Process: Implementation
    Client Need: Health Promotion/Maintenance

27. The nurse would be most correct in telling a client that when a colostomy is created in the area of the descending colon, the fecal consistency is generally
    1. liquid
    2. semi-liquid
    3. soft
    4. formed

    Nursing Process: Implementation
    Client Need: Safe, Effective Care Environment

28. Which one of the following descriptions is most correct concerning the function of a double barrel colostomy? Feces is expelled from
    1. both the proximal and the distal stomas
    2. the proximal stoma and mucus from the distal stoma
    3. the proximal stoma and mucus is expelled from the anus
    4. the distal stoma and mucus is expelled from the proximal stoma

    Nursing Process: Implementation
    Client Need: Safe, Effective Care Environment

29. A client would have a correct understanding of the reason a loop colostomy is opened after surgery if he said this practice
    1. promotes wound healing
    2. prevents stomal edema
    3. ensures a better stomal size
    4. enhances bowel elimination

    Nursing Process: Evaluation
    Client Need: Safe, Effective Care Environment

30. The nurse would be most correct in telling a client that when the segment of the exposed bowel is opened forming a loop colostomy,
    1. the client will not feel any pain
    2. the client will be given an analgesic
    3. a local anesthetic will be provided
    4. a sedative will be administered

    Nursing Process: Implementation
    Client Need: Safe, Effective Care Environment

31. Which one of the following would be essential to document in the nursing care plan of a client with a double barrel colostomy?
    1. date of the client's last normal bowel movement
    2. labeled diagram identifying the proximal and distal stomas
    3. measurement of the circumference around each stoma
    4. list of retailers who sell stomal care products

    Nursing Process: Implementation
    Client Need: Safe, Effective Care Environment

32. The best analogy the nurse could give for a colostomy irrigation is that it is similar to
    1. a urinary catheterization
    2. siphoning gas from a car
    3. a cleansing enema
    4. inflating a flat tire

    Nursing Process: Implementation
    Client Need: Safe, Effective Care Environment

33. The maximum volume of solution that should be instilled during a colostomy irrigation is no more than
    1. 500 mL
    2. 1000 mL
    3. 1500 mL
    4. 2000 mL

    Nursing Process: Implementation
    Client Need: Safe, Effective Care Environment

34. A client who has been instructed on colostomy irrigation repeats all of the following explanations for the causes of cramping. Which one indicates the client needs more teaching? The client says that cramping may indicate that the
    1. bowel is ready to evacuate
    2. irrigating solution is too cold
    3. solution is instilled too rapidly
    4. irrigation tip is too large

    Nursing Process: Evaluation
    Client Need: Health Promotion/Maintenance

35. The best evidence that a client knows the maximum distance that an irrigation tip can be inserted within a stoma during colostomy irrigation is when the client identifies the depth as no more than
    1. 6 inches
    2. 4 inches
    3. 2 inches
    4. 1 inch

    Nursing Process: Evaluation
    Client Need: Health Promotion/Maintenance

II. CRITICAL THINKING EXERCISES

1. Mr. Eugene Taylor, age 38, will have a total colectomy and conventional ileostomy. What preoperative activities would you explain to Mr. Taylor?

2. What information would be important to include in the teaching plan for a client with a conventional ileostomy?

3. Mr. Lawrence Baker, age 32, has an ileostomy. He is depressed about how its presence will affect sexual relationships. What information could the nurse provide?

4. What are the differences between single barrel, double barrel, and loop colostomies?

5. What instructions are appropriate when teaching a client to irrigate a colostomy?

6. What recommendations could the nurse make to a client whose colostomy irrigation solution does not drain after more than 30 minutes?

53/ Caring for Clients with Disorders of the Liver, Gallbladder, and Pancreas

Digestion is impaired without the added assistance of accessory organs like the liver, gallbladder, and pancreas. Though each participates in the digestive process, these organs also play a role in other physiological activities. When disorders in accessory organs occur, they can affect the homeostasis of many body systems.

The following questions deal with the content of Chapter 53.

I. MULTIPLE CHOICE QUESTIONS

Circle the number of the most appropriate answer.

1. If a client's jaundice is due to liver or biliary disease, the nurse would most likely see an elevation in which one of the following laboratory test results?
   1. unconjugated bilirubin
   2. conjugated bilirubin
   3. free bilirubin
   4. indirect bilirubin

   Nursing Process: Assessment
   Client Need: Physiological Integrity

2. The best explanation for why stool may appear clay-colored is that it lacks
   1. fiber content
   2. bile pigment
   3. moisture
   4. cellulose

   Nursing Process: Implementation
   Client Need: Health Promotion/Maintenance

3. During the end-of-shift report a nurse asks what causes Laennec's cirrhosis. The reporting nurse would be most correct in identifying which one of the following etiologies?
   1. obstruction of bile ducts
   2. right-sided heart failure
   3. constrictive pericarditis
   4. chronic alcohol abuse

   Nursing Process: Implementation
   Client Need: Safe, Effective Care Environment

4. If a client with cirrhosis is typical of others with the disease, he or she is likely to describe having
   1. nosebleeds
   2. leg cramps
   3. cold feet
   4. dry mouth

   Nursing Process: Assessment
   Client Need: Safe, Effective Care Environment

5. In a male client with cirrhosis, which one of the following physical findings would be considered *atypical*? The client has
   1. gynecomastia
   2. flat abdomen
   3. palmar erythema
   4. spider angiomata

   Nursing Process: Assessment
   Client Need: Safe, Effective Care Environment

6. The nurse would be most correct in explaining to a client with cirrhosis that the primary goal of medical management is
   1. finding a liver for transplantation
   2. restoring pre-disease liver function
   3. preserving existing liver function
   4. replacing the functions of the liver

   Nursing Process: Implementation
   Client Need: Safe, Effective Care Environment

7. When caring for a client with cirrhosis, the nurse might notice which one of the following assessment findings as one of the earliest signs of alcohol withdrawal?

   1. hypertension
   2. bradycardia
   3. nausea and vomiting
   4. chills and fever

   Nursing Process: Assessment
   Client Need: Psychosocial Integrity

8. The nurse would be most correct in explaining to a client with a cirrhotic liver that blood flow is often obstructed, leading to congestion in the

   1. inferior vena cava
   2. renal artery
   3. portal vein
   4. ascending aorta

   Nursing Process: Implementation
   Client Need: Health Promotion/Maintenance

9. The nurse reports that a client with cirrhosis has had a large weight gain and has pitting edema of the lower extremities. If the physician prescribes a diuretic, which one is the most likely choice?

   1. furosemide (Lasix), a loop diuretic
   2. chlorothiazide (Diuril), a thiazide diuretic
   3. mannitol (Osmitrol), an osmotic diuretic
   4. spironolactone (Aldactone), a potassium-sparing diuretic

   Nursing Process: Planning
   Client Need: Physiological Integrity

10. The physician prescribes a restricted sodium diet for a client with cirrhosis. The best reason the nurse can give the client for this medical order is that avoiding sodium will help to prevent edema and

    1. reduce blood volume
    2. slow the heart rate
    3. dilate blood vessels
    4. augment heart contraction

    Nursing Process: Implementation
    Client Need: Safe, Effective Care Environment

11. While discussing the care of a client with esophageal varices at a nursing team conference, the primary care nurse would be most correct in attributing the development of the varices to

    1. peptic ulcer disease
    2. portal hypertension
    3. a hiatal hernia
    4. gallstones

    Nursing Process: Implementation
    Client Need: Safe, Effective Care Environment

12. The best explanation for why esophageal varices bleed so easily is that they

    1. are easily traumatized by food and chemicals
    2. tend to be malformed due to a congenital weakness
    3. are buried deeply within the muscular layer of esophagus
    4. do not have the capacity to form collateral circulation

    Nursing Process: Implementation
    Client Need: Safe, Effective Care Environment

13. Which one of the following tubes would be important to have on hand if a client has esophageal varices?

    1. Dubhoff tube
    2. Harris tube
    3. Sengstaken-Blakemore tube
    4. Miller-Abbott tube

    Nursing Process: Planning
    Client Need: Physiological Integrity

14. A nurse is asked to prepare a client with ascites for a paracentesis. Which one of the following is essential to the safety of the client?

    1. administer a sedative
    2. listen to bowel sounds
    3. check the apical pulse
    4. have the client void

    Nursing Process: Implementation
    Client Need: Safe, Effective Care Environment

15. Which one of the following assessment findings is most likely due to ascites? The client is
    1. jaundiced
    2. short of breath
    3. constipated
    4. nauseous

    Nursing Process: Assessment
    Client Need: Physiological Integrity

16. A client who will undergo a peritoneal venous shunt (LeVeen shunt) to reduce ascites asks the nurse to clarify into which blood vessel the fluid is redirected. The correct answer is the
    1. portal vein
    2. jugular vein
    3. hepatic vein
    4. splenic vein

    Nursing Process: Implementation
    Client Need: Safe, Effective Care Environment

17. The best explanation for why encephalopathy develops among clients with liver failure is that it is due to the accumulation of
    1. fibrinogen
    2. prothrombin
    3. ammonia
    4. bilirubin

    Nursing Process: Implementation
    Client Need: Safe, Effective Care Environment

18. The most effective dietary means of reducing encephalopathy associated with liver failure is by limiting the client's intake of
    1. sodium
    2. potassium
    3. carbohydrates
    4. protein

    Nursing Process: Implementation
    Client Need: Physiological Integrity

19. When a colleague asks the nurse for the term that refers to a flapping tremor of the hands, the best answer is
    1. grand mal
    2. asterixis
    3. chorea
    4. palsy

    Nursing Process: Implementation
    Client Need: Safe, Effective Care Environment

20. When clarifying the prognosis of chronic active hepatitis to a client with this condition, the nurse would be correct in saying that
    1. most recover without liver damage
    2. liver damage continues to occur
    3. liver damage does not worsen
    4. all liver cells remain functional

    Nursing Process: Implementation
    Client Need: Health Promotion/Maintenance

21. Which one of the following nursing measures would be most appropriate for preventing the transmission of the hepatitis B virus (HBV)?
    1. using universal precautions
    2. obtaining immune globulin (IG)
    3. not sharing cigarettes
    4. not eating raw seafood

    Nursing Process: Implementation
    Client Need: Safe, Effective Care Environment

22. If the client with a primary, malignant liver tumor is similar to many others who develop this condition, which disorder is most likely to have occurred in the client's past medical history?
    1. ulcerative colitis
    2. irritable bowel syndrome
    3. cirrhosis of the liver
    4. hepatitis B infection

    Nursing Process: Assessment
    Client Need: Safe, Effective Care Environment

23. The nurse reviews the laboratory test results on a client suspected of having a primary liver tumor. If all of the following tests are elevated, which one supports the tentative diagnosis?

    1. uric acid
    2. creatinine
    3. carcinoembryonic antigen (CEA)
    4. alpha-fetoprotein (AFP)

    Nursing Process: Assessment
    Client Need: Physiological Integrity

24. After a liver biopsy is performed, the nurse should plan to keep the client in which one of the following positions?

    1. dorsal recumbent
    2. right lateral
    3. Trendelenburg
    4. high Fowler's

    Nursing Process: Planning
    Client Need: Safe, Effective Care Environment

25. Following a liver biopsy, the complication for which the nurse must monitor to detect is

    1. hemorrhage
    2. encephalopathy
    3. paralytic ileus
    4. bowel obstruction

    Nursing Process: Planning
    Client Need: Physiological Integrity

26. The client with ascites is likely to be most comfortable in which one of the following positions?

    1. Fowler's
    2. Sim's
    3. lithotomy
    4. supine

    Nursing Process: Implementation
    Client Need: Physiological Integrity

27. If a client receives albumin to mobilize fluid trapped within interstitial tissue or the peritoneum, which one of the following assessments would be the best indication of its effectiveness?

    1. lung sounds
    2. bowel sounds
    3. pulse rate
    4. urine output

    Nursing Process: Evaluation
    Client Need: Physiological Integrity

28. If a jaundiced client develops pruritus, which one of the following should the nurse plan to avoid?

    1. soap
    2. iodine
    3. peroxide
    4. oxygen

    Nursing Process: Planning
    Client Need: Physiological Integrity

29. If it is necessary to give a client with cirrhosis an intramuscular injection, which gauge needle would be most appropriate to use?

    1. 16-gauge
    2. 18-gauge
    3. 20-gauge
    4. 23-gauge

    Nursing Process: Implementation
    Client Need: Physiological Integrity

30. After giving an injection to a client with a liver disorder, the nurse would choose which one of the following actions as most appropriate?

    1. allow the swabbed area to air dry
    2. rub the injection site vigorously
    3. apply firm, prolonged pressure to the site
    4. swab the area with alcohol using a circular pat-

    Nursing Process: Implementation
    Client Need: Physiological Integrity

31. If a client with a liver disorder becomes disoriented and confused, which one of the following would be the best action to take first?

    1. obtain an order for a sedative drug, such as diazepam (Valium)
    2. obtain an order for and apply restraints to all extremities
    3. relocate the client to a room close to the nursing station
    4. tell the client to use the signal cord attached to the bed

    Nursing Process: Planning
    Client Need: Safe, Effective Care Environment

32. During the data-base assessment, the client with gallstones is most likely to tell the nurse that pain is experienced when

    1. fried foods are consumed
    2. the stomach is empty
    3. a meal contains whole grains
    4. the meal includes alcohol

    Nursing Process: Assessment
    Client Need: Physiological Integrity

33. If the pain associated with gallbladder disorders radiates, it is most likely to be felt in the

    1. arm
    2. jaw
    3. teeth
    4. back

    Nursing Process: Assessment
    Client Need: Physiological Integrity

34. Which one of the following assessment findings is most typical of an obstruction in the bile ducts?

    1. urine is dark brown
    2. stools are black
    3. skin is pale
    4. nailbeds are dusky

    Nursing Process: Assessment
    Client Need: Physiological Integrity

35. If a client has cholecystitis, which one of the following foods should the client avoid?

    1. cheddar cheese
    2. cottage cheese
    3. dill pickles
    4. canned tuna

    Nursing Process: Implementation
    Client Need: Health Promotion/Maintenance

36. Which one of the following drugs should be questioned if it is prescribed for a client with cholecystitis?

    1. meperidine (Demerol)
    2. ketorolac (Toradol)
    3. codeine sulfate
    4. morphine sulfate

    Nursing Process: Implementation
    Client Need: Physiological Integrity

37. If a client plans to have his gallbladder removed with a laparoscope, which one of the following statements indicates that the client needs more teaching? The client says, "I will

    1. have a T-tube for bile drainage"
    2. have three or four abdominal puncture sites"
    3. be able to go home in 24 to 48 hours"
    4. have only slight pain for a few days"

    Nursing Process: Evaluation
    Client Need: Safe, Effective Care Environment

38. During the immediate postoperative care of a client with a T-tube, which one of the following notations is appropriate to add to the care plan?

    1. clamp the T-tube for 2 hours and then release for 2 hours
    2. do not clamp the T-tube until there is a medical order
    3. keep the drainage collector above the operative site
    4. irrigate the T-tube with 30 mL of sterile normal saline

    Nursing Process: Implementation
    Client Need: Safe, Effective Care Environment

39. Which one of the following statements indicates that the client who has had the gallbladder removed needs more teaching?
    1. I will have to take bile replacements.
    2. bile will be in an unconcentrated form.
    3. I may eat fats again in moderation.
    4. my liver will produce sufficient bile.

    Nursing Process: Evaluation
    Client Need: Safe, Effective Care Environment

40. Which one of the following statements is the best evidence that a client with pancreatitis understands the etiology of his symptoms? The client says,
    1. "My pancreas is infected with pathogens"
    2. "My pancreas is being destroyed by digestive enzymes"
    3. "My pancreas is being attacked by destructive antibodies"
    4. "My pancreas is gangrenous from lack of arterial blood"

    Nursing Process: Evaluation
    Client Need: Health Promotion/Maintenance

41. When examining the stool of a client with pancreatitis, which one of the following characteristics is the nurse most likely to observe? The stool is
    1. liquid and green
    2. well formed and tarry
    3. frothy and foul smelling
    4. pencil-shaped and brown

    Nursing Process: Assessment
    Client Need: Physiological Integrity

42. When performing a physical assessment, which one of the following signs supports the diagnosis of acute pancreatitis? The nurse observes a
    1. bluish-gray skin discoloration about the umbilicus
    2. brown pigmented stripe down the center of the abdomen
    3. diagonal crease in both ear lobes
    4. raised yellow plaques about the eyelids

    Nursing Process: Assessment
    Client Need: Physiological Integrity

43. If the client with pancreatitis has a low serum calcium level, the nurse is most likely to observe
    1. evidence of previous pathological fractures
    2. spasm of the fingers when taking a blood pressure
    3. poor condition of the teeth
    4. fast, irregular heart beat

    Nursing Process: Assessment
    Client Need: Physiological Integrity

44. According to laboratory test results, the most diagnostic evidence for pancreatitis is an elevation of
    1. lactase
    2. maltase
    3. urokinase
    4. amylase

    Nursing Process: Assessment
    Client Need: Physiological Integrity

45. The nurse is most correct in explaining to the client with pancreatitis that the drug that has been pre-scribed to reduce the activity of the vagus nerve and thereby protect the pancreas is
    1. morphine sulfate, a narcotic analgesic
    2. atropine sulfate, a cholinergic blocker
    3. cimetidine (Tagamet), an H_2 antagonist
    4. chlorpromazine (Thorazine), an antiemetic

    Nursing Process: Implementation
    Client Need: Health Promotion/Maintenance

46. To detect complications from pancreatitis, the nurse should plan to monitor
    1. urine specific gravity
    2. capillary blood glucose
    3. stool for occult blood
    4. pH of gastric secretions

    Nursing Process: Planning
    Client Need: Physiological Integrity

47. A client with chronic pancreatitis is most likely to manifest
    1. anorexia and indigestion
    2. nausea and vomiting
    3. flatulence and diarrhea
    4. cramping and constipation

    Nursing Process: Assessment
    Client Need: Physiological Integrity

48. If pancreatic enzyme replacement therapy is prescribed, the best time for the nurse to administer it is
    1. with each meal
    2. before breakfast
    3. between meals
    4. before sleep

    Nursing Process: Planning
    Client Need: Physiological Integrity

49. Which one of the following assessments would provide the best evidence for evaluating the effectiveness of pancreatic enzyme replacement therapy?
    1. characteristics of stools
    2. level and location of pain
    3. color of skin and sclera
    4. amount and color of urine

    Nursing Process: Evaluation
    Client Need: Physiological Integrity

50. Which one of the following would be most appropriate to use around abdominal sump drains to prevent skin excoriation from fluid containing pancreatic enzymes?
    1. povidone iodine (Betadine) ointment
    2. nitroglycerin transdermal patch
    3. a collar about the drain made from cardboard
    4. a karaya disc with an ostomy appliance

    Nursing Process: Implementation
    Client Need: Physiological Integrity

II. CRITICAL THINKING EXERCISES

1. How would you explain portal hypertension to a client with cirrhosis of the liver?

2. How would you explain the purpose and procedure for a portocaval shunt?

3. When there is an outbreak of hepatitis in a community, a parent–teachers organization plans a meeting during which they are seeking a nurse who will speak about the types of hepatitis, modes of transmission, and how hepatitis may be prevented. If you were to volunteer as this program's speaker, what information would you include?

4. What information should the nurse include for a client who must take pancreatic enzyme replacements?

XII Caring for Clients with Endocrine Problems

54/ Introduction to the Endocrine System

Endocrine glands secrete their hormones directly into the bloodstream. Most disorders of the endocrine system are the result of overproduction or underproduction of the hormones that the glands secrete, causing a disturbance in the delicate balance that hormones normally maintain.

The following questions deal with the content of Chapter 54.

I. MULTIPLE CHOICE QUESTIONS

Circle the number of the most appropriate answer.

A series of team conferences are scheduled for discussion of endocrine disorders. The first conference focuses on the anatomy and physiology of the endocrine system.

1. When asked to give the function of adrenocorticotrophic hormone, the nurse states that this hormone controls
   1. secretions of the adrenal medulla and adrenal cortex
   2. the pituitary
   3. the growth, development, and function of the adrenal cortex
   4. all endocrine glands

   Nursing Process: Implementation
   Client Need: Safe, Effective Care Environment

2. When asked to give the function of antidiuretic hormone, the nurse's correct response is that this hormone controls the excretion of water by the kidneys by affecting
   1. potassium excretion by the kidneys
   2. the thirst mechanism of the thalamus
   3. calcium ions contained in urine
   4. the reabsorption of water from the kidney tubules

   Nursing Process: Implementation
   Client Need: Safe, Effective Care Environment

3. When asked to name two hormones produced by the thyroid gland, the nurse's correct response is
    1. tetraiodothyronine and triiodothyronine
    2. thyroid-releasing hormone and parathormone
    3. calcitonin and thyroid-inhibiting hormone
    4. thyroxine 4 and thyroxine 3

    Nursing Process: Implementation
    Client Need: Safe, Effective Care Environment

4. The nurse uses a textbook to review the anatomy of endocrine glands and finds that the known function of the thymus is the
    1. development of T lymphocytes
    2. production of antithymus hormone
    3. regulation of phosphorus metabolism
    4. regulation of the thyroid and parathyroids

    Nursing Process: Implementation
    Client Need: Safe, Effective Care Environment

5. The anatomy book also states that the adrenal cortex manufactures and secretes
    1. glucocorticoids, mineralocorticoids, and small amounts of sex hormones
    2. epinephrine, norepinephrine, and estrogen
    3. adrenal cortical-inhibiting hormone
    4. adrenocorticotrophic hormone and corticosteroids

    Nursing Process: Implementation
    Client Need: Safe, Effective Care Environment

6. When checking another reference, the nurse reads that the adrenal medulla produces
    1. corticosteroids
    2. epinephrine and norepinephrine
    3. adrenal medullary hormone
    4. antidiuretic hormone

    Nursing Process: Implementation
    Client Need: Safe, Effective Care Environment

7. When asked to name one function of the glucocorticoids, the nurse correctly answers
    1. increasing the production of thyroid hormone
    2. promoting inflammatory activities
    3. helping the body to withstand stress
    4. suppressing the function of the kidney tubules

    Nursing Process: Implementation
    Client Need: Safe, Effective Care Environment

8. When asked to give a function of the mineralocorticoids, the nurse correctly answers
    1. maintenance of water and electrolyte balances
    2. production of growth hormone
    3. suppression of inflammation
    4. metabolism of glucose

    Nursing Process: Implementation
    Client Need: Safe, Effective Care Environment

9. When asked to give one function of the sex glands (ovaries, testicles), the nurse correctly answers
    1. determination of the sex of the fetus
    2. development of secondary sex characteristics
    3. development of primary sex characteristics
    4. inhibition of adrenal hormone release

    Nursing Process: Implementation
    Client Need: Safe, Effective Care Environment

10. A client scheduled for a thyroid scan asks about the use of radioactive materials for the test. An explanation given to this client can include the fact that this test
    1. requires avoiding contact with others for 24 hours
    2. uses harmless radioactive materials
    3. requires staying in the hospital until radioactivity ceases
    4. ordinarily poses no danger to others

    Nursing Process: Implementation
    Client Need: Safe, Effective Care Environment

II. CRITICAL THINKING EXERCISES

1. Ms. Craig, who was seen in the medical outpatient clinic, is scheduled for thyroid function tests including a radioactive iodine uptake test and a thyroid scan. There are situations that can make these test invalid, and allergy to certain substances may require the tests be canceled. When obtaining a history, what specific questions would you ask Ms. Craig?

55/ Caring for Clients with Disorders of the Endocrine System

Endocrine glands secrete their hormones directly into the bloodstream because of the rich blood supply surrounding the glands and their hormone-secreting cells. A disorder of any one of the endocrine glands has the potential for a profound effect on other endocrine glands as well as many major body systems. When caring for clients with endocrine disorders, the nurse must consider not only the management of the endocrine disorder but also any effects of the disorder on other body organs and systems.

The following questions deal with the content of Chapter 55.

I. MULTIPLE CHOICE QUESTIONS

Circle the number of the most appropriate answer.

A series of team conferences and inservice programs are scheduled for all health team members. The first topic is endocrine disorders. Various health team members are assigned to be conference leaders throughout the series.

1. At a team conference the nurse is asked to describe what occurs when a client has diabetes insipidus. The most correct answer is that this disorder results in
    1. inadequate excretion of urine by the kidneys
    2. a copious output of urine
    3. extremely concentrated urine with a high specific gravity
    4. concentrated urine when fluids are limited

   Nursing Process: Implementation
   Client Need: Safe, Effective Care Environment

2. SIADH (syndrome of inappropriate antidiuretic hormone) is discussed and the nurse asks how this syndrome can be recognized. The conference leader states that SIADH is characterized by
    1. periods of apnea, diarrhea, dysuria
    2. muscle paralysis, anxiety, insomnia
    3. water retention, muscle cramps, excessive thirst
    4. difficulty swallowing, constipation, double vision

   Nursing Process: Implementation
   Client Need: Safe, Effective Care Environment

3. A nurse asks how SIADH may be treated. The most correct answer is administration of

   1. diuretics, intravenous hypertonic sodium chloride
   2. antidiuretic hormone, bedrest
   3. tranquilizers, forcing fluids
   4. antibiotics, corticosteroids

   Nursing Process: Implementation
   Client Need: Safe, Effective Care Environment

4. During an inservice program the lecturer asks if anyone can give the pathophysiology of Simmond's disease. The nurse correctly answers that this disorder is characterized by a(n)

   1. increase in pituitary hormonal activity
   2. decrease in thyroxine production
   3. increase in plasma cortisol levels
   4. absence of all pituitary hormonal activity

   Nursing Process: Implementation
   Client Need: Safe, Effective Care Environment

5. When asked to describe the treatment of cancer of the thyroid, the nurse correctly replies

   1. a total or subtotal thyroidectomy, administration of ^{131}I
   2. antithyroid drugs, corticosteroids
   3. thyroid and adrenal hormone replacement therapy
   4. iodine to suppress thyroid function, antibiotics

   Nursing Process: Implementation
   Client Need: Safe, Effective Care Environment

6. Conference members are asked to define the term *goitrogens*. The nurse replies that goitrogens are substances that

   1. destroy goiters
   2. are excreted by goiters
   3. are capable of causing a goiter
   4. are normally present in all persons

   Nursing Process: Implementation
   Client Need: Safe, Effective Care Environment

7. At an inservice lecture, those attending are asked to explain the result of overproduction of parathyroid hormone in those with hyperparathyroidism. The most correct response is

   1. decreased urinary excretion of phosphorus and calcium
   2. increase in calcium deposits in the bones
   3. decreased serum calcium, increased serum phosphorus
   4. increased urinary excretion of phosphorus, loss of calcium from the bones

   Nursing Process: Implementation
   Client Need: Safe, Effective Care Environment

Ms. Olson has hyperthyroidism and is being treated by her physician.

8. Ms. Olson is prescribed the antithyroid drug methimazole (Tapazole) and asks how this drug will help her. The nurse explains that this drug

   1. increases thyroid hormone production
   2. promotes the production of iodine by the thyroid gland
   3. increases the size of the thyroid gland
   4. blocks the production of thyroid hormone

   Nursing Process: Implementation
   Client Need: Health Promotion/Maintenance

9. When explaining drug therapy to Ms. Olson, the nurse explains that the

   1. effects of drug therapy may not be seen for several weeks
   2. drug is taken once every 3 days
   3. drug is only effective if taken with food
   4. effects of drug therapy will be seen in 2–3 days

   Nursing Process: Implementation
   Client Need: Health Promotion/Maintenance

10. Which one of the following can the nurse suggest to help relieve Ms. Olson's present symptoms of hyperthyroidism?
    1. drink hot liquids, wear extra clothing
    2. exercise frequently, eat frequent small meals
    3. drink cool liquids, keep the living area cool
    4. take frequent hot showers, avoid exposure to the sun

    Nursing Process: Implementation
    Client Need: Health Promotion/Maintenance

Ms. Shelby, age 28, has had symptoms of hyperthyroidism for 3 years. She is now admitted to the hospital for a thyroidectomy.

11. When obtaining a history from Ms. Shelby, the nurse identifies symptoms related to hyperthyroidism which usually include
    1. weight loss, intolerance to heat
    2. weight gain, sleepiness
    3. anorexia, dyspnea
    4. difficulty concentrating, intolerance to cold

    Nursing Process: Collecting Data
    Client Need: Physiological Integrity

12. During the preoperative history the nurse asks Ms. Shelby if she took the prescribed antithyroid drug for 2 weeks before surgery. This information is important because antithyroid therapy is used to
    1. increase the activity of the thyroid gland
    2. increase iodine uptake by the thyroid gland
    3. decrease the production of iodine
    4. decrease bleeding during surgery

    Nursing Process: Collecting Data
    Client Need: Physiological Integrity

13. Ms. Shelby returns from the recovery room. Once she is fully awake and responding, she is placed
    1. in a semi-Fowler's position
    2. flat and turned on her side
    3. in a full Fowler's position
    4. on her side with the head of the bed elevated

    Nursing Process: Implementation
    Client Need: Physiological Integrity

14. To detect a low serum calcium following a thyroidectomy, the nurse examines Ms. Shelby's
    1. extremities for tetany and spasm
    2. surgical dressing for evidence of bleeding
    3. face and neck for swelling
    4. abdomen for distention

    Nursing Process: Evaluation
    Client Need: Physiological Integrity

15. If Ms. Shelby complains of a sense of fullness in or around the neck, frequent evaluation is necessary to detect early signs of
    1. shock
    2. pulmonary embolus
    3. myocardial infarction
    4. airway obstruction

    Nursing Process: Evaluation
    Client Need: Physiological Integrity

16. Ms. Shelby complains of a feeling of fullness in her throat. On inspection, the surgical dressing is dry and intact. The next step is to
    1. check her chart and administer oxygen as ordered
    2. turn her on her side and slightly hyperextend her neck
    3. check for drainage on the pillow or bedding behind her neck
    4. have her cough and deep breathe

    Nursing Process: Evaluation
    Client Need: Physiological Integrity

17. During the postoperative period the nurse examines Ms. Shelby for injury to the recurrent laryngeal nerve by
    1. asking her to say a few words q2–4h
    2. auscultating the lungs q4h
    3. inspecting the surgical dressing q3–4h
    4. monitoring vital signs q4h

    Nursing Process: Implementation
    Client Need: Physiological Integrity

Ms. March is diagnosed as having hypothyroidism and is being treated in an outpatient clinic with thyroid hormone replacement.

18. Ms. March states that she does not like to take medications. The nurse explains that if her hypothyroidism is not treated it may lead to
    1. enlargement of the heart, an increased tendency toward atherosclerosis
    2. an increased heart rate, severe weight loss
    3. visual problems, arthritis
    4. liver enlargement, severe diarrhea

    Nursing Process: Implementation
    Client Need: Health Promotion/Maintenance

19. When Ms. March is seen in the clinic, the nurse observes her for adverse effects of thyroid replacement therapy, namely
    1. weight gain, bradycardia
    2. signs of hyperthyroidism
    3. lethargy, edema of the hands and feet
    4. signs of hypothyroidism

    Nursing Process: Evaluation
    Client Need: Physiological Integrity

20. Ms. March asks if her thyroid problem happened recently. The nurse can explain that hypothyroidism may go unnoticed for many years because
    1. there are few laboratory tests that can confirm the diagnosis
    2. there are no symptoms connected with this disorder
    3. the symptoms are the same as many other diseases or disorders
    4. many of the symptoms are very general and nonspecific

    Nursing Process: Implementation
    Client Need: Health Promotion/Maintenance

Mr. Williams, a 23-year-old factory worker, was discovered to have Addison's disease 2 years ago. He is now admitted to the hospital acutely ill and thought to be in adrenal crisis.

21. When performing an initial physical examination, the nurse checks Mr. Williams' skin. If he has Addison's disease his skin will appear
    1. abnormally dark and pigmented
    2. ruddy and oily
    3. puffy
    4. pale, dry, and scaly

    Nursing Process: Collecting Data
    Client Need: Physiological Integrity

22. Mr. Williams is observed for the gradual development of the early signs of adrenal crisis which usually include
    1. nausea, vomiting, intensification of hypotension
    2. constipation, abdominal distention, increased urinary output
    3. urinary retention, chest pain, numbness in the extremities
    4. headache, absence of bowel sounds, double vision

    Nursing Process: Collecting Data
    Client Need: Physiological Integrity

23. During a team conference the nurse explains that Mr. Williams developed adrenal crisis because there was a(n)
    1. increase in his blood cortisol levels
    2. sudden failure of his adrenal glands
    3. change in his blood pressure
    4. decrease in his potassium and sodium blood

    Nursing Process: Implementation
    Client Need: Safe, Effective Care Environment

24. The nurse prepares for the emergency treatment of adrenal crisis by checking for the immediate availability of
    1. an IV corticosteroid, IV normal saline and glucose
    2. IV normal saline, ACTH, and potassium
    3. IM ACTH and IV glucose
    4. an IV corticosteroid and oral potassium tablets

    Nursing Process: Implementation
    Client Need: Physiological Integrity

25. When planning discharge teaching, the nurse prepares to reinforce the physician's explanation of ongoing medical treatment which includes
    1. cortisone and thyroxine
    2. ACTH and corticotropin
    3. a medication possessing both glucocorticoid and mineralocorticoid properties
    4. a medication that will stimulate both the pituitary and adrenal glands

    Nursing Process: Planning
    Client Need: Health Promotion/Maintenance

26. When teaching Mr. Williams about management of his disorder, the nurse stresses that he must
    1. exercise daily and eat a low-carbohydrate diet
    2. avoid the use of salt and foods high in sodium
    3. add foods to his diet that are high in potassium
    4. avoid exposure to infections and stressful situations

    Nursing Process: Implementation
    Client Need: Health Promotion/Maintenance

27. During a teaching session the nurse also stresses that the prescribed corticosteroid
    1. must be taken as directed and never be omitted
    2. dosage can be decreased if infection occurs
    3. can be omitted if nausea occurs
    4. must be taken with meals or milk

    Nursing Process: Implementation
    Client Need: Health Promotion/Maintenance

Ms. Barnes, a 35-year-old housewife, works part-time as a clerk in a small dress shop. Three months ago she noticed she began to gain weight and developed other physical changes. Following a visit to her physician and many clinical tests, she was diagnosed as having Cushing's syndrome.

28. When explaining Cushing's syndrome during a team conference, the nurse states that this disorder is caused by a(n)
    1. decrease in the production of mineralocorticoids
    2. overproduction of adrenal cortical hormones
    3. decrease in glucocorticoid production
    4. cessation of pituitary stimulation of the adrenal glands

    Nursing Process: Implementation
    Client Need: Safe, Effective Care Environment

29. When performing a physical assessment, the nurse looks for signs of Cushing's syndrome which may include
    1. pale complexion, periods of apnea
    2. evidence of weight loss, hypotension
    3. tachycardia, dilated pupils
    4. moon face, muscle wasting

    Nursing Process: Collecting Data
    Client Need: Physiological Integrity

30. When obtaining a history from Ms. Barnes, the nurse identifies complaints that may be related to Cushing's disease which may include
    1. repeated infections, absence of menses
    2. increase in appetite, loss of weight
    3. diarrhea, burning on urination
    4. frequent urination, heavy menses

    Nursing Process: Collecting Data
    Client Need: Physiological Integrity

31. Ms. Barnes is scheduled for a bilateral adrenalectomy. When helping develop a plan of postoperative nursing management, the nurse suggests
    1. observing for problems associated with Cushing's syndrome
    2. monitoring vital signs q8h
    3. observing for signs of adrenal insufficiency
    4. changing the surgical dressing q4h

    Nursing Process: Implementation
    Client Need: Safe, Effective Care Environment

32. When doing client teaching, the nurse explains to Ms. Barnes that the dose of the prescribed corticosteroid drug
    1. will remain constant
    2. may need to be adjusted to meet her body's needs
    3. changes daily
    4. depends on her diet

    Nursing Process: Implementation
    Client Need: Health Promotion/Maintenance

Individual Questions

33. A client is scheduled to receive radioactive iodine as treatment for hyperthyroidism. The nurse can explain that this procedure
    1. increases the thyroid gland's ability to use iodine
    2. removes thyroid hormones from the gland
    3. destroys thyroid tissue
    4. increases the size of the thyroid gland

    Nursing Process: Implementation
    Client Need: Health Promotion/Maintenance

34. A nurse assistant asks the meaning of the term *endemic goiter*. The nurse describes this disorder as an enlargement of the thyroid
    1. usually without symptoms of thyroid dysfunction
    2. due to an increase of iodine in the diet
    3. due to a deficiency of thyroid-stimulating hormone
    4. seen in those under age 35

    Nursing Process: Implementation
    Client Need: Health Promotion/Maintenance

35. When a client has a goiter, which one of the following can be recommended to be included in the diet?
    1. foods high in iron
    2. iodized salt
    3. foods high in potassium
    4. salt substitutes

    Nursing Process: Implementation
    Client Need: Health Promotion/Maintenance

36. When a client is diagnosed as having thyrotoxic crisis,
    1. a warming blanket is used to raise the body temperature
    2. an incentive spirometer is used to increase respiratory rate and depth
    3. the temperature is monitored at frequent intervals
    4. oral fluids are withheld

    Nursing Process: Implementation
    Client Need: Physiological Integrity

37. Mr. Charles asks why his hyperparathyroidism requires surgery. The nurse explains that surgery is necessary since persons with this disorder have a tendency to develop
    1. malignant tumors
    2. severe anemia and weight loss
    3. lung tumors
    4. renal disease including kidney stones and pyelonephritis

    Nursing Process: Implementation
    Client Need: Health Promotion/Maintenance

38. When explaining long-term treatment to a client with hypoparathyroidism, the nurse explains that it will be necessary to
    1. eat a diet low in calcium
    2. take vitamins A, B$_1$, and C
    3. take vitamin D or D$_2$
    4. eat a diet high in phosphorus

    Nursing Process: Implementation
    Client Need: Health Promotion/Maintenance

39. Which one of the following is placed in the room if a client is admitted with severe hypocalcemia?
    1. IV potassium gluconate
    2. an emergency tracheostomy tray
    3. extra bed linens
    4. a nasogastric tube

    Nursing Process: Implementation
    Client Need: Physiological Integrity

40. If intravenous administration of a calcium salt is necessary to correct severe hypoparathyroidism, the client is observed for
    1. hypotension, abdominal distention, diarrhea
    2. flushing, cardiac arrhythmia, tingling in the extremities
    3. excessive salivation, difficulty swallowing, chest pain
    4. dyspnea, headache, diaphoresis

    Nursing Process: Evaluation
    Client Need: Physiological Integrity

41. When a client is receiving a corticosteroid drug over a prolonged period of time and the drug is to be discontinued, the nurse must make sure that the dosage on the medication cards is strictly followed since the dose of the drug
    1. is decreased over a period of 1 to 2 days
    2. must be tapered over a period of time
    3. must be discontinued after 3 days
    4. is increased before it is decreased

    Nursing Process: Implementation
    Client Need: Physiological Integrity

42. Nursing management of the client with a pheochromocytoma includes
    1. closely monitoring the blood pressure when therapy is initiated
    2. notifying the physician if the urinary output is below 1000 mL/day
    3. auscultating heart and lung sounds daily
    4. keeping the client on complete bedrest

    Nursing Process: Implementation
    Client Need: Physiological Integrity

43. Clients with hyperthyroidism are advised to
    1. avoid foods high in protein
    2. keep their caloric intake below 2000 calories a day
    3. avoid CNS stimulants such as caffeine and alcohol
    4. limit their carbohydrate and fat intake

    Nursing Process: Implementation
    Client Need: Health Promotion/Maintenance

II. CRITICAL THINKING EXERCISES

1. Your neighbor Ms. Hampton was diagnosed as hypothyroid and was started on thyroid replacement therapy. After 3 weeks of medication she tells you that she threw away her medication because it was not helping her. She also tells you that she is not going to call her doctor for another appointment. What advice or suggestions would you give Ms. Hampton?

2. Ms. Reese had a thyroidectomy yesterday. Today her voice is hoarse, and she is complaining of difficulty in breathing and swallowing. What nursing actions would you take?

3. Mr. Kerr is admitted with possible primary adrenal insufficiency (Addison's disease). Shortly after admission he develops severe hypotension, vomiting, and fever. He complains of abdominal pain and a headache. What immediate nursing measures are taken until the client is seen by a physician and treatment is instituted?

4. Ms. Timon developed diabetes insipidus following a severe head injury. She is admitted unconscious and, according to her family, had not been taking desmopressin (DDAVP) to control her urinary output. Intravenous fluid replacement will be necessary to correct her fluid imbalance. What specific nursing tasks are included in her plan of care?

56/ Caring for Clients with Diabetes Mellitus

The pancreas is both an endocrine and exocrine gland. *Diabetes mellitus* is a metabolic disorder of the pancreas in which glucose intolerance results from varying degrees of insulin insufficiency. Although no age group is exempt, diabetes is most frequently seen in people between ages 40 and 60.

The following questions deal with the content of Chapter 56.

I. MULTIPLE CHOICE QUESTIONS

Circle the number of the most appropriate answer.

During National Hospital Week, the American Diabetes Association conducted a detection service. Ms. Jacobs decided to have a small sample of blood taken from her finger for a screening test for diabetes. She was advised to see a physician because of the results of the test. Ms. Jacobs' physician orders a series of laboratory tests at the time of her first office visit.

1. When reviewing the results of the fasting blood glucose performed on Ms. Jacobs, the nurse is aware that the normal fasting blood glucose is ____ mg/dL.
    1. 60–80
    2. 70–110
    3. 100–150
    4. 100–200

    Nursing Process: Evaluation
    Client Need: Physiological Integrity

2. Which of the following symptoms obtained by the nurse during the initial history are most probably related to diabetes mellitus?
    1. weight gain, headache, diarrhea
    2. constipation, bloating, epigastric distress
    3. loss of appetite, weight loss, swelling of the ankles
    4. excessive thirst, excessive urine production, hunger

    Nursing Process: Collecting Data
    Client Need: Physiological Integrity

3. Ms. Jacobs asks why the body needs insulin. The most correct response is insulin is used to
    1. aid in the use of glucose by the body
    2. reduce the amount of fat stored in the liver
    3. change carbohydrates to glucose
    4. decrease cellular metabolism

    Nursing Process: Implementation
    Client Need: Health Promotion/Maintenance

4. Mrs. Jacobs requires insulin to control her diabetes. The physician prescribes 36 units of insulin daily, and she will be using insulin labeled as U100. When explaining the label on the insulin bottle, the nurse is most correct in saying that
    1. the entire bottle contains 100 units of insulin
    2. 1 mL contains 100 units of insulin
    3. 1 mL contains 36 units of insulin
    4. 1 mL contains 50 units of insulin

    Nursing Process: Implementation
    Client Need: Health Promotion/Maintenance

5. Since Ms. Jacobs is taking insulin, she is taught about insulin lipoatrophy which occurs when
    1. insulin doses are skipped
    2. regular insulin is used
    3. repeated insulin injections are given into the same area
    4. her diet is high in fats

    Nursing Process: Implementation
    Client Need: Health Promotion/Maintenance

6. Ms. Jacobs is also made aware of the fact that she
    1. must eat a diet high in protein and fats
    2. must self-monitor her blood glucose level 30 minutes after each meal
    3. cannot take many antibiotic preparations because these drugs interact with insulin
    4. is susceptible to infection, especially of the skin and subcutaneous tissues

    Nursing Process: Implementation
    Client Need: Health Promotion/Maintenance

Mr. Terry is admitted to the hospital with the diagnosis of diabetic ketoacidosis (DKA).

7. When performing an initial assessment on Mr. Terry, the nurse looks for the signs and symptoms of DKA which include
    1. severe anxiety, hypertension, abdominal distention
    2. drowsiness, dry skin, hypotension
    3. pale skin, cyanosis, dyspnea
    4. restlessness, diarrhea, pronounced bradycardia

    Nursing Process: Collecting Data
    Client Need: Physiological Integrity

8. Ms. Terry asks what caused her husband's problem. The nurse correctly replies that his problem was caused by
    1. taking too little insulin
    2. taking too much insulin
    3. eating a diet high in fat
    4. eating a diet low in carbohydrates

    Nursing Process: Implementation
    Client Need: Health Promotion/Maintenance

9. When helping to develop a plan of nursing management, the nurse knows that treatment of Mr. Terry will most likely include
    1. a high-carbohydrate diet
    2. administration of glycogen
    3. a salt-restricted, low-protein diet
    4. administration of insulin

    Nursing Process: Planning
    Client Need: Safe, Effective Care Environment

10. Because of poor compliance to his treatment regimen, Mr. Terry is referred to a diabetic teaching program. During the program, the nurse discusses the complications of diabetes. Which of the following problems have an increased incidence in those with diabetes mellitus?

    1. circulatory disturbances, DKA, diabetic retinopathy
    2. coronary artery disease, diarrhea, stomatitis
    3. diverticulitis, pathological fractures, cirrhosis
    4. ileitis, polycythemia, pneumonia

    Nursing Process: Implementation
    Client Need: Health Promotion/Maintenance

A team conference is held to review the pathophysiology, treatment, and nursing management of clients with diabetes mellitus.

11. A nurse assistant attending the conference asks where insulin comes from. The most correct response is that insulin is

    1. secreted by ß cells in the pancreas
    2. manufactured by the liver and secreted by the pancreas
    3. present in and manufactured by all body cells
    4. secreted by special cells in the liver

    Nursing Process: Implementation
    Client Need: Safe, Effective Care Environment

12. A nurse asks, "After a person eats, when does the blood glucose level normally return close to a fasting level?" The most correct response is in approximately

    1. 30 minutes
    2. 2 hours
    3. 4 hours
    4. 6 hours

    Nursing Process: Implementation
    Client Need: Safe, Effective Care Environment

13. A nurse assistant asks what the term *ketone bodies* means. The most correct response is ketone bodies are

    1. formed when the body is unable to metabolize proteins
    2. the result of glucose metabolism
    3. stored in the liver and used for energy
    4. chemical intermediate products in the metabolism of fat

    Nursing Process: Implementation
    Client Need: Safe, Effective Care Environment

14. The importance of diet in the management of diabetes mellitus is discussed. The conference leader asks what happens if the carbohydrate intake is more than can be used or stored. The most correct response is

    1. hypoglycemia
    2. hyperkalemia
    3. ketoacidosis
    4. acidosis

    Nursing Process: Implementation
    Client Need: Safe, Effective Care Environment

15. A nurse asks when diabetes mellitus cannot be treated with one of the oral hypoglycemic agents. The most correct response is that these agents cannot be used in a client who

    1. is overweight
    2. has too much pancreatic insulin-secreting activity
    3. is elderly
    4. has little or no pancreatic insulin-secreting activity

    Nursing Process: Implementation
    Client Need: Safe, Effective Care Environment

16. A nurse assistant asks how an oral hypoglycemic agent helps control diabetes mellitus. The most correct response is that these agents

    1. stimulate the ß cells of the pancreas to secrete more insulin
    2. increase insulin levels in the cell
    3. are broken down into insulin in the stomach
    4. dilate the pancreatic duct thereby helping in the release of insulin

    Nursing Process: Implementation
    Client Need: Safe, Effective Care Environment

Individual Questions

17. When charting respirations that are fast, deep, and labored as seen in those with diabetic acidosis, the nurse correctly uses the term
    1. irregular respirations
    2. Cheyne-Stokes respirations
    3. Kussmaul respirations
    4. Trousseau's respirations

    Nursing Process: Implementation
    Client Need: Safe, Effective Care Environment

18. When a postprandial glucose is ordered, the nurse makes sure that a blood sample is drawn
    1. 1 hour before eating a normal meal
    2. 2 hours after eating a high-carbohydrate meal
    3. 1 hour after eating a high-fat meal
    4. 4 hours after eating a high-carbohydrate meal

    Nursing Process: Implementation
    Client Need: Safe, Effective Care Environment

19. Diabetic clients who are acutely ill are observed for the signs and symptoms of hyperosmolar hyperglycemic nonketotic syndrome (HNKS) which include
    1. hypotension, mental changes, dehydration, tachycardia
    2. diarrhea, peripheral edema, abdominal pain, diaphoresis
    3. abdominal distention, epigastric pain, hypothermia, headache
    4. hypertension, decreased urine output, bradycardia, fever

    Nursing Process: Collecting Data
    Client Need: Physiological Integrity

20. When a client with known diabetes mellitus is admitted to a hospital unit, the nurse must make sure that
    1. all insulins are kept in a warm place away from light
    2. intravenous glucagon is kept refrigerated
    3. the client receives a glass of orange juice at bedtime
    4. a quick-acting carbohydrate is always available

    Nursing Process: Implementation
    Client Need: Safe, Effective Care Environment

II. CRITICAL THINKING EXERCISES

1. The symptoms of hyperinsulinism may vary from client to client and also be dependent on the degree of hyperinsulinism. You suspect Mr. Howard may be having an "insulin reaction" (hyperinsulinism). What signs and symptoms would you look for? If you believe that he is having an insulin reaction, what steps would you take?

2. Mr. Leigh is admitted for treatment of an ulcer on his left heel. At the time he is giving an admission history, Mr. Leigh tells you that he is a diabetic. What questions related to his diabetes would you ask during the initial history? In addition to inspecting the ulcer on his heel, what physical assessments would you make at this time?

3. Mr. Walters was admitted for treatment of severe diabetic ketoacidosis. Mr. Walters admits to not following the recommendations of his physician regarding diet, monitoring his blood glucose, and taking insulin daily. Prior to his discharge from the hospital you plan to begin teaching this client about his diabetes and the importance of controlling the disorder. The physician has told Mr. Walters that after discharge from the hospital he will benefit from attending a diabetic teaching program. What would you include in the discharge teaching of this client? What would you strongly emphasize during a teaching session?

XIII Disturbances of Sexual Structures or Reproductive Function

57/ Introduction to the Female and Male Reproductive Systems and Related Structures

Reproduction is the primary function of the female and male reproductive systems. While the nervous system plays a principal role in sexual response, pituitary and gonadal hormones regulate the reproductive process.

The following questions deal with the content of Chapter 57.

I. MULTIPLE CHOICE QUESTIONS

Circle the number of the most appropriate answer.

A series of inservice programs are scheduled for health team members with the programs given by various members of the health care team. All those attending the inservice programs are encouraged to participate, ask questions, and answer questions. The topic of the first inservice program is the anatomy and physiology of the female reproductive system.

1. The nurse presenting the anatomy and physiology of the female reproductive system is correct in stating that the ovarian follicle matures under the influence of

    1. luteinizing hormone
    2. oxytocin
    3. vasopressin
    4. follicle-stimulating hormone

    Nursing Process: Implementation
    Client Need: Safe, Effective Care Environment

2. A nurse asks what hormone influences the rupture of the mature ovarian follicle. The inservice program leader is correct in answering

    1. luteinizing hormone
    2. vasopressin
    3. prolactin
    4. oxytocin

    Nursing Process: Implementation
    Client Need: Safe, Effective Care Environment

3. After the ovum is released from the ovary, the ruptured follicle is transformed into a small body filled with yellow fluid. The inservice program leader is correct in stating that this small body is called the
   1. ovulatory zonus
   2. mature follicle
   3. estrogen follicle
   4. corpus luteum

   Nursing Process: Implementation
   Client Need: Safe, Effective Care Environment

4. A nurse assistant asks what hormone controls the development of the uterine endometrium. A nurse is correct in stating that the development of the uterine endometrium is governed by
   1. progesterone
   2. estrogen
   3. follicle-stimulating hormone
   4. luteinizing hormone

   Nursing Process: Implementation
   Client Need: Safe, Effective Care Environment

5. A nurse asks where progesterone is produced. The inservice program leader is correct in stating that this hormone is produced by the
   1. corpus luteum
   2. ovum
   3. ovary
   4. pituitary

   Nursing Process: Implementation
   Client Need: Safe, Effective Care Environment

6. The inservice program leader is correct in stating that lactation is stimulated by
   1. estrogen
   2. progesterone and prolactin
   3. luteinizing hormone and follicle-stimulating hormone
   4. the endometrium

   Nursing Process: Implementation
   Client Need: Safe, Effective Care Environment

The topic of the second inservice program is the anatomy and physiology of the male reproductive system.

7. The nurse presenting the anatomy and physiology of the male reproductive system is correct in stating that one function of the testes is the
   1. manufacture of prostatic fluid
   2. release of prolactin
   3. manufacture of testosterone
   4. regulation of the production of seminal fluid

   Nursing Process: Implementation
   Client Need: Safe, Effective Care Environment

8. A nurse asks where spermatozoa are stored. The inservice program leader is correct in answering that spermatozoa are stored in the
   1. vas deferens
   2. seminal vesicles
   3. epididymides
   4. prostate gland

   Nursing Process: Implementation
   Client Need: Safe, Effective Care Environment

9. The inservice program leader asks if anyone can describe the location of the prostate gland. A nurse correctly responds that the prostate is located
   1. below the outlet of the bladder
   2. behind the urethra
   3. in front of the urethra
   4. near the ureters

   Nursing Process: Implementation
   Client Need: Safe, Effective Care Environment

10. A nurse asks what can be recommended when the client has moderate to severe pain after a digital examination of the prostate. The most correct reply is
    1. two tablets of acetaminophen every 8 hours
    2. a sitz bath
    3. a soothing rectal ointment
    4. aspirin every 12 hours

    Nursing Process: Implementation
    Client Need: Safe, Effective Care Environment

A team conference is scheduled for all members working on a clinical unit that specializes in gynecologic disorders. The topic of the conference is to discuss the various tests performed for the diagnosis of disorders related to the female reproductive system.

11. A nurse assistant asks, "What is the Papanicolaou (Pap) test used for?" A nurse correctly answers that this test is used mainly to
    1. identify the length of the menstrual cycle
    2. detect endometriosis
    3. detect early cancer of the cervix
    4. identify sexually transmitted diseases

    Nursing Process: Implementation
    Client Need: Safe, Effective Care Environment

12. A nurse asks how the diagnosis of endometrial carcinoma may be made. The conference leader correctly states that one method of diagnosing endometrial cancer is by
    1. laboratory determination of urine hormone levels
    2. a fallopian smear
    3. taking blood samples for tumor cells
    4. an endometrial smear and biopsy

    Nursing Process: Implementation
    Client Need: Safe, Effective Care Environment

13. A student nurse attending the conference asks why a culdoscopy is performed. Another nurse answers that this procedure may be performed to
    1. obtain a breast biopsy
    2. visualize the uterus, broad ligaments, and fallopian tubes
    3. inspect the anterior and posterior vaginal walls
    4. determine pituitary hormone levels

    Nursing Process: Implementation
    Client Need: Safe, Effective Care Environment

14. The conference leader asks if anyone can describe the purpose of hysterosalpingography. A nurse correctly answers that this procedure is a(n)
    1. radiographic examination that visualizes the uterus and fallopian tubes
    2. study performed to obtain a biopsy of the cervix or uterus
    3. endoscopic examination of the uterus, ovary, and fallopian tubes
    4. panendoscopic examination of the fallopian tubes

    Nursing Process: Implementation
    Client Need: Safe, Effective Care Environment

15. A conference leader asks for an explanation of an incisional biopsy. The nurse is most correct in stating that when an incisional biopsy of a breast lesion is performed,
    1. one or more sections of tissue are removed
    2. the entire lesion is removed
    3. a needle is inserted to remove small sections of tissue
    4. a trocar with a cannula is inserted to remove tissue

    Nursing Process: Implementation
    Client Need: Safe, Effective Care Environment

II. CRITICAL THINKING EXERCISES

1. Ms. Sims, age 67, has made an appointment with an outpatient clinic specializing in diagnosing and treating gynecologic disorders. What questions would you include in her initial history?

2. Ms. Taylor is scheduled for a cervical biopsy. What explanation regarding the procedure would you give to this client?

3. Mr. Best is scheduled for a transrectal ultrasound examination. How would you explain this procedure to this client?

58/ Caring for Clients with Disorders of the Female Reproductive System and Related Structures

The presence of a functional female reproductive system is not essential to life but is essential to the continuation of the species. Diseases or disorders of the female reproductive system can have a profound effect on an individual's sexuality and in some instances present a danger to the life and well-being of the individual.

The following questions deal with the content of Chapter 58.

I. MULTIPLE CHOICE QUESTIONS

Circle the number of the most appropriate answer.

A series of team conferences are held for discussing the nursing management of various types of gynecologic disorders.

1. When discussing PMS at a team conference, the nurse correctly states that treatment depends on the
    1. hormone levels of the client
    2. severity and type of symptoms
    3. type of menstrual flow
    4. results of a biopsy

    Nursing Process: Implementation
    Client Need: Safe, Effective Care Environment

2. When asked to define the term *menorrhagia,* the nurse correctly answers
    1. severe pain during menstruation
    2. an absence of the menstrual flow
    3. irregular menses
    4. a heavy menstrual flow

    Nursing Process: Implementation
    Client Need: Safe, Effective Care Environment

3. A nurse asks how severe menorrhagia is treated. The most correct answer is
    1. administration of an analgesic
    2. hormone therapy to produce menses
    3. hormone therapy to increase the menstrual flow
    4. by dilatation and curretage

    Nursing Process: Implementation
    Client Need: Safe, Effective Care Environment

4. A nurse assistant asks what the term *therapeutic abortion* means. The nurse replies that a therapeutic abortion is
    1. the intentional termination of pregnancy with the consent of the client
    2. one performed to save the life of the mother
    3. only performed after 16 weeks of gestation
    4. a procedure required when some products of pregnancy are retained

    Nursing Process: Implementation
    Client Need: Safe, Effective Care Environment

5. When asked how the combination oral contraceptives inhibit ovulation, the nurse correctly answers by suppressing
    1. follicle-stimulating and luteinizing hormones
    2. prolactin and luteinizing hormone
    3. estrogen and progesterone
    4. progesterone only

    Nursing Process: Implementation
    Client Need: Safe, Effective Care Environment

6. When asked to explain the purpose of an abortifacient drug, the nurse replies that the drug is used
   1. to prevent an abortion
   2. to induce an abortion
   3. after the fetus has been expelled
   4. to aid in expelling the placenta after a missed abortion

   Nursing Process: Implementation
   Client Need: Safe, Effective Care Environment

7. When asked to describe what an ectopic pregnancy is, the nurse explains that when an ectopic pregnancy occurs, the fertilized ovum
   1. is implanted outside of the uterus
   2. cannot develop because of an absence of a placenta
   3. undergoes changes that result in an abortion
   4. degenerates

   Nursing Process: Implementation
   Client Need: Safe, Effective Care Environment

Ms. Sherman, age 40, is admitted to the hospital for a subtotal abdominal hysterectomy. She has had uterine fibroids for approximately 6 years but recently experienced symptoms related to the fibroids.

8. When obtaining a history from Ms. Sherman, the nurse questions her about her symptoms. The most common symptom of fibroids of the uterus is
   1. moderate to severe pain
   2. amenorrhea
   3. menorrhagia
   4. fever

   Nursing Process: Collecting Data
   Client Need: Physiological Integrity

9. During a team conference held to develop a plan of care for Ms. Sherman, the nurse explains that this surgery involves removal of
   1. the uterus and cervix
   2. the uterus only, with a stump of the cervix left intact
   3. all female reproductive organs
   4. the uterus and ovaries

   Nursing Process: Implementation
   Client Need: Safe, Effective Care Environment

10. A nurse assistant asks why Ms. Sherman needs a catheter. The nurse explains that an indwelling catheter is inserted preoperatively to
    1. measure bladder capacity before and after surgery
    2. help the surgeon identify the uterus
    3. keep the bladder empty during and after surgery
    4. make it easier to measure urinary output after surgery

    Nursing Process: Implementation
    Client Need: Safe, Effective Care Environment

11. Following surgery, Ms. Sherman's indwelling catheter is connected to closed drainage. The intake and output is closely monitored since oliguria, anuria, or the sudden onset of back pain may indicate
    1. renal shutdown due to the sudden hormonal changes
    2. edema of the cervical stump
    3. a vaginal infection
    4. a surgical injury to a ureter or a ligated ureter

    Nursing Process: Evaluation
    Client Need: Physiological Integrity

12. Ms. Sherman had antiembolic stockings applied preoperatively. During the postoperative period these stockings are removed and reapplied
    1. every 2 hours
    2. every 8 hours
    3. daily
    4. every other day

    Nursing Process: Implementation
    Client Need: Physiological Integrity

13. When Ms. Sherman's indwelling urethral catheter is removed, the nurse
    1. measures and records the urine output after each voiding
    2. encourages her to void in the bathroom
    3. instructs her to save all urine in a 24-hour collection container
    4. measures and records the total urine output every 8 hours

    Nursing Process: Implementation
    Client Need: Physiological Integrity

14. Which one of the following can the nurse plan to include in a discharge teaching plan for Ms. Sherman?
    1. limit fluid intake for the next 2 weeks
    2. avoid heavy lifting until permitted to do so
    3. eat a diet low in fiber and high in protein
    4. take a laxative or enema daily

    Nursing Process: Planning
    Client Need: Health Promotion/Maintenance

A hospital has initiated a program for the women in the community to help them understand treatment of diseases and disorders of the female reproductive tract. The program is held weekly. Nurses working in the hospital are asked to lecture and discuss various topics with those attending the program.

15. When discussing disorders of the female reproductive tract with women attending the conference, the nurse explains that the most common early symptom of cancer of the endometrium is
    1. pain
    2. bleeding
    3. absence of menses
    4. enlargement of inguinal lymph nodes

    Nursing Process: Implementation
    Client Need: Health Promotion/Maintenance

16. A woman asks, "What are the early signs of cancer of the cervix?" The nurse replies that the early stage of cancer of the cervix
    1. usually has no symptoms
    2. has symptoms of pain, bleeding, and a yellow discharge
    3. most often causes abdominal and back pain or discomfort
    4. has symptoms of fever, pain, and abdominal distention

    Nursing Process: Implementation
    Client Need: Health Promotion/Maintenance

17. A major role of the nurse is educating women in the early detection of cancer of the cervix by recommending
    1. reading pamphlets from the American Cancer Society
    2. health checkups every 2 years
    3. regular Pap smears
    4. avoiding estrogen for the treatment of the symptoms of menopause

    Nursing Process: Implementation
    Client Need: Health Promotion/Maintenance

18. Another woman asks about malignant tumors of the ovary. The nurse states that malignant tumors of the ovary
    1. are frequently far advanced and inoperable by the time they are diagnosed
    2. respond well to radiation and chemotherapy
    3. are easily detected because symptoms appear early
    4. are usually curable

    Nursing Process: Implementation
    Client Need: Health Promotion/Maintenance

19. A woman asks, "What has the highest success rate of any single birth control method?" The nurse answers
    1. the IUD
    2. condoms
    3. the vaginal sponge
    4. oral contraceptives

    Nursing Process: Implementation
    Client Need: Health Promotion/Maintenance

Individual Questions

20. When teaching a client about oral contraceptives, the nurse instructs the client to start taking the drug
    1. immediately after the prescription is filled
    2. 10 days after the start menstruation
    3. on the 5th day of menstruation
    4. on the 1st day of the month

    Nursing Process: Implementation
    Client Need: Health Promotion/Maintenance

21. The nurse instructs the client taking an oral contraceptive that it is important that the drug is
    1. taken every other day
    2. used with an estrogen-stimulating drug
    3. taken at the same time each day, preferably in the evening
    4. not used with other birth control measures

    Nursing Process: Implementation
    Client Need: Health Promotion/Maintenance

22. When discussing the termination of a pregnancy with a group attending classes held in an outpatient clinic, the nurse explains that in medicine the term *abortion* is used to describe an interruption of pregnancy
    1. anytime after 3 months of gestation
    2. before 9 months of gestation
    3. by a physician
    4. before the fetus weighs more than 500 g (about 20 weeks of gestation)

    Nursing Process: Implementation
    Client Need: Health Promotion/Maintenance

23. A nurse assistant asks what the term *incomplete abortion* means. The nurse explains that this term is used when
    1. some of the products of pregnancy are retained
    2. the fetus is born alive but unable to survive
    3. the loss of the products of pregnancy is due to a malformed fetus
    4. the placenta is always expelled first

    Nursing Process: Implementation
    Client Need: Safe, Effective Care Environment

24. A client asks how she could tell if she has a vaginal infection. The nurse explains that a prominent symptom of a vaginal infection is
    1. pain
    2. absence of menses
    3. heavy menses
    4. an abnormal vaginal discharge

    Nursing Process: Implementation
    Client Need: Health Promotion/Maintenance

25. Ms. Reid is prescribed metronidazole (Flagyl) to treat a *Trichomonas* infection. The nurse tells her that usually sexual partners
    1. do not develop the infection or require treatment
    2. are treated even though they are asymptomatic
    3. only require 1 day of treatment with this drug
    4. are required, by law, to examined by a physician

    Nursing Process: Implementation
    Client Need: Health Promotion/Maintenance

26. When explaining chronic cervicitis to another nurse, treatment may be described as including
    1. electrocautery
    2. subtotal hysterectomy and salpingectomy
    3. insertion of a pessary
    4. corticosteroids

    Nursing Process: Implementation
    Client Need: Safe, Effective Care Environment

27. A client asks the nurse, "What are the symptoms of pelvic inflammatory disease?" The nurse tells the client that symptoms may include
    1. headache, absence of menstruation, double vision
    2. constipation, a clear and watery vaginal discharge, shaking chills
    3. a malodorous vaginal discharge, abdominal and pelvic pain, fever
    4. weight loss, swelling of the legs, pain around the umbilicus

    Nursing Process: Implementation
    Client Need: Health Promotion/Maintenance

28. When a vaginal or cervical smear is to be taken to identify an infectious disorder of the female reproductive tract, the client is told
    1. to douche before the examination
    2. not to douche before being examined
    3. not to shower for 24 hours before the examination
    4. to withhold food and fluids after midnight

    Nursing Process: Implementation
    Client Need: Safe, Effective Care Environment

29. Ms. Cross was told she has endometriosis and asks what this word means. The nurse describes the endometrium as the lining of the uterus and endometriosis as a condition in which
    1. the endometrium is shed at times other than during the menstrual cycle
    2. the endometrium becomes spongy and thick, resulting in a scant menses
    3. there is an overgrowth of endometrium in the uterus, resulting in painful menstruation
    4. tissue that resembles the endometrium is found outside the uterus

    Nursing Process: Implementation
    Client Need: Health Promotion/Maintenance

30. Which of the following may be included in a plan of care for the preoperative preparation of a client scheduled for surgery for a vaginal or uterine disorder?
    1. enema, a cleansing vaginal irrigation
    2. a high-caloric high-residue diet, insertion of an indwelling catheter
    3. clear fluids for 6 days prior to surgery,
    4. penicillin, shaving of the operative area

    Nursing Process: Planning
    Client Need: Safe, Effective Care Environment

31. Nursing management of the client admitted with a possible threatened abortion includes
    1. preparing the client for abdominal surgery
    2. saving all large clots and tissue for examination
    3. advising the client to walk to relieve cramping and pain
    4. keeping the client NPO

    Nursing Process: Implementation
    Client Need: Physiological Integrity

II. CRITICAL THINKING EXERCISES

1. Your friend Mary Beth tells you that she is pregnant and is considering having an abortion. What advice can you give to Mary Beth regarding the medical and psychological implications of this procedure?

2. A large vaginal fistula causes the client distress because of odor and the constant leakage of fecal material or urine. What suggestions could you give to reduce odors associated with this problem?

3. Ms. Leonard had a hysterectomy yesterday. Today she is complaining of severe back and abdominal pain. What assessments would you perform before you contact her physician?

59/ Caring for Clients with Disorders of the Breast

Both malignant and benign lesions of the breast are common in all age groups. The most common breast disorder is cystic disease, and breast cancer is the most common malignancy of the female reproductive system. While some breast disorders are benign in nature, others are serious and can be life-threatening.

The following questions deal with the content of Chapter 59.

I. MULTIPLE CHOICE QUESTIONS

Circle the number of the most appropriate answer.

Ms. Howard, age 56, sees her physician because of a lump she discovered in her right breast. She was admitted for an incisional breast biopsy, followed by a mastectomy if the lesion is malignant. After microscopic examination of the removed tissue, the lesion is found to be malignant.

1. On Ms. Howard's surgical record it is noted that a radical mastectomy and skin grafting was performed. When developing a plan of postoperative care, the nurse is aware of the fact that this surgery involves removal of the breast and the

   1. axillary lymph nodes and pectoral muscles
   2. pectoralis major and pectoralis minor
   3. axillary nodes and fascia covering the pectoral muscles
   4. axillary and sternal lymph nodes

   Nursing Process: Planning
   Client Need: Physiological Integrity

2. During the immediate postoperative period, vital signs are monitored every 30 to 60 minutes. The blood pressure and pulse are taken on
   1. either arm
   2. the left arm only
   3. the right arm only
   4. with the stethoscope over the popliteal artery

   Nursing Process: Implementation
   Client Need: Physiological Integrity

3. When checking Ms. Howard's dressing, the nurse not only checks the top of the dressing but also looks for hidden drainage
   1. on top of the sheets
   2. on the first layers of the surgical dressing
   3. underneath the client's upper body
   4. on or near the incision

   Nursing Process: Evaluation
   Client Need: Physiological Integrity

4. The physician orders Ms. Howard's arm on the operative side elevated on a pillow. Since she had a skin graft to close the wide surgical incision it is important that her arm not be allowed to
   1. adduct
   2. abduct
   3. lay close to her chest
   4. bent at the elbow

   Nursing Process: Implementation
   Client Need: Physiological Integrity

5. When developing a plan of care for Ms. Howard, the nurse considers that arm exercises on the operative side are usually not instituted until
   1. the second postoperative day
   2. 3 months after surgery
   3. 1 year after surgery
   4. the graft site has healed

   Nursing Process: Planning
   Client Need: Physiological Integrity

6. The wearing of a breast prosthesis is discussed during discharge teaching. Ms. Howard can be told that
   1. a prosthesis can be worn beginning 1 year after surgery
   2. only a foam rubber prosthesis is medically approved
   3. the physician determines when a prosthesis can be worn
   4. she can be fitted for a prosthesis before she is discharged from the hospital

   Nursing Process: Implementation
   Client Need: Health Promotion/Maintenance

Individual Questions

7. When doing health teaching, the nurse can explain that an important method of early detection of breast cancer is
   1. yearly examination of the breasts by a physician
   2. monthly BSE
   3. mammograms every 3 years
   4. blood test for estrogen levels every 2 years

   Nursing Process: Implementation
   Client Need: Health Promotion/Maintenance

8. At an inservice program the nurse discusses fibrocystic breast disease and the most common symptom, which is
   1. painful, tender breasts especially before menstruation
   2. painful and bloody drainage from the nipples
   3. a feeling of fullness in the breasts
   4. tenderness in the breasts after menstruation

   Nursing Process: Implementation
   Client Need: Safe, Effective Care Environment

9. A nurse assistant asks what causes a breast abscess. The nurse explains that breast abscesses occur more frequently as a
   1. result of hormonal changes following a menstrual period
   2. result of cystic mastitis
   3. complication of a mastectomy
   4. postpartum complication

   Nursing Process: Implementation
   Client Need: Safe, Effective Care Environment

10. When a client has had a simple mastectomy, the nurse assists her in exercises of the arm of the operative side to prevent
    1. contractures of joints, loss of muscle tone
    2. excessive scarring of the incision, edema
    3. metastasis, muscle hypertrophy
    4. loss of strength, stretching of the shoulder muscles

    Nursing Process: Implementation
    Client Need: Physiological Integrity

11. When discussing the long-term effects of a radical mastectomy at a team conference, the nurse states that the client may develop
    1. an inability to move the arm on the operative side
    2. total loss of feeling in the arm on the operative side
    3. lymphedema
    4. lymphosarcoma

    Nursing Process: Implementation
    Client Need: Safe, Effective Care Environment

12. A nurse asks if additional surgery may be performed in the premenopausal woman who has had a mastectomy and known lymph node metastasis. The nurse states that the surgeon may decide to perform a
    1. pelvic lymph node dissection
    2. bilateral oophorectomy
    3. periaortic lymph node dissection
    4. hysterectomy

    Nursing Process: Implementation
    Client Need: Safe, Effective Care Environment

II. CRITICAL THINKING EXERCISES

1. Ms. Keefe is brought to the emergency department with a history of severe nausea and vomiting for 16 hours. Her husband tells you that his wife "had breast cancer, had her breast removed and several other surgeries after that." Is there anything in this statement by Mr. Keefe that the nurse immediately investigate? What serious or life-threatening situation may be occurring?

2. Ms. Wilson has discovered a lump in her breast. She tells you that she is afraid to go to a doctor because she is sure she has cancer. What could you say to Ms. Wilson to relieve her anxiety?

3. Ms. Dodge had a left radical mastectomy 6 months ago and has developed lymphedema. What suggestions or recommendations could you give her regarding care of her arm and hand as well as tasks that may reduce her lymphedema?

60/ Caring for Clients with Disorders of the Male Reproductive System

Several structures of the male reproductive system are parts of the urinary tract as well as the reproductive system. Structures of the male reproductive system include the prostate, vas deferans, testes and adjacent structures, and the penis. Diseases of the male reproductive system not only may influence reproductive ability but also may affect the urinary tract.

The following questions deal with the content of Chapter 60.

I. MULTIPLE CHOICE QUESTIONS

Circle the number of the most appropriate answer.

Mr. Greene, age 69, is admitted to the hospital for surgical treatment of benign prostatic hypertrophy (BPH).

1. When obtaining an initial history from Mr. Greene, the nurse questions him about his symptoms which may include
   1. scrotal swelling, skin rash
   2. narrowing of the urinary stream, urinary frequency
   3. chills and fever, voiding large amounts of urine
   4. lower abdominal pain, diarrhea

   Nursing Process: Collecting Data
   Client Need: Physiological Integrity

2. After Mr. Greene returns to his room following a suprapubic prostatectomy, it is noted that he has two catheters, a cystostomy catheter and a urethral catheter. Usually the indwelling urethral catheter
   1. is not inflated
   2. has a balloon filled with 30 mL of fluid
   3. is kept clamped
   4. is connected to suction

   Nursing Process: Collecting Data
   Client Need: Physiological Integrity

3. During the immediate postoperative period both catheters are inspected for the presence of clots which can cause
   1. an increase in urine output, thrombophlebitis
   2. further bleeding, difficulty urinating
   3. pain, bladder spasms
   4. hemorrhagic cystitis, fever

   Nursing Process: Collecting Data
   Client Need: Physiological Integrity

4. During the process of monitoring vital signs in the postoperative period, Mr. Greene's temperature is taken
   1. orally
   2. rectally
   3. every 8 hours
   4. hourly

   Nursing Process: Collecting Data
   Client Need: Physiological Integrity

5. Two hours after surgery the surgeon orders irrigation of the urethral catheter. It is most important that the surgeon's orders be followed regarding this procedure since irrigating the catheter too frequently may result in
   1. bladder spasms and further bleeding
   2. an increase in urinary output
   3. difficulty measuring intake and output
   4. nausea and vomiting

   Nursing Process: Implementation
   Client Need: Physiological Integrity

6. Twelve hours after surgery the surgeon examines Mr. Greene and orders a continuous irrigation system connected to both catheters to
   1. reduce the possibility of a postoperative bladder infection
   2. prevent clots from forming in the bladder
   3. control the pain caused by the surgery
   4. help establish urinary continence once the catheters are removed

   Nursing Process: Implementation
   Client Need: Physiological Integrity

7. After Mr. Greene's cystostomy tube is removed by the surgeon, the suprapubic wound is closely monitored since it
   1. will bleed for 1 to 2 days
   2. will close in 2 to 3 hours
   3. will most likely be painful for several weeks
   4. frequently leaks urine for a few days

   Nursing Process: Collecting Data
   Client Need: Physiological Integrity

8. Following removal of the urethral catheter, Mr. Greene is checked for
   1. severe pain for 2 to 3 hours
   2. some dribbling of urine
   3. severe bleeding
   4. excessive urinary output

   Nursing Process: Collecting Data
   Client Need: Physiological Integrity

9. Mr. Greene is to be discharged from the hospital. He tells you that he is retired but wonders if he can do any lifting after he goes home. Clients who have had a prostatectomy are told
   1. there are no restrictions on lifting
   2. generally no lifting or straining is allowed until permitted by the surgeon
   3. any object under 20 pounds can be lifted safely
   4. to lift any object that does not cause discomfort in the operative area

   Nursing Process: Implementation
   Client Need: Health Promotion/Maintenance

A team conference is held to discuss prostate diseases and disorders.

10. A nurse asks, "What are the symptoms of prostatitis?" The most correct response is symptoms may include
    1. low back pain, urinary urgency and frequency
    2. dysphagia, abdominal pain
    3. bloody urine, abdominal distention
    4. diarrhea, scrotal pain

    Nursing Process: Implementation
    Client Need: Safe, Effective Care Environment

11. The conference leader states that a prostatic malignancy is spread by the bloodstream and lymphatics to the
    1. lungs
    2. pelvic lymph nodes and bones
    3. stomach
    4. brain

    Nursing Process: Implementation
    Client Need: Safe, Effective Care Environment

12. A student nurse asks what symptoms the client might notice if a prostatic malignancy has metastasized. A nurse answers that the first symptoms may be
    1. chest pain, cough
    2. back pain, pain down the legs
    3. anorexia, nausea
    4. headache, double vision

    Nursing Process: Implementation
    Client Need: Safe, Effective Care Environment

13. When discussing malignant testicular tumors, the nurse states that the success of treatment depends on the
    1. type of testicular tumor and extent of metastasis
    2. size of the tumor and response to testosterone therapy
    3. dose of antineoplastic drugs and age of the client
    4. response to estrogen therapy and length of treatment

    Nursing Process: Implementation
    Client Need: Safe, Effective Care Environment

Individual Questions

14. Following a vasectomy the client is told that the ejaculatory fluid
    1. is free from sperm in 4 to 7 days
    2. contains sperm for a period of time after surgery
    3. no longer contains sperm
    4. will appear clear for 1 to 2 months after surgery

    Nursing Process: Implementation
    Client Need: Health Promotion/Maintenance

15. If a client is admitted with the diagnosis of torsion of the spermatic cord, the nurse develops a short-term plan of care since this condition will require immediate
    1. application of heat to prevent swelling
    2. incision and drainage of the vas deferens
    3. application of ice to prevent testicular swelling
    4. surgery

    Nursing Process: Implementation
    Client Need: Physiological Integrity

16. The client receiving treatment for prostatitis can be advised to
    1. remain quiet in a chair or bed for 2 to 3 days
    2. limit his fluid intake until discomfort is relieved
    3. avoid taking a tub bath or shower until discomfort is relieved
    4. avoid prolonged periods of sitting

    Nursing Process: Implementation
    Client Need: Health Promotion/Maintenance

17. When reviewing a newly admitted client's laboratory tests performed prior to admission, the nurse notes that the PSA is markedly elevated. This alerts the nurse to the fact that the client most probably has
    1. cancer of the prostate
    2. benign prostatic hypertrophy
    3. prostatitis
    4. epididymitis

    Nursing Process: Evaluation
    Client Need: Safe, Effective Care Environment

18. The client receiving Proscar (finasteride) for benign prostatic hypertrophy can be told that
    1. the drug is taken once a week for 6 weeks
    2. effects of the drug are usually seen immediately
    3. it may take about 6 months before results are seen
    4. the drug must be given by injection

    Nursing Process: Implementation
    Client Need: Health Promotion/Maintenance

19. When labeling the catheters of the client who has had a suprapubic prostatectomy, the catheter inserted into the bladder through the abdominal incision is labeled as a ____ catheter.
    1. urethral
    2. cystostomy
    3. ureteral
    4. cystectomy

    Nursing Process: Implementation
    Client Need: Safe, Effective Care Environment

20. When reviewing the record of a client returning from surgery, the nurse notes that the surgical procedure is listed as an orchiopexy. The nurse can develop a plan of postoperative management for a client having surgery for
    1. removal of a testicle
    2. a urethral stricture
    3. an undescended testicle
    4. an abscess of the testicle

    Nursing Process: Planning
    Client Need: Physiological Integrity

21. When assessing the client with epididymo-orchitis, the nurse looks for
    1. drainage from the urethra
    2. scrotal pain and tenderness
    3. suprapubic pain and tenderness
    4. pain over the kidney area

    Nursing Process: Collecting Data
    Client Need: Physiological Integrity

22. During the postoperative period the client having extensive surgery for a malignant tumor of the testes is closely observed for complications, which may include
    1. gastric dilatation, severe diarrhea, headache
    2. paralytic ileus, thrombophlebitis, gout
    3. hemorrhage, shock, wound infection
    4. septicemia, pathological fractures, aplastic anemia

    Nursing Process: Collecting Data
    Client Need: Physiological Integrity

II. CRITICAL THINKING EXERCISES

1. Mr. Locke, age 78, is scheduled for a transcystoscopic urethroplasty. His wife states that she really doesn't know what the surgeon is going to do and is concerned that her husband will have a big incision in his abdomen. How would you explain this procedure to Ms. Locke?

2. Yesterday, Mr. Crane had a suprapubic prostatectomy. Today, the output from his urethral catheter is less than 75 mL over the past 2 hours. What specific observations would you make at this time? What information do you need in order to make a decision regarding any nursing interventions?

3. Mr. Roth, age 77, had a retropubic prostatectomy 2 days ago. He tells you, "I have to go to the bathroom and when I do, I have a lot of pain." What assessments would you make? What suggestions or explanations would you give to Mr. Roth?

61/ Caring for Clients with Sexually Transmitted Diseases

Sexually transmitted diseases (STDs) are a diverse group of infections acquired through sexual activity with an infected person. Examples of STDs are the venereal diseases syphilis, gonorrhea, chancroid, and granuloma inguinale as well as such diseases as human papillomavirus, herpes simplex virus, chlamydial infections, and trichomonal vaginitis. Acquired immunodeficiency syndrome (AIDS) is not a true STD but one method of transmission is by sexual intercourse.

The following questions deal with the content of Chapter 61.

I. MULTIPLE CHOICE QUESTIONS

Circle the number of the most appropriate answer.

1. When obtaining a history from a client with gonorrhea, the nurse must also be alert to the signs and symptoms of another common coexisting STD, namely
   1. lymphogranuloma
   2. granuloma inguinale
   3. chlamydia
   4. chancroid

   Nursing Process: Collecting Data
   Client Need: Safe, Effective Care Environment

2. When doing client teaching, the nurse emphasizes that treatment failure of some STDs is usually due to
   1. failure to report symptoms accurately
   2. inadequate laboratory testing
   3. inaccurate determination of the type of STD
   4. reinfection and noncompliance

   Nursing Process: Implementation
   Client Need: Health Promotion/Maintenance

3. When obtaining a history from Mr. Hull who has possible gonorrhea, the nurse asks questions related to symptoms of this STD which include
   1. a urethral discharge, pain on urination
   2. urinary retention, diarrhea
   3. blood in the urine, abdominal pain
   4. fever, nausea, and vomiting

   Nursing Process: Collecting Data
   Client Need: Physiological Integrity

4. At a team conference a nurse assistant asks why HSV infections recur. The most correct answer is that recurrence is due to the
   1. inability of antibiotics to kill the virus
   2. virus remaining dormant in nerve ganglia
   3. endemic occurrence of the virus
   4. transmission of the infection by autoinnoculation

   Nursing Process: Implementation
   Client Need: Safe, Effective Care Environment

5. The client with periodic recurrences of an HSV-2 infection is instructed to
   1. take acyclovir to prevent future recurrences
   2. wash the lesions with an antiseptic
   3. apply a topical antibiotic to prevent spread of the infection
   4. use a condom at all times

   Nursing Process: Implementation
   Client Need: Health Promotion/Maintenance

6. When discussing genital warts at a team conference, the nurse correctly states that this STD is caused by
   1. a herpes simplex virus
   2. the human papillomavirus
   3. a cytomegalovirus
   4. a mycoplasma

   Nursing Process: Implementation
   Client Need: Safe, Effective Care Environment

7. When teaching the client with an STD who has received a prescription for the infection, the nurse emphasizes the importance of
   1. completing the course of therapy
   2. taking the drug before having sexual intercourse
   3. stopping the drug if symptoms are relieved
   4. stopping the drug if symptoms become worse

   Nursing Process: Implementation
   Client Need: Health Promotion/Maintenance

8. When examining the client with a known or suspected STD, the nurse
   1. uses aseptic technique
   2. wears a gown and mask
   3. observes universal precautions
   4. covers the area to be examined with sterile drapes

   Nursing Process: Implementation
   Client Need: Safe, Effective Care Environment

9. Female clients with a chlamydia infection are instructed to
   1. take the prescribed drug for 5 days
   2. douche daily until treatment is completed
   3. insert a medicated vaginal sponge before intercourse
   4. refrain from sexual activity until the infection is eradicated

   Nursing Process: Implementation
   Client Need: Health Promotion/Maintenance

10. Since the virus is endemic, the nurse looks for HSV infections which often occur in those who
    1. are immunocompromised
    2. recently have had surgery
    3. are malnourished
    4. reside in crowded living areas

    Nursing Process: Collecting Data
    Client Need: Physiological Integrity

11. At a team conference a nurse asks what type of drug is used to treat candidiasis. The most correct answer is a(n)
    1. broad-spectrum antibiotic
    2. topical antiseptic
    3. antifungal agent
    4. antiviral agent

    Nursing Process: Implementation
    Client Need: Safe, Effective Care Environment

II. CRITICAL THINKING

1. When discussing sexually transmitted diseases with a group of women attending a health information seminar, one woman asks about genital warts. How would you explain the cause and treatment of this STD?

2. Mr. Carson has gonorrhea and tells you that he refuses to tell any of his recent sexual contacts that he has the infection. What arguments could you give to persuade Mr. Carson to have him tell these individuals that he has been infected with gonorrhea?

XIV Caring for Clients with Urinary and Renal Problems

62/ Introduction to the Urinary Tract

The urinary tract consists of the kidneys, ureter, bladder, and urethra. The urinary tract is one of several systems by which the body rids itself of the waste products of metabolism.

The following questions deal with the content of Chapter 62.

I. MULTIPLE CHOICE QUESTIONS

Circle the number of the most appropriate answer.

A team conference is held to discuss and review the anatomy and physiology of the urinary tract.

1. The conference leader asks for one function of the kidneys. A nurse correctly answers
   1. excretion of old blood cells
   2. excretion of plasma angiotensin
   3. maintenance of acid-base balance
   4. manufacture of red blood cells

   Nursing Process: Implementation
   Client Need: Safe, Effective Care Environment

2. A nurse asks, "What is the function of the hormone erythropoietin, which is produced by the kidneys?" The most correct answer is that erythropoietin
   1. regulates the excretion of potassium
   2. regulates red blood cell production
   3. controls the production of angiotensin
   4. inhibits white blood cell production

   Nursing Process: Implementation
   Client Need: Safe, Effective Care Environment

3. When asked to name the smallest functioning unit of the kidney, the nurse correctly answers
   1. the afferent arteriole
   2. Bowman's capsule
   3. Henle's loop
   4. the nephron

   Nursing Process: Implementation
   Client Need: Safe, Effective Care Environment

4. When asked where the removal of waste products, electrolytes, and water from the blood takes place, the nurse correctly answers in
    1. the glomerulus
    2. Henle's loop
    3. the efferent arteriole
    4. the proximal convoluted tubules

    Nursing Process: Implementation
    Client Need: Safe, Effective Care Environment

5. When asked to explain an intravenous pyelogram (IVP), the nurse correctly states that this diagnostic test is a radiographic study based on the ability of the kidneys to excrete
    1. creatinine
    2. glucose
    3. a radiopaque dye
    4. proteins

    Nursing Process: Implementation
    Client Need: Safe, Effective Care Environment

6. When asked to explain why a cystoscopy may be performed, the nurse correctly answers to
    1. directly visualize the bladder and urethra
    2. treat tumors of the kidney by electrosurgery
    3. directly visualize the kidney pelvis
    4. test the ability of the kidneys to excrete glucose

    Nursing Process: Implementation
    Client Need: Safe, Effective Care Environment

7. When asked one purpose of retrograde pyelograms, the nurse correctly answers to
    1. inject 25 or more mL of air
    2. collect separate specimens of urine from each kidney
    3. visualize the renal pelvis
    4. outline the urethra

    Nursing Process: Implementation
    Client Need: Safe, Effective Care Environment

8. When asked to describe a cystourethrogram, the nurse correctly states that this procedure involves
    1. instillation of water to determine bladder capacity
    2. measuring bladder size by instilling blue dye
    3. emptying the bladder before taking radiographs
    4. instillation of a radiopaque dye into the bladder through a urethral catheter

    Nursing Process: Implementation
    Client Need: Safe, Effective Care Environment

9. When asked to give the purpose of the creatinine clearance test, the nurse replies that this test is used to determine
    1. the dietary intake of glucose and protein
    2. kidney function
    3. the metabolic breakdown of fats and proteins
    4. the ability of the kidneys to reabsorb sodium

    Nursing Process: Implementation
    Client Need: Safe, Effective Care Environment

Individual Questions

10. When a schedule of a specific amount of fluid intake is planned,
    1. one-half of the total intake is given before noon
    2. three-quarters or more of the total intake is given during daytime hours
    3. three-quarters of the total intake is given between lunch and dinner
    4. one-half of the intake is given during nighttime hours

    Nursing Process: Planning
    Client Need: Physiological Integrity

11. When explaining the preparation for an IVP, the nurse can tell the client that an enema and a laxative are necessary to
    1. provide clear radiograph pictures of the kidneys
    2. increase the concentration of the dye in the kidneys
    3. keep the stomach empty
    4. decrease the concentration of dye in the bladder

    Nursing Process: Implementation
    Client Need: Safe, Effective Care Environment

12. Following a cystoscopy with retrograde pyelograms, the nurse can advise the client to
    1. limit the fluid intake for 24 hours
    2. take a hot bath to relieve pain and discomfort
    3. eat a soft diet for 2 days
    4. rest in bed for the next 48 hours

    Nursing Process: Implementation
    Client Need: Safe, Effective Care Environment

13. When reviewing a client's chart prior to developing a plan of care, the nurse knows that there is a deterioration in renal function when there is a(n)
    1. increase in the CBC and sedimentation rate
    2. decrease in the creatinine levels
    3. rise in the blood urea nitrogen and creatinine values
    4. increase in the urine specific gravity

    Nursing Process: Planning
    Client Need: Physiological Integrity

14. When the client has a nephrostomy tube,
    1. drainage must be continuous and unobstructed
    2. the end of the tube is connected to suction
    3. a dressing is not placed around the point of insertion
    4. the distal end of the tube is placed in an open container

    Nursing Process: Collecting Data
    Client Need: Physiological Integrity

15. A common amount for a single irrigation of a urethral catheter is
    1. 500 mL
    2. 30 mL
    3. 100 mL
    4. 5 mL

    Nursing Process: Implementation
    Client Need: Physiological Integrity

II. CRITICAL THINKING EXERCISES

1. Mr. Shelby is scheduled for an IVP. How would you explain how the test will be performed? What special instructions regarding preparation for the test are explained to Mr. Shelby?

2. Mr. Hull is scheduled for a diagnostic test that uses radiopaque dye. At times, he appears confused and you believe that his admission history may be unreliable. What steps would you take to obtain a more reliable medical history? What particular areas would you attempt to explore?

63/   Caring for Clients with Disorders of the Kidneys and Ureters

The kidneys are basically a filtering system that constantly monitor the water and electrolyte content of the blood. Any disorder that interferes with the urinary tract's ability to filter, remove, and excrete waste products, electrolytes, and water can be serious unless the situation is corrected.

The following questions deal with the content of Chapter 63.

I. MULTIPLE CHOICE QUESTIONS

Circle the number of the most appropriate answer.

Mr. Abbott is a 52-year-old truck driver. Several weeks ago he experienced severe pain in his right side that radiated to his groin. Two days later the pain disappeared. This morning he experienced severe chills and fever along with severe flank pain. He is examined in his physician's office and referred to a urologist, followed by admission to the hospital with a possible stone in his right ureter.

1. When developing a plan of care for Mr. Abbott, the nurse is aware of the fact that Mr. Abbott's acute pain may be due to
    1. retention of urine in the bladder
    2. ureteral dilatation and pressure below the stone
    3. infection in the lower urinary tract
    4. violent contractions and spasms of the ureter

    Nursing Process: Planning
    Client Need: Physiological Integrity

2. It is possible that Mr. Abbott will pass the stone. One way of detecting whether the stone has been passed is to
    1. strain all urine through gauze and inspect the gauze for the stone
    2. hold the container of urine next to a strong light and look for the stone
    3. add Evans blue dye to each voided specimen
    4. obtain a specimen for urinalysis each day

    Nursing Process: Evaluation
    Client Need: Physiological Integrity

3. Surgery will be necessary to remove Mr. Abbott's stone, which is in the middle third of the right ureter. Following surgery Mr. Abbott is assessed for development of the main complication associated with surgery on the ureter which is
   1. failure of the ureter to transport urine from the kidney to the bladder
   2. pneumonia
   3. failure of the bladder to empty fully with each voiding
   4. infection in the kidney of the unoperative side

   Nursing Process: Collecting Data
   Client Need: Physiological Integrity

4. To detect the main complication associated with ureteral surgery, the nurse
   1. measures the output from the ureteral catheter
   2. auscultates his lungs every 2 hours
   3. catheterizes him for residual urine
   4. obtains samples for daily culture and sensitivity tests

   Nursing Process: Collecting Data
   Client Need: Physiological Integrity

5. If Mr. Abbott complains of excessive abdominal pain during the immediate postoperative period, the physician is notified because
   1. there may be an infection in the bladder or urethra
   2. an infection in the lungs may have spread to the GU tract
   3. urine may be leaking from the ureter into the peritoneal cavity
   4. pain may indicate a hypertensive crisis

   Nursing Process: Evaluation
   Client Need: Physiological Integrity

6. Mr. Abbott's discharge teaching plan will include methods of preventing further stone formation and include instructions to
   1. keep physical activity to a minimum
   2. eat foods high in carbohydrates
   3. increase his daily fluid intake
   4. limit fluids during the morning hours

   Nursing Process: Implementation
   Client Need: Health Promotion/Maintenance

Individual Questions

7. Which one of the following is included in a plan of care for the client with acute pyelonephritis?
   1. restriction of the fluid intake
   2. warming blankets to control hypothermia
   3. force fluids
   4. drugs to combat hypotension

   Nursing Process: Planning
   Client Need: Physiological Integrity

8. When obtaining a history from the client with suspected acute glomerulonephritis, it would be important to know if the client
   1. has an allergy to sulfonamides
   2. had an upper respiratory infection about 2 weeks prior to the onset of symptoms
   3. had been receiving antibiotics 6 months prior to symptoms
   4. has benign prostatic hypertrophy

   Nursing Process: Collecting Data
   Client Need: Physiological Integrity

9. The plan of care for the client with acute glomerulonephritis includes
   1. encouraging intake of foods high in carbohydrates
   2. restricting the fluid intake
   3. restricting foods high in vitamins
   4. encouraging intake of foods high in protein

   Nursing Process: Planning
   Client Need: Physiological Integrity

10. When a client is admitted to the hospital with the diagnosis of chronic glomerulonephritis, the plan of nursing management must take into consideration that this kidney disorder often results in
    1. irreversible damage to the nephrons
    2. hypotension
    3. absence of protein in the urine
    4. increase in serum proteins

    Nursing Process: Planning
    Client Need: Physiological Integrity

11. When reviewing laboratory tests of the client with chronic glomerulonephritis, the nurse looks for
    1. decreased blood urea nitrogen
    2. decreased serum creatinine
    3. elevated red blood cell count
    4. proteinuria

    Nursing Process: Evaluation
    Client Need: Physiological Integrity

12. Clients in the nephrotic stage of chronic glomerulonephritis are assessed for
    1. signs and symptoms of hypokalemia
    2. decreased respiratory rate
    3. generalized edema
    4. signs of dehydration

    Nursing Process: Collecting Data
    Client Need: Physiological Integrity

13. The nursing care plan of the client with an infectious or inflammatory disorder of the upper urinary tract includes
    1. encouraging a diet high in protein
    2. determining the ratio of intake to output
    3. encouraging a diet high in potassium
    4. determining the pulse deficit

    Nursing Process: Planning
    Client Need: Physiological Integrity

14. When teaching the client who must restrict the protein intake, the nurse can recommend that protein be obtained from
    1. high biological value sources such as eggs, milk, and meat
    2. protein drinks available from health food stores
    3. cheese, beans, and chicken
    4. low biological value sources such as vegetable proteins

    Nursing Process: Implementation
    Client Need: Health Promotion/Maintenance

15. At a team conference a nurse asks why extracorporeal shock wave lithotripsy is used. The most correct answer is that this procedure is used to
    1. treat glomerulonephritis
    2. break up kidney stones
    3. remove small, soft stones in the bladder
    4. remove urethral stones

    Nursing Process: Implementation
    Client Need: Safe, Effective Care Environment

16. Following lithotripsy, the client is assessed for pain or discomfort in the back or flank which may be due to
    1. an inflammatory process in the bladder or urethra
    2. the prolonged immobility necessary for the procedure
    3. infection due to a lack of aseptic technique during the procedure
    4. small, broken pieces of stone being passed down the ureter

    Nursing Process: Collecting Data
    Client Need: Physiological Integrity

17. During a team conference a nurse asks, "What is one of the first signs of a malignant tumor of the kidney?" The most correct response is
    1. flank pain
    2. lower abdominal pain
    3. painless hematuria
    4. cloudy urine

    Nursing Process: Implementation
    Client Need: Safe, Effective Care Environment

18. Following surgery on the kidney, the client is assessed for moderate to severe pain in the operative site due to
    1. removal of fat around the kidney
    2. urinary retention
    3. the large incision
    4. spasm of the ureter on the unoperative side

    Nursing Process: Collecting Data
    Client Need: Physiological Integrity

19. Clients with a nephrostomy tube
    1. can be placed in a position of comfort
    2. can be placed on the operative or unoperative side
    3. are not given narcotic analgesics
    4. are not turned on the operative side

    Nursing Process: Implementation
    Client Need: Physiological Integrity

20. During a team conference the nurse describes uremia as a toxic state characterized by
    1. hypotension, anemia
    2. a marked accumulation of urea and other nitrogenous wastes in the blood
    3. nausea, vomiting, decrease in the serum creatinine
    4. increased serum creatinine, decreased blood urea nitrogen

    Nursing Process: Implementation
    Client Need: Safe, Effective Care Environment

21. Nurses can contribute to the prevention of acute renal failure by
    1. increasing a client's oral fluid intake
    2. preventing urinary retention
    3. encouraging a diet high in protein and low in fat
    4. encouraging ambulation

    Nursing Process: Implementation
    Client Need: Physiological Integrity

22. The nurse may identify early signs of acute renal failure by noting when the
    1. client's blood pressure shows a marked decrease
    2. urinary output is less than 400–500 mL/24 hr
    3. client complains of abdominal discomfort
    4. urine appears dilute

    Nursing Process: Evaluation
    Client Need: Physiological Integrity

23. When asked to explain at a team conference why edema is often present in chronic renal failure, the nurse correctly states that edema may result from
    1. an increase in serum creatinine
    2. failure of the kidneys to excrete water and sodium
    3. chronic urinary retention
    4. hyperkalemia

    Nursing Process: Implementation
    Client Need: Safe, Effective Care Environment

24. A nurse assistant notes a white film on the face of a client and is told that this is uremic frost which is composed of
    1. electrolytes and sweat
    2. waste products excreted by the skin instead of the failing kidneys
    3. proteins that cannot be excreted by the failing kidneys
    4. water, electrolytes, and minerals

    Nursing Process: Implementation
    Client Need: Safe, Effective Care Environment

25. Which of the following assessments or observations may detect the complications associated with renal failure?
    1. vital signs, observing for electrolyte imbalances
    2. checking the urine for hematuria
    3. weekly weights, observing for signs of hypokalemia
    4. auscultation of the abdomen, checking weekly laboratory reports

    Nursing Process: Collecting Data
    Client Need: Physiological Integrity

26. When asked at a team conference to explain the basic composition of the dialysate fluid used in hemodialysis, the nurse responds that the fluid is

    1. composed of potassium and trace vitamins
    2. similar to the electrolyte composition of normal human plasma
    3. similar to the composition of normal urine
    4. composed primarily of glucose and electrolytes

    Nursing Process: Implementation
    Client Need: Safe, Effective Care Environment

27. Following hemodialysis the client is observed for bleeding which may occur because of

    1. stress related to the procedure
    2. anemia
    3. the administration of antibiotics before the procedure
    4. the administration of heparin during dialysis

    Nursing Process: Collecting Data
    Client Need: Physiological Integrity

28. When the nurse is instilling the dialysate for peritoneal dialysis, the solution is

    1. injected with a special 50 mL syringe
    2. infused by means of a volumetric infusion pump
    3. allowed to flow in by gravity
    4. injected with a special syringe using positive pressure

    Nursing Process: Implementation
    Client Need: Physiological Integrity

29. The client having peritoneal dialysis is assessed for a major complication of this procedure which is

    1. hypertension
    2. anemia
    3. peritonitis
    4. pneumonia

    Nursing Process: Collecting Data
    Client Need: Physiological Integrity

30. When teaching the client on continuous ambulatory peritoneal dialysis (CAPD), the nurse explains that the cycle or exchange is usually performed

    1. once a day
    2. twice a day
    3. 4 times a day
    4. weekly

    Nursing Process: Implementation
    Client Need: Health Promotion/Maintenance

II. CRITICAL THINKING EXERCISES

1. Mr. Jones requires daily cycles of CAPD for renal failure. What explanations would you use when starting a teaching program for this client?

2. Ms. Keppler is in renal failure and requires peritoneal dialysis. What information do you need to know before starting the procedure?

3. A client is to be discharged on CAPD. He asks you how he can keep the bag containing the dialysate elevated until it infuses. What suggestions, based on an average home, could you give this client?

64/ Caring for Clients with Disorders of the Bladder and Urethra

The kidneys selectively filter more than 50 gallons of plasma daily. All but a quart or so of this volume is resorbed back into the circulation every 24 hours. The ureters transport the urine produced by the kidneys to the bladder, where urine is stored until it is eliminated.

The following questions deal with the content of Chapter 64.

I. MULTIPLE CHOICE QUESTIONS

Circle the number of the most appropriate answer.

Mr. Yates is incontinent of urine following a cerebrovascular accident. He is presently in a skilled nursing facility undergoing rehabilitation. He is cooperative and oriented and ambulates by using a walker.

1. When explaining incontinence to a nurse assistant, the nurse states that incontinence in many clients is primarily due to
   1. damage to the bladder mucosa
   2. a relaxation of the urinary sphincters
   3. abdominal distention
   4. ignoring the need to void

   Nursing Process: Implementation
   Client Need: Safe, Effective Care Environment

2. The use of which one of the following is avoided when it is necessary to control odors due to incontinence?
   1. electric room deodorizers
   2. incontinence briefs
   3. perfumed or scented powders, lotions, or sprays
   4. use of plastic to cover the mattress

   Nursing Process: Implementation
   Client Need: Health Promotion/Maintenance

3. Ammonia dermatitis may be prevented by applying
   1. a light dusting of an absorbent powder
   2. incontinence briefs
   3. an antibiotic to the perineum
   4. a corticosteroid to reddened areas

   Nursing Process: Implementation
   Client Need: Physiological Integrity

4. The physician orders insertion of the indwelling urethral catheter. In an effort to establish a voiding reflex, the catheter is unclamped for 5 to 15 minutes every
   1. 15 minutes
   2. 1 to 2 hours
   3. 4 to 6 hours
   4. 12 hours

   Nursing Process: Implementation
   Client Need: Health Promotion/Maintenance

5. In 3 weeks Mr. Yates' urethral catheter is removed and he is instructed to
   1. void every 4 to 6 hours
   2. avoid drinking fluids during the morning hours
   3. try and void every hour
   4. stay in bed until he has the urge to void

   Nursing Process: Implementation
   Client Need: Health Promotion/Maintenance

Ms. Phillips is a 73-year-old housewife who is admitted to the hospital for treatment of a possible malignant tumor of the bladder.

6. When obtaining a history from Ms. Phillips, the nurse must be alert to the most common first symptom of a malignant tumor of the bladder which is
   1. pelvic pain
   2. foul odor to the urine
   3. diarrhea
   4. painless hematuria

   Nursing Process: Collecting Data
   Client Need: Physiological Integrity

7. When discussing treatment of Ms. Phillips with other health team members, the nurse is correct in stating that the physician bases the type of treatment for Ms. Phillips on
   1. her willingness to cooperate with treatment
   2. her symptoms
   3. whether she has pain
   4. the grade and stage of the tumor

   Nursing Process: Implementation
   Client Need: Safe, Effective Care Environment

8. Ms. Phillips is found to have a small, superficial tumor. When developing a plan of care, the nurse takes into consideration that this type of tumor most likely will be treated by
   1. resection or coagulation of the tumor
   2. removal of the entire bladder
   3. removal of a segment of the bladder and the ureter and kidney
   4. a permanent cystostomy tube

   Nursing Process: Planning
   Client Need: Safe, Effective Care Environment

9. When developing a teaching plan for Ms. Phillips, the nurse will discuss the importance of
   1. 1 year of chemotherapy
   2. weekly urinalysis for 1 year
   3. frequent cystoscopic examinations for the rest of her life
   4. yearly retrograde pyelograms for the next 5 years

   Nursing Process: Implementation
   Client Need: Health Promotion/Maintenance

Individual Questions

10. At a team conference the nurse describes a neurogenic bladder as one that
    1. does not receive adequate nerve stimulation
    2. cannot hold more than 150 mL of urine
    3. cannot be emptied
    4. holds more than 500 mL of urine

    Nursing Process: Implementation
    Client Need: Safe, Effective Care Environment

11. When obtaining a history from a client with chronic urinary retention and a large residual urine, it is important to determine the
    1. amount and types of fluids ingested daily
    2. type of diet normally eaten
    3. client's usual daily activities
    4. client's voiding pattern

    Nursing Process: Collecting Data
    Client Need: Physiological Integrity

12. When teaching the client with chronic urinary retention to use Credé's maneuver to aid in emptying a bladder, the nurse indicates that the hands are placed on top of one another
    1. just below the umbilicus and pressed firmly inward and downward
    2. just above the umbilicus with pressure exerted upward towards the chest
    3. on the umbilicus with pressure exerted towards the back
    4. on one side of the abdomen and pushed towards the center

    Nursing Process: Implementation
    Client Need: Health Promotion/Maintenance

13. If catheterization for residual urine is used for those with chronic urinary retention, the client is catheterized after each voiding until the residual urine is
    1. 30 mL or less
    2. between 50 and 100 mL
    3. less than 10 mL
    4. between 30 and 80 mL

    Nursing Process: Implementation
    Client Need: Physiological Integrity

14. If a client has cystitis, making the urine acidic provides a less favorable climate for bacterial growth. To accomplish this the nurse can suggest drinking
    1. milk
    2. orange juice
    3. cranberry juice
    4. distilled water

    Nursing Process: Implementation
    Client Need: Health Promotion/Maintenance

15. When a client has interstitial cystitis, the nurse can suggest
    1. drinking extra fluids when the pain is severe
    2. trying anything that appears to relieve symptoms
    3. including fruit juices in the fluid intake
    4. taking oral vitamin C

    Nursing Process: Implementation
    Client Need: Health Promotion/Maintenance

16. When a client has urethritis, the nurse can suggest
    1. adding fruit juices to the fluid intake
    2. remaining in bed until the infection is controlled
    3. warm sitz baths to relieve discomfort
    4. increasing the carbohydrate intake

    Nursing Process: Implementation
    Client Need: Health Promotion/Maintenance

17. Following urethral dilatation for a urethral stricture the client is told
    1. not to drink fluids for 6 hours after the procedure
    2. to rest in bed for the next 12 hours
    3. to eat a soft diet for the next 24 hours
    4. to be aware that the urine may be blood-tinged for 1–2 days

    Nursing Process: Implementation
    Client Need: Health Promotion/Maintenance

18. When discussing malignant bladder tumors at a team conference, the nurse is correct in saying that metastasis usually has not occurred as long as
    1. the urine output from both kidneys is adequate
    2. the muscle wall of the bladder has not been penetrated by the tumor
    3. fever and chills have not occurred
    4. the client is free of pain

    Nursing Process: Implementation
    Client Need: Safe, Effective Care Environment

19. When discussing a cutaneous ureterostomy at a team conference, the nurse explains that the ureters are
    1. amputated from the bladder and brought to the surface of the skin
    2. implanted in the sigmoid colon
    3. anastomosed to a section of amputated ileum
    4. reanastomosed to a different area of the bladder

    Nursing Process: Implementation
    Client Need: Safe, Effective Care Environment

20. When a client has a urinary diversion procedure, one of the most important postoperative nursing tasks is
    1. assessing for pain
    2. auscultating the lungs
    3. checking the abdomen for distention
    4. accurately measuring the urinary output

    Nursing Process: Implementation
    Client Need: Physiological Integrity

21. Once healing has occurred, the continent ileal reservoir is drained by insertion of a catheter approximately every
    1. 30 to 60 minutes
    2. 2 to 3 hours
    3. 12 hours
    4. 24 hours

    Nursing Process: Implementation
    Client Need: Physiological Integrity

22. One recommendation that can be given during discharge teaching of the client who has had a urinary diversion procedure is to keep the urine acidic, which helps
    1. prevent skin breakdown around the stoma
    2. maintain acid-base balance
    3. prevent urinary tract infections
    4. prevent electrolyte imbalances

    Nursing Process: Implementation
    Client Need: Health Promotion/Maintenance

23. When developing a plan of care for the client having a ureterosigmoidostomy, the nurse considers that these clients are
    1. likely to have frequent bouts of constipation
    2. prone to fluid and electrolyte imbalances
    3. prone to skin breakdown at the site of the ureteral anastomoses
    4. usually instructed to eliminate salt from their diets

    Nursing Process: Planning
    Client Need: Physiological Integrity

II. CRITICAL THINKING EXERCISES

1. The physician recommends that Ms. Barnes perform Kegel exercises to control her incontinence. How would you explain these exercises to Ms. Barnes?

2. What suggestions could you give to family members regarding the home care of the incontinent client?

3. Mr. Billings had a cutaneous ureterostomy performed for cancer of the bladder. How would you explain the care and placement of the drainage system to Ms. Billings who will help Mr. Billings with the care of his drainage system?

4. Mr. Kerr has developed bladder stones several times in the past 5 years. Four days ago he required open surgery for removal of a large bladder stone. What suggestions would you include in Mr. Kerr's teaching plan that may prevent future development of bladder stones?

XV Caring for Clients with Musculoskeletal Problems

65. *Introduction to the Musculoskeletal System*
66. *Caring for Clients with Orthopedic and Connective Tissue Disorders*

65/ Introduction to the Musculoskeletal System

Clients with musculoskeletal disorders may be assessed in the emergency department, on an outpatient basis, or following admission for medical or surgical treatment. The nurse implements any protocols necessary for preparing the clients for diagnostic examinations, identifies and sends collected specimens to the laboratory, and manages the client's safe recovery after invasive procedures.

The following questions deal with the content of Chapter 65.

I. MULTIPLE CHOICE QUESTIONS

Circle the number of the most appropriate answer.

1. The most correct term for the nurse to use when referring to the type of light, porous bone that is found at the ends of long bones is ____ bone.
   1. pulpy
   2. dense
   3. compact
   4. cancellous

   Nursing Process: Implementation
   Client Need: Health Promotion/Maintenance

2. A nurse would be correct in identifying the process by which immature bone cells become hardened as
   1. refraction
   2. accommodation
   3. ossification
   4. diffusion

   Nursing Process: Implementation
   Client Need: Health Promotion/Maintenance

3. When explaining normal skeletal physiology to a client, the cells that help remodel bone by absorbing bony tissue that has already formed are most accurately called
   1. T cells
   2. B cells
   3. osteoclasts
   4. osteoblasts

   Nursing Process: Implementation
   Client Need: Health Promotion/Maintenance

4. If the physician intended to aspirate red bone marrow, the nurse would be accurate in explaining that the potential sites would include either the
   1. sternum or ilium
   2. femur or humerus
   3. ilium or femur
   4. humerus or sternum

   Nursing Process: Implementation
   Client Need: Safe, Effective Care Environment

5. When explaining a joint disorder to a client, the nurse would be correct in saying that a diarthrotic joint is one that is
   1. slightly moveable
   2. freely moveable
   3. inflexible
   4. degenerative

   Nursing Process: Implementation
   Client Need: Health Promotion/Maintenance

6. The best evidence that a client has understood the nurse's explanation of a ball and socket joint is if the client cites as an example the joint located in the
   1. hip
   2. wrist
   3. elbow
   4. finger

   Nursing Process: Evaluation
   Client Need: Health Promotion/Maintenance

7. It would be most correct for a nurse to identify the type of cartilage that covers diarthrotic joints as ____ cartilage.
   1. costal
   2. articular
   3. semilunar
   4. fibrous

   Nursing Process:
   Client Need:

8. Immediately after a musculoskeletal injury, the primary focus of assessment is acquiring information about
   1. the client's past health history
   2. when and how the injury occurred
   3. whether a similar injury ever occurred
   4. the client's drug and allergy history

   Nursing Process: Assessment
   Client Need: Safe, Effective Care Environment

9. If a client with a musculoskeletal injury has an open wound, it is most essential for the nurse to ask
   1. if the next-of-kin has been notified
   2. the date of the last tetanus injection
   3. if the client was ever admitted previously
   4. the name of the client's insurance carrier

   Nursing Process: Implementation
   Client Need: Safe, Effective Care Environment

10. The best technique for assessing joint function is to
    1. check each joint's range of motion
    2. look for abnormal joint appearance
    3. test muscle strength and resistance
    4. watch the client's gait pattern

    Nursing Process:[au: missing]
    Client Need:[au: missing]

11. If a client sustained recent musculoskeletal trauma in which there was a suspicion that the ribs had been injured, which other assessment would be most pertinent to obtain at this time?
    1. capillary refill
    2. peripheral pulses
    3. lung sounds
    4. pupil response

    Nursing Process: Assessment
    Client Need: Physiological Integrity

12. If a client has correctly understood the physician's explanation of an arthroscopy, the client will state that this test involves
    1. removing tissue for cell examination
    2. instilling a radioactive substance
    3. placing an instrument inside the joint
    4. taking radiographs of the joint

    Nursing Process: Evaluation
    Client Need: Safe, Effective Care Environment

13. Following an arthroscopy, it would be most appropriate for the nurse to tell the client to
    1. rest the extremity for several days
    2. apply heat to prevent swelling
    3. expect extensive bloody drainage
    4. immediately resume all activities

    Nursing Process: Implementation
    Client Need: Health Promotion/Maintenance

14. The nurse would be most correct in telling a client that immediately before the physician injects medication, such as a corticosteroid, into a joint, a(n) ____ will be performed.
    1. arthroscopy
    2. arthrogram
    3. arthrocentesis
    4. bone scan

    Nursing Process: Implementation
    Client Need: Safe, Effective Care Environment

15. If a client is scheduled to have synovial fluid aspirated, the medical record is most likely to indicate that the client has a disorder like
    1. a sprain
    2. a fracture
    3. osteoporosis
    4. arthritis

    Nursing Process: Assessment
    Client Need: Safe, Effective Care Environment

16. If the physician orders all of the following laboratory tests on a client with musculoskeletal symptoms, which one would the nurse be most correct in telling colleagues is performed to determine if the client has a bone tumor?
    1. serum calcium
    2. serum uric acid
    3. alkaline phosphatase
    4. antinuclear antibodies

    Nursing Process: Implementation
    Client Need: Safe, Effective Care Environment

II. CRITICAL THINKING EXERCISES

1. If a client sustained trauma to an extremity, what could the nurse do to relieve the client's discomfort before and during the time that a radiographic examination is being performed?

2. What nursing approaches would be helpful in relieving the anxiety of a client who is undergoing diagnostic tests of the musculoskeletal system?

3. What kinds of discharge instructions would be important to provide after a client has undergone a diagnostic test or invasive treatment procedure involving the musculoskeletal system?

66/ Caring for Clients with Orthopedic and Connective Tissue Disorders

The musculoskeletal system consists of structures that the body uses for support and movement. Disorders affecting the tissues that are components of this system affect an individual's ability to perform activities of daily living, remain active and mobile, and stay physically fit.

The following questions deal with the content of Chapter 66.

I. MULTIPLE CHOICE QUESTIONS

Circle the number of the most appropriate answer.

1. A nurse would be most correct in explaining to a client with a strain that this type of injury involves trauma to the
   1. skeletal muscles
   2. articular cartilage
   3. ligaments
   4. tendons

   Nursing Process: Implementation
   Client Need: Health Promotion/Maintenance

2. The best advice the nurse could give a client who suspects that a sprain has been incurred is to apply a
   1. splint
   2. bandage
   3. cold pack
   4. hot pack

   Nursing Process: Implementation
   Client Need: Physiological Integrity

3. It would be appropriate for the nurse to warn a client that the consequence of continuing to use a sprained extremity may be a(n)
    1. avulsion fracture
    2. unstable joint
    3. hematoma
    4. ecchymosis

    Nursing Process: Implementation
    Client Need: Health Promotion/Maintenance

4. The best explanation of a dislocation is that it is a
    1. separation at the joint surfaces
    2. break in the continuity of a bone
    3. degeneration of the articular cartilage
    4. fibrous ankylosis between two bones

    Nursing Process: Implementation
    Client Need: Health Promotion/Maintenance

5. If a client with a neck sprain asked why the physician has prescribed that he wear a soft cervical collar, it would be correct for the nurse to say it is used to
    1. limit motion
    2. reduce swelling
    3. maintain alignment
    4. improve circulation

    Nursing Process: implementation
    Client Need: Health Promotion/Maintenance

6. It would be most accurate to explain to a client that one of the leading causes of joint instability following a dislocation is
    1. inadequate amounts of calcium
    2. inactivity of osteoclastic cells
    3. insufficient deposition of collagen
    4. impaired mononuclear phagocytes

    Nursing Process: Implementation
    Client Need: Health Promotion/Maintenance

7. When the nurse is gathering subjective data from a client who is suspected of having a dislocation, the client is most likely to describe that at the time of the injury he
    1. lost muscular strength
    2. felt an electrical shock
    3. became weak and dizzy
    4. heard a popping sound

    Nursing Process: Assessment
    Client Need: Safe, Effective Care Environment

8. When performing a physical examination of a client with a dislocation, the most diagnostic finding in the extremity with the injury is that the
    1. client has no palpable peripheral pulses
    2. extremity is shorter than the one uninjured
    3. muscles are weak and atrophied
    4. deep tendon reflexes are absent

    Nursing Process: Assessment
    Client Need: Physiological Integrity

9. When performing a neurovascular assessment, after compressing and releasing the nailbed, color should return in ____ second(s) or less.
    1. 1
    2. 2
    3. 3
    4. 4

    Nursing Process: Assessment
    Client Need: Physiological Integrity

10. The nurse would be correct in explaining to colleagues that compartment syndrome is ultimately the result of inadequate
    1. circulation
    2. nutrition
    3. clotting
    4. exercise

    Nursing Process: Implementation
    Client Need: Safe, Effective Care Environment

11. Which one of the following assessments is essential for detecting compartment syndrome?
    1. moving each joint through its range of motion
    2. measuring the circumference of an injured extremity
    3. checking the results of radiographs
    4. monitoring neurovascular status

    Nursing Process: Implementation
    Client Need: Physiological Integrity

12. A nurse would be negligent if assessment for compartment syndrome were omitted from the care of a client with a fracture of the
    1. vertebrae
    2. ribs
    3. phalanges
    4. radius

    Nursing Process: Assessment
    Client Need: Physiological Integrity

13. In response to a question from a nursing assistant, the term that refers to a fracture in which the broken bone pierces through the skin is
    1. displaced
    2. compound
    3. greenstick
    4. impacted

    Nursing Process: Implementation
    Client Need: Safe, Effective Care Environment

14. If all of the following clients are examined by the nurse following a fall, which one is most likely to have sustained a greenstick fracture?
    1. Ms. Quentin, who is 65 years old
    2. Mr. Paulson, who is 36 years old
    3. Kyla Adams, who is 18 years old
    4. Jerry Taylor, who is 7 years old

    Nursing Process: Assessment
    Client Need: Physiological Integrity

15. A nurse would be most correct in referring to the calcium deposit that forms between and around the broken ends of bones as
    1. phallus
    2. pannus
    3. callus
    4. crepitus

    Nursing Process: Implementation
    Client Need: Safe, Effective Care Environment

16. A client asks the nurse how long it will take for his fracture to heal. The best answer is that it will take an average of ____ months before the bone regains its former structural strength.
    1. 3
    2. 6
    3. 9
    4. 12

    Nursing Process: Implementation
    Client Need: Health Promotion/Maintenance

17. Within 24 hours following a fracture of the femur, a client has severe chest pain and dyspnea. The nurse would be most correct in suspecting that the symptoms are due to
    1. fat embolism
    2. compartment syndrome
    3. thrombophlebitis
    4. myocardial infarction

    Nursing Process: Assessment
    Client Need: Physiological Integrity

18. A client asks the nurse why the physician has ordered a bone scan when the radiographic examination following an injury 2 weeks ago demonstrated negative results. The best answer is that a bone scan is better for identifying
    1. nondisplaced and stress fractures
    2. greenstick and compression fractures
    3. impacted and avulsion fractures
    4. pathologic and displaced fractures

    Nursing Process: Implementation
    Client Need: Safe, Effective Care Environment

19. Before placing a client with a fractured femur in traction, the nurse would be correct in explaining that traction is used for all of the following reasons *except*

    1. immobilizing an injury
    2. aligning fractured bones
    3. relieving muscle spasm
    4. shortening rehabilitation

    Nursing Process: Implementation
    Client Need: Safe, Effective Care Environment

20. When assigned to a client in skeletal leg traction, which one of the following would be most appropriate to add to the plan for care?

    1. cleanse the pin or nail sites daily
    2. roll the client from side to side q2h
    3. remove the traction to facilitate exercise
    4. decrease the traction weight by 5 lbs each day

    Nursing Process: Planning
    Client Need: Safe, Effective Care Environment

21. When the nurse inspects the client in traction, which one of the following must be corrected to provide effective treatment?

    1. The ropes move through all pulleys.
    2. The weights rest on the floor.
    3. The body part is aligned with the pull of traction.
    4. The prescribed amount of weight has been applied.

    Nursing Process: Assessment
    Client Need: Safe, Effective Care Environment

22. When caring for a client in traction, which one of the following would be best to implement to preserve muscle tone?

    1. isometric exercises
    2. maintain alignment
    3. range of motion
    4. position changes

    Nursing Process: Implementation
    Client Need: Physiological Integrity

23. Which one of the following would be the best evidence that a client's peroneal nerve is becoming irritated from traction applied to the lower leg? The client has difficulty

    1. plantarflexing his foot
    2. dorsiflexing his foot
    3. flexing his knee
    4. extending his knee

    Nursing Process: Assessment
    Client Need: Physiological Integrity

24. A client who is undergoing a closed reduction to repair a fracture demonstrates an accurate understanding of the procedure if he says that

    1. the bone ends will be manipulated manually into place
    2. the bone ends will be aligned during a surgical procedure
    3. a metal device will be attached to the bone for stabilization
    4. there will be metal pins protruding from the skin surface

    Nursing Process: Evaluation
    Client Need: Safe, Effective Care Environment

25. If a cast is applied immediately following a fracture of the tibia, the nurse can expect that its length will include the area

    1. below the knee to above the ankle
    2. from the thigh to the middle of the foot
    3. below the shoulder to above the wrist
    4. above the hips and one or both legs

    Nursing Process: Planning
    Client Need: Safe, Effective Care Environment

26. When assisting with a cast application, the nurse should plan to hold the injured extremity in a position of slight

    1. flexion
    2. extension
    3. abduction
    4. adduction

    Nursing Process: Planning

Client Need: Safe, Effective Care Environment

27. It would be appropriate for the nurse to inform a client that while the cast is applied, the area being covered by the cast will feel
    1. warm
    2. cold
    3. numb
    4. tight

    Nursing Process: Implementation
    Client Need: Safe, Effective Care Environment

28. A nurse observes a colleague caring for a client just after a leg cast has been applied. For which action would it be appropriate to intervene?
    1. The leg is elevated on pillows.
    2. The client wiggles all his toes.
    3. The leg is covered by a thermal blanket.
    4. A cold pack is over the injured area.

    Nursing Process: Evaluation
    Client Need: Safe, Effective Care Environment

29. One of the best indications that there is tissue necrosis beneath a leg cast is that there is
    1. swelling of the toes
    2. an odor from the cast
    3. pain beneath the cast
    4. prolonged capillary refill

    Nursing Process: Assessment
    Client Need: Physiological Integrity

30. If the nurse noted that the cast edges are crumbling, which nursing action is most appropriate?
    1. report it to the physician
    2. reinforce the edges with tape
    3. wash the exposed skin
    4. bivalve the cast

    Nursing Process: Implementation
    Client Need: Physiological Integrity

31. If a client whose fractured jaw was reduced and immobilized with wire loops is in imminent danger of vomiting, which one of the following measures would be most appropriate?
    1. have the client take deep breaths
    2. suction the client's mouth
    3. cut the wires with scissors
    4. take sips of a carbonated drink

    Nursing Process: Implementation
    Client Need: Physiological Integrity

32. If a figure-of-eight bandage is used to treat a fractured clavicle, it would be most appropriate for the nurse to tell the client to
    1. remove the bandage during the night
    2. wash and replace the bandage daily
    3. pad the axilla with soft cloth
    4. elevate the arms overhead q2h

    Nursing Process: Implementation
    Client Need: Health Promotion/Maintenance

33. A client with a hanging arm cast demonstrates an accurate understanding for the purpose of a hanging cast if he says it is used to
    1. realign the fractured bone
    2. immobilize the reduced fracture
    3. prevent compartment syndrome
    4. reduce the potential for infection

    Nursing Process: Evaluation
    Client Need: Safe, Effective Care Environment

34. When the nurse is instructing a client on how to apply an arm sling, which one of the following is correct information?
    1. keep the wrist higher than the elbow
    2. keep the wrist even with the elbow
    3. keep the elbow higher than the wrist
    4. keep the wrist lower than the elbow

    Nursing Process: Implementation
    Client Need: Health Promotion/Maintenance

35. If an older adult sustained a fracture, which disorder is most likely a contributing factor?
    1. osteomyelitis
    2. osteoporosis
    3. pellegra
    4. rickets

    Nursing Process: Assessment
    Client Need: Safe, Effective Care Environment

36. A client with a halo brace demonstrates an accurate understanding of its use with the statement, "I will
    1. need to wear this brace except when sleeping"
    2. be able to walk, but my spine will be immobile"
    3. be confined to bed until my spinal fracture heals"
    4. have a plaster cast from my neck to my hips"

    Nursing Process: Evaluation
    Client Need: Safe, Effective Care Environment

37. When examining a client who has fallen, which one of the following findings suggests that the client has fractured a hip? The injured leg is shortened and
    1. externally rotated
    2. internally rotated
    3. abducted
    4. adducted

    Nursing Process: Assessment
    Client Need: Physiological Integrity

38. When the nurse is turning a client following the repair of a fractured hip, the best technique to use is to
    1. turn the client on the unoperative side with pillows between the legs
    2. turn the client on the unoperative side without any pillows between the legs
    3. turn the client on the operative side with pillows between the legs
    4. turn the client on the operative side without any pillows between the legs

    Nursing Process: Implementation
    Client Need: Physiological Integrity

39. If all of the following clients experience an inflammatory condition of the joints, which one is most likely to have rheumatoid arthritis?
    1. Ms. Inez Klein, 75 years old
    2. Mr. Edward Wiggins, 59 years old
    3. Mr. Horace Grayson, 42 years old
    4. Ms. Janice Beutter, 25 years old

    Nursing Process: Assessment
    Client Need: Safe, Effective Care Environment

40. When explaining the pathophysiology to a client with rheumatoid arthritis, the nurse would be correct in saying that this is a disorder that
    1. mainly affects the knee and ankle joints
    2. results in changes in the shafts of bones
    3. is manifested by inflamed connective tissue
    4. affects most adults as they become older

    Nursing Process: Implementation
    Client Need: Health Promotion/Maintenance

41. If the physician indicated that a client had Heberden's nodes, the nurse would be most correct in assuming that the client has
    1. rheumatoid arthritis
    2. osteoarthritis
    3. gouty arthritis
    4. ankylosing spondylitis

    Nursing Process: Assessment
    Client Need: Safe, Effective Care Environment

42. If a client made all of the following statements, which one is accurate concerning rheumatoid arthritis?
    1. The distal finger joints are most commonly affected.
    2. There is often a pattern of remissions and exacerbations.
    3. Once the symptoms appear, they become continuously worse.
    4. The joints become inflamed, but they remain functional.

    Nursing Process: Evaluation
    Client Need: Health Promotion/Maintenance

43. What information is appropriate to give a client with arthritis who is advised to take aspirin on a regular basis?
    1. alternate the aspirin with acetaminophen
    2. never stop taking the aspirin abruptly
    3. take the aspirin with food, meals, or milk
    4. report if your stools become clay-colored

    Nursing Process: Implementation
    Client Need: Health Promotion/Maintenance

44. When explaining the etiology of osteoarthritis to a client who has this disorder, it would be most correct to say it is due to
    1. an autoimmune response
    2. an infectious microorganism
    3. a degenerative process
    4. a traumatic injury

    Nursing Process: Implementation
    Client Need: Health Promotion/Maintenance

45. When planning the care of a client following a total hip replacement, the most important positions to maintain are hip extension and
    1. adduction
    2. abduction
    3. external rotation
    4. internal rotation

    Nursing Process: Implementation
    Client Need: Safe, Effective Care Environment

46. Which one of the following would be most important for the client with a total hip replacement to use for bowel elimination?
    1. a bedside commode
    2. a conventional bedpan
    3. a raised toilet seat
    4. a suppository

    Nursing Process: Implementation
    Client Need: Health Promotion/Maintenance

47. If a client with a total hip replacement makes all of the following statements, which one indicates that he needs more teaching?
    1. "I should do deep knee bends to maintain joint flexibility."
    2. "I should not bend over to pick things up from the floor."
    3. "I should use an elevated toilet seat for elimination."
    4. "I should not cross my legs in bed or while sitting."

    Nursing Process: Evaluation
    Client Need: Health Promotion/Maintenance

48. A nurse would be most correct in explaining to a client with a total knee replacement that the primary use for continuous passive motion (CPM) device is to
    1. promote healing and increase circulation
    2. limit active movement until healing occurs
    3. prevent atrophy of muscles in the operative leg
    4. decrease the potential for thrombophlebitis

    Nursing Process: Implementation
    Client Need: Safe, Effective Care Environment

49. When reviewing the laboratory test results of a client with gout, the most significant finding is that the client has
    1. hyperuricemia
    2. hyperkalemia
    3. hypernatremia
    4. hypercalcemia

    Nursing Process: Assessment
    Client Need: Physiological Integrity

50. When assessing the client with gout, the nurse is most likely to find that the client experiences
    1. stiffness in the joints, especially in the morning
    2. anorexia, nausea, and vomiting, especially after a meal
    3. urinary frequency and urgency
    4. sudden, acute joint pain

    Nursing Process: Assessment
    Client Need: Physiological Integrity

51. A client with gout has an accurate understanding of the current treatment of the disorder when stating that it cannot be cured, but the symptoms can be controlled with drugs that
    1. reduce immunoglobulin formation
    2. inhibit production of prostaglandin
    3. decrease the formation of sodium urate
    4. block histamine (H_2) receptor sites

    Nursing Process: Evaluation
    Client Need: Health Promotion/Maintenance

52. If a client has ankylosing spondylitis, the symptoms would most likely occur in the
    1. shoulders
    2. legs
    3. spine
    4. fingers

    Nursing Process: Assessment
    Client Need: Physiological Integrity

53. The client with ankylosing spondylitis may delay the crippling effects of the disorder if the following advice is given.
    1. sleep on a firm mattress
    2. avoid eating organ meats
    3. abstain from drinking alcohol
    4. take vitamin E on a daily basis

    Nursing Process: Implementation
    Client Need: Health Promotion/Maintenance

54. Which one of the following is the most characteristic sign manifested by a client who has lupus erythematosus?
    1. butterfly rash about the cheeks
    2. dark circles about the eyes
    3. brown, furry tongue
    4. thick, pink lips

    Nursing Process: Assessment
    Client Need: Physiological Integrity

55. A client with osteoporosis may delay the consequences of the disorder by
    1. increasing calcium intake
    2. increasing potassium intake
    3. decreasing sodium intake
    4. decreasing magnesium intake

    Nursing Process: Implementation
    Client Need: Health Promotion/Maintenance

56. When a nurse is informed to expect a client with osteomyelitis, which one of the following measures may be considered as part of the client's plan for care?
    1. following isolation precautions
    2. monitoring urinary output
    3. placing the client on fluid restrictions
    4. keeping an accurate record of bowel elimination

    Nursing Process: Planning
    Client Need: Safe, Effective Care Environment

57. One of the common characteristics of clients with Paget's disease is
    1. weak arms
    2. small body
    3. large skull
    4. missing toes

    Nursing Process: Assessment
    Client Need: Physiological Integrity

58. Which of the following suggestions would be most appropriate for a client with hallux valgus?
    1. consume foods high in calcium
    2. go barefoot as much as possible
    3. wear comfortably fitting shoes
    4. trim all toenails straight across

    Nursing Process: Implementation
    Client Need: Health Promotion/Maintenance

59. If a client has carpal tunnel syndrome, which one of the following is likely to cause immediate pain and numbness?
    1. crossing the legs
    2. raising the arms
    3. waving the hands
    4. bending the wrist

    Nursing Process: Assessment
    Client Need: Physiological Integrity

60. Which one of the following may be beneficial for relieving the symptoms associated with carpal tunnel syndrome?
    1. doing active hand exercises
    2. applying an ice pack
    3. suspending the arm in a sling
    4. wearing a hand splint

    Nursing Process: Implementation
    Client Need: Physiological Integrity

61. A nurse would be most accurate in stating that the most common metastatic site associated with a malignant bone tumors is the
    1. lungs
    2. brain
    3. liver
    4. kidneys

    Nursing Process: Implementation
    Client Need: Health Promotion/Maintenance

62. Which one of the following should the nurse plan to place at the bedside of a client who has undergone an amputation?
    1. tracheostomy set
    2. suction machine
    3. rubber tourniquet
    4. cardiac defibrillator

    Nursing Process: Planning
    Client Need: Physiological Integrity

63. A client with an amputation says, "It feels like my foot is still there." What response from the nurse would be most appropriate?
    1. The mind has a strange way of playing tricks.
    2. The feeling is probably due to the walking pylon.
    3. This may be a complication for which you may require additional surgery.
    4. That is a common phenomenon which you will probably learn to ignore.

    Nursing Process: Implementation
    Client Need: Health Promotion/Maintenance

64. Which of the following should be discouraged during the postoperative period following an AK amputation?
    1. coughing to remove secretions
    2. sitting up in bed or a chair
    3. isometric exercises with the stump
    4. using crutches to ambulate

    Nursing Process: Implementation
    Client Need: Physiological Integrity

65. Which one of the following approaches would be best for helping the client with an amputation cope with his surgery?
    1. allow the client to be as independent as possible
    2. leave the client alone to deal with his grief in private
    3. discuss current events to distract the client from feeling sad
    4. offer to help the client with bathing, dressing, and grooming

    Nursing Process: Planning
    Client Need: Psychosocial Integrity

II. CRITICAL THINKING EXERCISES

1. What suggestions might you have for providing diversional activities for a client who is confined to bed while being treated with traction or a hip spica cast?

2. What measures would facilitate drying a plaster cast?

3. How could a nurse assess for hemorrhage when caring for a client with an open reduction and cast application?

4. What would be the best way to protect the anal opening in a hip spica cast from becoming damp from urine or soiled from feces?

5. If a client experiences itching beneath a cast, what suggestions could be offered?

6. What instructions would be appropriate following a total hip replacement?

7. What suggestions might the nurse make to help a client with a rheumatic disorder remain independent in performing activities of daily living?

8. What principles of body mechanics might the nurse give a client who has low back pain?

9. What factors affect the level at which a limb is amputated?

10. What principles are followed when wrapping a stump?

XVI Caring for Clients with Integumentary Problems

67. *Introduction to the Integumentary System*
68. *Caring for Clients with Integumentary Disorders*

67/ Introduction to the Integumentary System

The skin, the largest body organ, is a protective barrier between the body's internal and external environments. Because the skin is in constant contact with the environment, it is often subject to injury and irritation. Diseases and disorders of the skin *(integumentum)* are called *integumentary* disorders.

The following questions deal with the content of Chapter 67.

I. MULTIPLE CHOICE QUESTIONS

Circle the number of the most appropriate answer.

In preparation for the opening of a unit to care for clients with severe burns, a team conference is held for review of the anatomy and physiology of the integumentary system and the various methods used in the treatment of skin disorders.

1. When asked to give one method by which heat is lost by the body, the nurse answers by

   1. reduction
   2. radiation
   3. collection
   4. production

   Nursing Process: Implementation
   Client Need: Safe, Effective Care Environment

2. When asked for the function of melanin, the nurse answers

   1. production of oil to lubricate the skin
   2. manufacture of melanocytes
   3. manufacture of keratin
   4. skin color

   Nursing Process: Implementation
   Client Need: Safe, Effective Care Environment

3. When discussing the use of corticosteroids for the treatment of skin disorders, the nurse states that these drugs

   1. produce few systemic effects when used topically
   2. are used primarily to relieve minor skin disorders
   3. relieve symptoms only when used systemically
   4. are rarely effective for most skin disorders

   Nursing Process: Implementation
   Client Need: Safe, Effective Care Environment

4. When discussing the use of antihistamines in treating skin disorders, the nurse states that these drugs are used
   1. when an allergy is causing the skin disorder
   2. to relieve the pain associated with some skin disorders
   3. when other drugs fail to relieve symptoms
   4. when burning is the major symptom of the disorder

   Nursing Process: Implementation
   Client Need: Safe, Effective Care Environment

5. The nurse defines a keratolytic as a drug that
   1. dissolves thickened, cornified skin
   2. softens dry skin
   3. prevents sunburn
   4. reduces itching

   Nursing Process: Implementation
   Client Need: Safe, Effective Care Environment

6. When describing the application of wet dressing, the nurse states that this type of dressing is
   1. applied tightly
   2. applied loosely
   3. used only when the skin is dry and rough
   4. generally ineffective in the treatment of skin disorders

   Nursing Process: Implementation
   Client Need: Safe, Effective Care Environment

7. A nurse assistant asks why solutions, powders, and oils are sometimes added to a client's bath water. The nurse replies that these substances may be used to
   1. aid in the removal of crusts and scales
   2. slow the healing of open lesions
   3. kill viruses on the skin
   4. increase water loss from skin cells

   Nursing Process: Implementation
   Client Need: Safe, Effective Care Environment

8. When asked to define cryosurgery, the nurse states that this form of treatment for skin disorders uses
   1. heat
   2. external radiation
   3. an electrical current
   4. extreme cold

   Nursing Process: Implementation
   Client Need: Safe, Effective Care Environment

9. When asked to name the skin disorder for which photochemotherapy is used, the nurse answers
   1. contact dermatitis
   2. melanomas
   3. psoriasis
   4. superficial skin cancers

   Nursing Process: Implementation
   Client Need: Safe, Effective Care Environment

10. A nurse assistant asks why diet is important in the treatment of skin disorders. The nurse answers that
    1. the skin requires a well-balanced diet high in vitamins
    2. lack of certain minerals can result in skin infections
    3. certain foods may cause skin disorders in some individuals
    4. individuals with allergic skin disorders must avoid foods high in protein

    Nursing Process: Implementation
    Client Need: Safe, Effective Care Environment

II. CRITICAL THINKING

1. Mr. Williams, who had a suprapubic prostatectomy 2 days ago, complains of severe itching. What specific steps would you take in investigating this problem?

2. Ms. Adams, an outpatient in a dermatology clinic, requires wet dressings to a skin lesion. How would you explain this treatment to Ms. Adams? What materials would you suggest that she obtain?

68/ Caring for Clients with Integumentary Disorders

The skin is in constant contact with the environment and is frequently subject to injury and irritation. Nurses are in a strategic position to help others maintain a normal, healthy skin. Serious injuries to the skin may occur, as, for example, the client sustaining a burn injury. A person who sustains serious burns is confronted with problems resulting from pain, mutilation, fear of death, disfigurement, separation, immobilization, helplessness, and possible abandonment.

The following questions deal with the content of Chapter 68.

I. MULTIPLE CHOICE QUESTIONS

Circle the number of the most appropriate answer.

An inservice program is held to present the nursing management of various skin disorders.

1. When asked for the type of drug use to treat tinea pedis, the nurse answers a(n)
   1. topical antifungal agent
   2. oral corticosteroid
   3. a topical pediculicide
   4. topical antibiotic

   Nursing Process: Implementation
   Client Need: Safe, Effective Care Environment

2. The nurse presenting the inservice defines a pigmented nevus as a
   1. malignant skin lesion
   2. mole
   3. basal cell carcinoma
   4. lesion due to exposure to sunlight

   Nursing Process: Implementation
   Client Need: Safe, Effective Care Environment

3. When asked what may be used to treat angiomas, the nurse answers
   1. methotrexate
   2. photochemotherapy
   3. the argon laser
   4. cryosurgery

   Nursing Process: Implementation
   Client Need: Safe, Effective Care Environment

4. When asked to define seborrheic keratosis, the nurse describes this skin lesion as a
   1. malignant tumor found in or near oil glands
   2. benign tumor of sweat glands
   3. malignant tumor arising from epidermal cells
   4. benign growth composed of immature epithelial cells

   Nursing Process: Implementation
   Client Need: Safe, Effective Care Environment

5. When discussing factors that predispose the skin to malignant changes, the nurse includes
   1. prolonged exposure to ultraviolet light
   2. excessive use of cosmetics
   3. exposure to heat
   4. the development of corns and calluses

   Nursing Process: Implementation
   Client Need: Safe, Effective Care Environment

6. When asked to discuss a malignant melanoma, the nurse describes it as a
   1. benign lesion that may become malignant
   2. low-grade malignant lesion that rarely spreads to other parts of the body
   3. malignant lesion that is most always seen in elderly clients
   4. highly malignant, rapidly spreading lesion

   Nursing Process: Implementation
   Client Need: Safe, Effective Care Environment

7. When asked to discuss squamous cell carcinoma of the skin, the nurse describes it as a
   1. a low-grade malignant tumor of the skin that rarely metastasizes
   2. dangerous lesion because it tends to metastasize to the internal organs
   3. premalignant lesion related to malignant melanomas
   4. malignant tumor arising from the dermis

   Nursing Process: Implementation
   Client Need: Safe, Effective Care Environment

8. When asked to discuss a basal cell carcinoma, the nurse describes it as
   1. a rare tumor most always seen in young adults
   2. the most common type of skin cancer
   3. a highly malignant tumor that spreads to the internal organs
   4. a tumor arising from dermal cells

   Nursing Process: Implementation
   Client Need: Safe, Effective Care Environment

9. When discussing the treatment of basal cell carcinomas, the nurse includes
   1. electrodessication
   2. application of a high temperature probe
   3. topical application of methotrexate
   4. radical excision of the tumor and adjacent lymph nodes

   Nursing Process: Implementation
   Client Need: Safe, Effective Care Environment

10. When discussing stasis ulcers, the nurse explains that they are skin manifestations resulting from
    1. psychiatric problems such as stress and depression
    2. diabetes mellitus
    3. inadequate or poor circulation in the legs
    4. multiple sclerosis

    Nursing Process: Implementation
    Client Need: Safe, Effective Care Environment

11. The nurse describes the primary objectives of treatment of stasis ulcers which include
    1. controlling infection and promoting healing
    2. decreasing the blood supply to the area and promoting good skin turgor
    3. increasing the elasticity of subcutaneous tissues and improving circulation
    4. promoting collateral and peripheral circulation

    Nursing Process: Implementation
    Client Need: Safe, Effective Care Environment

Hal Brock was cleaning and repairing his car in his garage. In one corner of the garage, he had an open can of gasoline. Working in a closed area caused a build-up of fumes, and an explosion and fire occurred, apparently caused by a spark. His clothing was on fire and he appeared to have suffered severe burns.

12. Clothing about Hal's head and neck is on fire and he is
    1. sprayed with water
    2. placed in a horizontal position and covered with plastic sheeting
    3. rolled in a blanket and kept standing if at all possible
    4. sprayed with a flame-retardant foam mixed with water and kept in a vertical position

    Nursing Process: Implementation
    Client Need: Physiological Integrity

13. The nurse prepares for the most important initial steps in the management of Hal which are
    1. establishing and maintaining a patent airway
    2. determining the amount of fluid lost
    3. evaluating his level of consciousness
    4. evaluating his mental status

    Nursing Process: Implementation
    Client Need: Physiological Integrity

14. If Hal is burned around the face and neck, he must be closely observed for
    1. excessive salivation
    2. excessive fluid loss
    3. bleeding
    4. respiratory difficulty

    Nursing Process: Collecting Data
    Client Need: Physiological Integrity

15. Hal is observed for signs of a fluid volume deficit because in the burned client fluid is lost from the burned area in the forms of
    1. water vapor and seepage
    2. potassium and bicarbonate ions
    3. plasma and fluid moving away from the burned area
    4. necrotic muscle and fat tissue

    Nursing Process: Collecting Data
    Client Need: Physiological Integrity

16. The physician wants to give Hal an intravenous narcotic for his severe pain. The nurse prepares the narcotic immediately because severe pain can cause
    1. hypotension
    2. respiratory difficulty
    3. pooling of blood in the extremities
    4. unconsciousness when he must be alert to cooperate with initial treatment

    Nursing Process: Implementation
    Client Need: Physiological Integrity

17. Since both of Hal's arms are burned, his blood pressure
    1. cannot be taken
    2. is only taken every 4 hours
    3. can be taken by use of an electronic device
    4. is not taken until some healing has occurred

    Nursing Process: Implementation
    Client Need: Physiological Integrity

18. After 2 or 3 days the nurse observes the areas of a third-degree or full-thickness burn for the formation of a leathery crust charted as

    1. epithelial skin
    2. eschar
    3. debrided skin
    4. denuded skin

    Nursing Process: Collecting Data
    Client Need: Physiological Integrity

19. If mafenide (Sulfamylon) is used for treatment, the previous applications of the drug are removed by

    1. using a tongue blade to scrape off the cream
    2. tubbing—usually in a Hubbard tank
    3. wiping the area with sterile gauze
    4. dissolving the cream with a weak alkali solution

    Nursing Process: Implementation
    Client Need: Physiological Integrity

20. When first applying mafenide, the nurse tells Hal

    1. to lie still
    2. hold his breath while the drug is applied
    3. to place his arms across his chest
    4. that a stinging or burning sensation may be noted

    Nursing Process: Implementation
    Client Need: Physiological Integrity

Individual Questions

21. To relieve dryness of the skin the nurse can recommend

    1. wearing rubber gloves when using soaps and detergents
    2. applying a keratolytic to the skin
    3. using detergents that do not contain phosphates
    4. avoiding the use of an antiperspirant containing perfumes

    Nursing Process: Implementation
    Client Need: Health Promotion/Maintenance

22. To relieve pruritus the nurse can recommend the use of

    1. starch baths
    2. a keratolytic
    3. an antiseborrheic
    4. an antiseptic

    Nursing Process: Implementation
    Client Need: Health Promotion/Maintenance

23. Clients with pediculosis are instructed to

    1. apply a scabicide each morning for 3 days
    2. avoid ironing clothes
    3. launder clothes in hot water
    4. clean the affected areas with alcohol

    Nursing Process: Implementation
    Client Need: Health Promotion/Maintenance

24. When performing a physical assessment on a client with possible scabies, the nurse looks for

    1. weeping lesions of the skin
    2. burrows under the skin
    3. dry, scaly, shiny patches of cornified skin
    4. raised, red areas filled with exudate

    Nursing Process: Collecting Data
    Client Need: Physiological Integrity

25. When instructing the client with scabies, the nurse emphasizes the fact that the scabies mite can

    1. cause a viral infection
    2. only be killed by an alcohol antiseptic
    3. travel to vital organs
    4. be transmitted by close personal contact

    Nursing Process: Implementation
    Client Need: Health Promotion/Maintenance

26. When reviewing the physician's suggestions regarding the application of a medication for seborrheic dermatitis, the nurse advises the client that
    1. the product must be used for 5 consecutive days
    2. gloves must be worn since the condition is infectious
    3. close personal contact may result in a spread of the infection to others
    4. overuse or heavy applications will not improve the problem

    Nursing Process: Implementation
    Client Need: Health Promotion/Maintenance

27. When assessing the client with an allergic contact dermatitis, the nurse looks for
    1. redness and swelling
    2. appearance of silver scales over the lesions
    3. scarring and changes in skin pigmentation
    4. deep lesions with raised edges

    Nursing Process: Collecting Data
    Client Need: Physiological Integrity

28. Until the substance causing an allergic contact dermatitis is identified, the nurse can advise the client to
    1. apply a corticosteroid ointment to the area
    2. use a second rinse cycle when laundering
    3. apply a drying ointment to the skin
    4. apply a topical antibiotic to the affected areas

    Nursing Process: Implementation
    Client Need: Health Promotion/Maintenance

29. Women who are prescribed isotretinoin (Accutane) for acne vulgaris are advised to
    1. use effective contraceptive measures during therapy
    2. apply the drug in large amounts to affected areas
    3. use a hair spray to prevent reinfection of the area
    4. stop use of an oral contraceptive during therapy

    Nursing Process: Implementation
    Client Need: Health Promotion/Maintenance

30. When performing a physical examination on the client with psoriasis, the nurse looks for
    1. raised, red lesions covered with crusts
    2. deep lesions covered by weeping crusts
    3. patches of erythema covered with silvery scales
    4. infected sebaceous cysts covered with cornified plaques

    Nursing Process: Collecting Data
    Client Need: Physiological Integrity

31. The client receiving photochemotherapy for psoriasis is instructed to
    1. apply a softening ointment prior to treatment
    2. avoid exposure to sunlight for 8 hours after treatment
    3. apply a corticosteroid ointment between treatments
    4. fast from food and fluids for 4 hours before treatment

    Nursing Process: Implementation
    Client Need: Health Promotion/Maintenance

32. When an oily substance or drug is added to the bath water, the client must be assisted in and out of the tub because the
    1. bath additive leaves a slippery residue on the tub surface
    2. client's skin is oily and must be patted dry
    3. bath water cannot be emptied until the client is out of the tub
    4. client is usually elderly and therefore needs assistance getting out of a tub

    Nursing Process: Implementation
    Client Need: Safe, Effective Care Environment

33. Clients with one or more furuncles are advised
    1. to apply alcohol to the lesion
    2. not to pick or squeeze the lesion
    3. to apply a topical corticosteroid to the lesion
    4. use an astringent on the skin around the lesion

    Nursing Process: Implementation
    Client Need: Health Promotion/Maintenance

34. When a client has severe pruritus, the nurse can
    1. have the client wear white cotton gloves if scratching occurs during sleep
    2. apply alcohol to the affected area
    3. apply an aromatic dusting powder
    4. use a room deodorant

    Nursing Process: Implementation
    Client Need: Safe, Effective Care Environment

35. When evaluating the effectiveness of continuous wet dressings, the nurse must look for problems such as
    1. skin softening and ultimate maceration of the skin
    2. changes in skin pigmentation
    3. hardening of the skin under the dressings
    4. cornification of the skin

    Nursing Process: Evaluation
    Client Need: Physiological Integrity

36. When a member of the family has an infectious skin disorder, the family is instructed to
    1. discard all used towels and washcloths
    2. presoak towels and washcloths in undiluted laundry soap and then wash
    3. wash towels and washcloths in cold water followed by a warm water rinse
    4. soak towels and washcloths in bleach and wash in hot water separate from other laundry

    Nursing Process: Implementation
    Client Need: Health Promotion/Maintenance

37. Nurses can tell persons with warts that self-treatment with nonprescription products
    1. usually is effective
    2. may be effective but the warts will return
    3. can result in the development of a malignant tumor
    4. can result in serious injury to superficial and subcutaneous tissues

    Nursing Process: Implementation
    Client Need: Health Promotion/Maintenance

38. Client teaching following removal of a superficial malignant skin lesion includes
    1. allowing the scab to dry and fall off
    2. soaking the scab with warm water to facilitate removal
    3. applying a topical anesthetic to relieve pain
    4. applying moist heat to speed healing

    Nursing Process: Implementation
    Client Need: Health Promotion/Maintenance

39. Pressure ulcers can be prevented by
    1. application of a drying agent to ulcerated areas
    2. position changes every 2 hours
    3. forcing fluids
    4. encouraging a diet high in vitamins and minerals

    Nursing Process: Implementation
    Client Need: Physiological Integrity

40. When a client with herpes zoster has pain and itching, the nurse can advise the client to
    1. apply ice to the area
    2. wash the area with a mild detergent
    3. apply cool or warm compresses to the area
    4. dab alcohol on the area

    Nursing Process: Implementation
    Client Need: Health Promotion/Maintenance

41. When performing a physical assessment on a client with suspected pemphigus, the nurse looks for
    1. bullae randomly distributed on the body surface or mucous membranes
    2. a rash on the trunk of the body
    3. raised, red lesions over bony prominences
    4. scaly lesions found anywhere on the body surface

    Nursing Process: Collecting Data
    Client Need: Physiological Integrity

42. When performing a physical assessment on the client with suspected exfoliative dermatitis, the nurse looks for
    1. oozing and drainage from small pustules scattered over the trunk and head
    2. swelling and erythema of subcutaneous tissues
    3. peeling, scaling, and redness of the upper layers of the skin
    4. callus formation on upper layers of the skin

    Nursing Process: Collecting Data
    Client Need: Physiological Integrity

43. To prevent an impairment of skin integrity when the client has a severe skin disorder, the nurse can
    1. allow the wet dressings to dry before they are removed
    2. warm the solution applied to the dressing to 120°F
    3. apply tincture of benzoin to denuded areas
    4. apply and remove dressings gently

    Nursing Process: Implementation
    Client Need: Safe, Effective Care Environment

44. Clients with an extensive and severe skin disorders may develop hypothermia. Nursing methods to correct hypothermia include
    1. cooling the solution used for wet dressings to 80°F
    2. decreasing the temperature of the room
    3. administering an antipyretic agent
    4. covering areas not affected with extra blankets

    Nursing Process: Implementation
    Client Need: Physiological Integrity

II. CRITICAL THINKING EXERCISES

1. Mr. Matthews has pemphigus. What two major problems associated with this disease are incorporated into a nursing care plan?

2. Mr. Dalton is recovering from 2nd and 3rd degree burns over 30% of his body. Presently, he is undergoing skin grafting and physical therapy and he tells you that he is bored. What diversional therapies could be used to decrease his boredom?

3. You have been asked to participate in a team conference. The topic is "Care of the Client with Burns." What reasons or explanations would you give for the importance of 1) preventing wound infection and 2) accurately measuring the urinary intake and output?

Appendix/Answers

The answers to the multiple-choice questions for each chapter are given in this section. All critical thinking exercises are taken from the material contained in each chapter. The answers can be found by reviewing the material in the chapters.

CHAPTER 1

I. MULTIPLE CHOICE

1. 1
2. 4
3. 2
4. 3
5. 1
6. 3
7. 1
8. 3
9. 4
10. 3

CHAPTER 2

I. MULTIPLE CHOICE

1. 2
2. 3
3. 3
4. 1
5. 2
6. 4
7. 3
8. 4
9. 2
10. 4
11. 2

CHAPTER 3

I. MULTIPLE CHOICE

1. 2
2. 1
3. 3
4. 2
5. 2
6. 1
7. 3
8. 3
9. 3
10. 3
11. 2
12. 1
13. 1
14. 4

CHAPTER 4

I. MULTIPLE CHOICE

1. 2
2. 3
3. 1

4. 1
5. 4
6. 3
7. 3
8. 2
9. 2
10. 2
11. 3
12. 1
13. 2
14. 2
15. 2
16. 4
17. 3
18. 4

CHAPTER 5

I. MULTIPLE CHOICE

1. 4
2. 1
3. 3
4. 2
5. 2
6. 3
7. 3
8. 1
9. 3
10. 4
11. 3

CHAPTER 6

I. MULTIPLE CHOICE

1. 1
2. 3
3. 1
4. 3
5. 4
6. 2
7. 4
8. 1
9. 1
10. 2
11. 2
12. 2
13. 3
14. 1
15. 2
16. 3
17. 2

CHAPTER 7

I. MULTIPLE CHOICE

1. 4
2. 2
3. 1
4. 2
5. 1
6. 3
7. 1
8. 3
9. 4
10. 2
11. 3
12. 3
13. 2
14. 4
15. 2
16. 3
17. 2
18. 2
19. 4
20. 2
21. 1
22. 1
23. 3
24. 4
25. 1
26. 2
27. 2
28. 3
29. 2
30. 1

CHAPTER 8

I. MULTIPLE CHOICE

1. 3
2. 1
3. 2
4. 1
5. 4
6. 2
7. 3
8. 3
9. 2
10. 4
11. 2
12. 4
13. 2
14. 1
15. 3
16. 2

17. 2
18. 3
19. 1
20. 3

CHAPTER 9

I. MULTIPLE CHOICE

1. 1
2. 2
3. 2
4. 1
5. 2
6. 1
7. 3
8. 1
9. 4
10. 4
11. 3
12. 1
13. 4
14. 3
15. 4

CHAPTER 10

I. MULTIPLE CHOICE

1. 2
2. 1
3. 3
4. 4
5. 4
6. 1
7. 3
8. 4
9. 3
10. 1
11. 3
12. 3
13. 2
14. 2
15. 2
16. 4
17. 2
18. 1
19. 2
20. 1

CHAPTER 11

I. MULTIPLE CHOICE

1. 3
2. 1
3. 4
4. 3
5. 2
6. 3
7. 1
8. 1
9. 4
10. 1
11. 4
12. 1
13. 3
14. 4
15. 2

CHAPTER 12

I. MULTIPLE CHOICE

1. 4
2. 1
3. 2
4. 1
5. 4
6. 4
7. 1
8. 4
9. 3
10. 4
11. 2
12. 3
13. 1
14. 1
15. 3

CHAPTER 13

I. MULTIPLE CHOICE

1. 4
2. 2
3. 3
4. 3
5. 4
6. 1
7. 3
8. 1
9. 1
10. 3

CHAPTER 14

I. MULTIPLE CHOICE

1. 4
2. 1
3. 2
4. 2
5. 4
6. 1
7. 3
8. 3
9. 2
10. 4
11. 1
12. 2
13. 1
14. 4
15. 2

CHAPTER 15

1. 4
2. 4
3. 2
4. 1
5. 4
6. 3
7. 2
8. 4
9. 3
10. 3
11. 3
12. 1
13. 2
14. 1
15. 3
16. 3

17. 2
18. 4
19. 2
20. 4
21. 2
22. 3
23. 1
24. 1

CHAPTER 16

1. 1
2. 3
3. 2
4. 3
5. 1
6. 1
7. 4
8. 1
9. 3
10. 1
11. 4
12. 2
13. 3
14. 2
15. 3
16. 4
17. 2
18. 4
19. 3
20. 1
21. 2
22. 4
23. 2

CHAPTER 17

1. 1
2. 1
3. 3
4. 4
5. 4
6. 2
7. 3
8. 3
9. 2

CHAPTER 18

1. 1
2. 4
3. 3
4. 1
5. 3
6. 1
7. 3
8. 4
9. 3
10. 1

CHAPTER 19

1. 2
2. 1
3. 2
4. 4
5. 3
6. 2
7. 3
8. 1
9. 4
10. 3

11. 2
12. 3
13. 1
14. 1
15. 2
16. 4
17. 4
18. 1
19. 3
20. 4

CHAPTER 20

1. 4
2. 3
3. 1
4. 3
5. 2
6. 2
7. 4
8. 2
9. 3
10. 4
11. 2
12. 4
13. 1
14. 1

CHAPTER 21

1. 2
2. 4
3. 1
4. 2
5. 3
6. 1
7. 3
8. 3
9. 3
10. 2
11. 2
12. 3
13. 2
14. 1
15. 2

CHAPTER 22

1. 2
2. 3
3. 4
4. 1
5. 4
6. 1
7. 4
8. 3
9. 2
10. 3
11. 1
12. 4
13. 3
14. 3
15. 2
16. 1
17. 3

CHAPTER 23

1. 3
2. 3
3. 4
4. 3

5. 1
6. 1
7. 2
8. 1
9. 2
10. 4
11. 2
12. 3
13. 3
14. 2
15. 4
16. 1
17. 1

CHAPTER 24

1. 1
2. 4
3. 2
4. 1
5. 2
6. 3
7. 4
8. 2
9. 4
10. 4
11. 1
12. 3
13. 3
14. 2
15. 4
16. 3
17. 2
18. 3

CHAPTER 25

1. 3
2. 1
3. 2
4. 3
5. 4
6. 1
7. 3
8. 2
9. 1
10. 4
11. 2
12. 2
13. 3
14. 2
15. 1
16. 1
17. 1
18. 4
19. 3
20. 1
21. 2
22. 4
23. 1
24. 3
25. 2
26. 4
27. 4
28. 1

CHAPTER 26

1. 2
2. 4
3. 3

4. 1
5. 2
6. 4
7. 2
8. 2
9. 4
10. 3
11. 1
12. 4
13. 2
14. 3
15. 1
16. 2
17. 1
18. 3
19. 2
20. 4
21. 2
22. 1
23. 4
24. 2
25. 1
26. 1
27. 3
28. 4
29. 2
30. 4
31. 1
32. 3
33. 2
34. 1
35. 3
36. 3
37. 2
38. 4
39. 4

CHAPTER 27

1. 4
2. 1
3. 4
4. 3
5. 3
6. 2
7. 1
8. 2
9. 4
10. 1
11. 4

CHAPTER 28

I. MULTIPLE CHOICE

1. 3
2. 4
3. 3
4. 1
5. 3
6. 2
7. 2
8. 4
9. 2
10. 2
11. 3
12. 4
13. 4
14. 2
15. 1
16. 2
17. 2

18. 1
19. 3
20. 3
21. 2
22. 1
23. 2
24. 4
25. 2
26. 1
27. 4
28. 2
29. 1
30. 2
31. 2
32. 3
33. 4
34. 2
35. 4
36. 2
37. 1
38. 1
39. 4
40. 2

CHAPTER 29

I. MULTIPLE CHOICE

1. 1
2. 3
3. 2
4. 1
5. 4
6. 4
7. 4
8. 4
9. 3
10. 1
11. 3
12. 3
13. 2
14. 3
15. 3
16. 3
17. 3
18. 4
19. 1
20. 1
21. 2
22. 1
23. 2
24. 2
25. 1
26. 4
27. 2
28. 2
29. 1
30. 2
31. 4
32. 3
33. 1
34. 3

CHAPTER 30

I. MULTIPLE CHOICE

1. 1
2. 2
3. 4
4. 3
5. 2

6. 4
7. 1
8. 1
9. 1
10. 4
11. 2
12. 2
13. 1
14. 1
15. 1
16. 2
17. 4
18. 3
19. 2
20. 1

CHAPTER 31

I. MULTIPLE CHOICE

1. 2
2. 4
3. 3
4. 1
5. 1
6. 2
7. 2
8. 3
9. 3
10. 4
11. 4
12. 3
13. 1
14. 1
15. 2
16. 3
17. 2
18. 2
19. 1
20. 2
21. 4
22. 1
23. 3
24. 4
25. 2
26. 1
27. 2
28. 2
29. 1
30. 2
31. 4
32. 3
33. 1
34. 3
35. 2
36. 3
37. 3

CHAPTER 32

I. MULTIPLE CHOICE

1. 1
2. 2
3. 3
4. 2
5. 3
6. 3
7. 3
8. 1
9. 3
10. 2

11. 1
12. 4
13. 1.
14. 4
15. 1
16. 2
17. 4
18. 1
19. 4
20. 3
21. 1
22. 2
23. 3
24. 1
25. 2
26. 1

CHAPTER 33

I. MULTIPLE CHOICE

1. 2
2. 2
3. 3
4. 1
5. 3
6. 1
7. 4
8. 2
9. 4
10. 3
11. 4
12. 1
13. 3
14. 1
15. 3
16. 4
17. 1
18. 3
19. 2
20. 2
21. 3

CHAPTER 34

I. MULTIPLE CHOICE

1. 1
2. 3
3. 4
4. 1
5. 2
6. 2
7. 2
8. 2
9. 4
10. 3
11. 1
12. 1
13. 3
14. 1
15. 2
16. 1
17. 1
18. 1
19. 2
20. 4
21. 3
22. 2
23. 1
24. 1
25. 1

26. 1
27. 1
28. 2
29. 1
30. 4
31. 1
32. 3

CHAPTER 35

I. MULTIPLE CHOICE

1.   3
2.   1
3.   1
4.   4
5.   3
6.   4
7.   1
8.   3
9.   4
10. 2
11. 3
12. 1
13. 2
14. 4
15. 3
16. 3
17. 2
18. 2
19. 1
20. 2
21. 1
22. 3
23. 3
24. 3

CHAPTER 36

I. MULTIPLE CHOICE

1.   2
2.   3
3.   1
4.   3
5.   4
6.   1
7.   2
8.   2
9.   4
10. 2

CHAPTER 37

I. MULTIPLE CHOICE

1.   2
2.   3
3.   1
4.   1
5.   2
6.   2
7.   3
8.   3
9.   4
10. 1
11. 2
12. 3
13. 1
14. 3
15. 4
16. 2
17. 1

18. 2
19. 1
20. 1
21. 1
22. 3
23. 4
24. 1
25. 1
26. 3
27. 2
28. 2
29. 3

CHAPTER 38

I. MULTIPLE CHOICE

1.   4
2.   2
3.   3
4.   3
5.   1
6.   1
7.   2
8.   3

CHAPTER 39

I. MULTIPLE CHOICE

1.   4
2.   2
3.   1
4.   2
5.   3
6.   2
7.   1
8.   4
9.   2
10. 3

CHAPTER 40

I. MULTIPLE CHOICE

1.   2
2.   1
3.   3
4.   3
5.   4
6.   1
7.   3
8.   1
9.   2
10. 2
11. 4

CHAPTER 41

I. MULTIPLE CHOICE

1.   4
2.   3
3.   1
4.   2
5.   2
6.   3
7.   1
8.   1
9.   3
10. 2

CHAPTER 42

I. MULTIPLE CHOICE

1.   2
2.   4
3.   3
4.   2
5.   4
6.   1
7.   4
8.   4
9.   2
10. 1
11. 3
12. 2
13. 2
14. 3
15. 4
16. 1

CHAPTER 43

I. MULTIPLE CHOICE

1.   4
2.   2
3.   1
4.   2
5.   1
6.   2
7.   1
8.   1
9.   3
10. 2
11. 4
12. 1
13. 1
14. 4
15. 2
16. 1
17. 3
18. 4
19. 1
20. 4
21. 3
22. 4
23. 1
24. 2
25. 2
26. 4
27   2
28. 3
29. 1
30. 1
31. 2
32. 3
33. 4
34. 3
35. 1

CHAPTER 44

I. MULTIPLE CHOICE

1.   3
2.   3
3.   4
4.   2
5.   2
6.   1
7.   3
8.   1

9. 2
10. 4
11. 2
12. 4
13. 2
14. 4
15. 1
16. 3
17. 2
18. 1
19. 2
20. 1
21. 1
22. 3

CHAPTER 45

I. MULTIPLE CHOICE

1. 1
2. 2
3. 1
4. 3
5. 2
6. 3
7. 1
8. 2
9. 3
10. 3
11. 1
12. 4
13. 2
14. 3
15. 1
16. 1
17. 2
18. 2
19. 2
20. 4
21. 4
22. 1
23. 3
24. 3
25. 1
26. 4
27. 2
28. 3
29. 4
30. 2
31. 1

CHAPTER 46

I. MULTIPLE CHOICE

1. 2
2. 3
3. 2
4. 1
5. 3
6. 4
7. 1
8. 3
9. 2
10. 4
11. 3
12. 2
13. 2
14. 2
15. 4
16. 1
17. 1
18. 3

CHAPTER 47

I. MULTIPLE CHOICE

1. 4
2. 3
3. 2
4. 4
5. 3
6. 1
7. 3
8. 1
9. 1
10. 2
11. 3
12. 1
13. 2
14. 3
15. 3
16. 4
17. 2
18. 3
19. 1
20. 4
21. 1
22. 1
23. 1
24. 3
25. 1
26. 3
27. 2

CHAPTER 48

I. MULTIPLE CHOICE

1. 3
2. 3
3. 4
4. 2
5. 2
6. 1
7. 3
8. 1
9. 3
10. 2
11. 4
12. 3
13. 2
14. 1
15. 2
16. 4
17. 1
18. 2
19. 4
20. 3
21. 3
22. 3
23. 2
24. 3
25. 4
26. 2
27. 1
28. 3
29. 4
30. 2
31. 1
32. 4
33. 3
34. 3
35. 1
36. 3
37. 1

38. 1
39. 3
40. 1
41. 1
42. 3
43. 2
44. 1
45. 3
46. 3
47. 1
48. 2
49. 1
50. 3

CHAPTER 49

I. MULTIPLE CHOICE

1. 2
2. 3
3. 4
4. 1
5. 3
6. 2
7. 1
8. 3
9. 4
10. 3
11. 3
12. 2
13. 3
14. 3
15. 3
16. 4
17. 2
18. 2
19. 1
20. 2
21. 1
22. 2
23. 3
24. 3
25. 3
26. 4

CHAPTER 50

I. MULTIPLE CHOICE

1. 4
2. 4
3. 1
4. 4
5. 1
6. 1
7. 2
8. 3
9. 3
10. 3
11. 1
12. 2
13. 1
14. 1
15. 2
16. 2
17. 3
18. 2
19. 2
20. 3
21. 3
22. 1
23. 2
24. 2

25. 3
26. 3
27. 4
28. 3
29. 1
30. 3
31. 2
32. 2
33. 1
34. 3
35. 3
36. 4
37. 1
38. 2

CHAPTER 51

I. MULTIPLE CHOICE

1. 1
2. 3
3. 4
4. 2
5. 3
6. 1
7. 3
8. 1
9. 3
10. 3
11. 2
12. 3
13. 2
14. 2
15. 3
16. 2
17. 1
18. 3
19. 3
20. 2
21. 1
22. 4
23. 3
24. 2
25. 2
26. 3
27. 4
28. 1
29. 3
30. 2
31. 3
32. 3
33. 4
34. 3
35. 4

CHAPTER 52

I. MULTIPLE CHOICE

1. 3
2. 4
3. 1
4. 2
5. 1
6. 2
7. 3
8. 1
9. 2
10. 3
11. 4
12. 2
13. 1
14. 1

15. 3
16. 1
17. 2
18. 4
19. 4
20. 1
21. 3
22. 4
23. 3
24. 2
25. 1
26. 2
27. 3
28. 3
29. 1
30. 1
31. 2
32. 3
33. 4
34. 4
35. 1

CHAPTER 53

I. MULTIPLE CHOICE

1. 2
2. 2
3. 4
4. 1
5. 2
6. 3
7. 1
8. 3
9. 4
10. 1
11. 2
12. 1
13. 3
14. 4
15. 2
16. 2
17. 3
18. 4
19. 2
20. 2
21. 1
22. 4
23. 4
24. 2
25. 1
26. 1
27. 4
28. 1
29. 4
30. 3
31. 3
32. 1
33. 4
34. 1
35. 1
36. 4
37. 1
38. 2
39. 1
40. 2
41. 3
42. 1
43. 2
44. 4
45. 2
46. 2

47. 3
48. 1
49. 1
50. 4

CHAPTER 54

I. MULTIPLE CHOICE

1. 3
2. 4
3. 1
4. 1
5. 1
6. 2
7. 3
8. 1
9. 2
10. 4

CHAPTER 55

I. MULTIPLE CHOICE

1. 2
2. 3
3. 1
4. 4
5. 1
6. 3
7. 4
8. 4
9. 1
10. 3
11. 1
12. 4
13. 1
14. 1
15. 4
16. 3
17. 1
18. 1
19. 2
20. 4
21. 1
22. 1
23. 2
24. 3
25. 3
26. 4
27. 1
28. 2
29. 4
30. 1
31. 3
32. 2
33. 3
34. 1
35. 2
36. 3
37. 4
38. 3
39. 2
40. 2
41. 2
42. 1
43. 3

CHAPTER 56

I. MULTIPLE CHOICE

1. 2
2. 4
3. 1
4. 2
5. 3
6. 4
7. 2
8. 1
9. 4
10. 1
11. 1
12. 2
13. 4
14. 3
15. 4
16. 1
17. 3
18. 2
19. 1
20. 4

CHAPTER 57

I. MULTIPLE CHOICE

1. 4
2. 1
3. 4
4. 2
5. 1
6. 2
7. 3
8. 2
9. 1
10. 2
11. 3
12. 4
13. 2
14. 1
15. 1

CHAPTER 58

I. MULTIPLE CHOICE

1. 2
2. 4
3. 4
4. 1
5. 1
6. 2
7. 1
8. 3
9. 2
10. 3
11. 4
12. 2
13. 1
14. 2
15. 2
16. 1
17. 3
18. 1
19. 4
20. 3
21. 3
22. 4
23. 1
24. 4

25. 2
26. 1
27. 3
28. 2
29. 4
30. 1
31. 2

CHAPTER 59

I. MULTIPLE CHOICE

1. 1
2. 2
3. 3
4. 2
5. 4
6. 3
7. 2
8. 1
9. 4
10. 1
11. 3
12. 2

CHAPTER 60

I. MULTIPLE CHOICE

1. 2
2. 2
3. 3
4. 1
5. 1
6. 2
7. 4
8. 2
9. 2
10. 1
11. 2
12. 2
13. 1
14. 2
15. 4
16. 4
17. 1
18. 3
19. 2
20. 3
21. 2
22. 3

CHAPTER 61

I. MULTIPLE CHOICE

1. 3
2. 4
3. 1
4. 2
5. 4
6. 2
7. 1
8. 3
9. 4
10. 1
11. 3

CHAPTER 62

I. MULTIPLE CHOICE

1. 3
2. 2

3. 4
4. 1
5. 3
6. 1
7. 2
8. 4
9. 2
10. 2
11. 1
12. 2
13. 3
14. 1
15. 2

CHAPTER 63

I. MULTIPLE CHOICE

1. 4
2. 1
3. 1
4. 1
5. 3
6. 3
7. 3
8. 2
9. 1
10. 1
11. 4
12. 3
13. 2
14. 1
15. 2
16. 4
17. 3
18. 3
19. 4
20. 2
21. 1
22. 2
23. 2
24. 2
25. 1
26. 2
27. 4
28. 3
29. 3
30. 3

CHAPTER 64

I. MULTIPLE CHOICE

1. 2
2. 3
3. 1
4. 2
5. 3
6. 4
7. 4
8. 1
9. 3
10. 1
11. 4
12. 1
13. 1
14. 3
15. 2
16. 3
17. 4
18. 2
19. 1

20.	4
21.	2
22.	3
23.	2

CHAPTER 65

I. MULTIPLE CHOICE

1.	4
2.	3
3.	3
4.	1
5.	2
6.	1
7.	2
8.	2
9.	2
10.	1
11.	3
12.	3
13.	1
14.	3
15.	4
16.	3

CHAPTER 66

I. MULTIPLE CHOICE

1.	3
2.	3
3.	2
4.	1
5.	1
6.	3
7.	4
8.	2
9.	3
10.	1
11.	4
12.	4
13.	2
14.	4
15.	3
16.	4
17.	1
18.	1
19.	4
20.	1
21.	2
22.	1
23.	2

24.	1
25.	2
26.	1
27.	1
28.	3
29.	2
30.	2
31.	3
32.	3
33.	1
34.	1
35.	2
36.	2
37.	1
38.	1
39.	4
40.	3
41.	2
42.	2
43.	3
44.	3
45.	2
46.	3
47.	1
48.	1
49.	1
50.	4
51.	3
52.	3
53.	1
54.	1
55.	1
56.	1
57.	3
58.	3
59.	4
60.	4
61.	1
62.	3
63.	4
64.	2
65.	1

CHAPTER 67

I. MULTIPLE CHOICE

1.	2
2.	4
3.	1
4.	1
5.	1
6.	2

7.	1
8.	4
9.	3
10.	3

CHAPTER 68

I. MULTIPLE CHOICE

1.	1
2.	2
3.	3
4.	4
5.	1
6.	4
7.	2
8.	3
9.	1
10.	3
11.	1
12.	3
13.	1
14.	4
15.	1
16.	1
17.	3
18.	2
19.	2
20.	4
21.	1
22.	1
23.	3
24.	2
25.	4
26.	4
27.	1
28.	2
29.	1
30.	3
31.	2
32.	1
33.	2
34.	1
35.	1
36.	4
37.	4
38.	1
39.	2
40.	3
41.	1
42.	3
43.	4
44.	4